FIFTH EDITION

Documentation Manual for Occupational Therapy

FIFTH EDITION

Documentation Manual for Occupational Therapy

CRYSTAL A. GATELEY, PhD, OTR/L

Associate Chair and Teaching Professor
Department of Occupational Therapy
University of Missouri—College of Health Sciences
Columbia, Missouri

SHERRY BORCHERDING, MA, OTR/L

Clinical Associate Professor (Retired)
University of Missouri
Columbia, Missouri

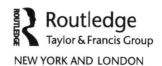

Routledge
Taylor & Francis Group

NEW YORK AND LONDON

Instructors: *Documentation Manual for Occupational Therapy, Fifth Edition*, includes ancillary materials specifically available for faculty use. Included is an *Instructor's Manual*. Please visit www.routledge.com/9781638220602 to obtain access.

First published 2024 by SLACK Incorporated

Published 2024 by Routledge
605 Third Avenue, New York, NY 10158

and by Routledge
4 Park Square, Milton Park, Abingdon, Oxon OX14 4RN

Routledge is an imprint of the Taylor & Francis Group, an informa business

Cover Artist: Tinhouse Design

Library of Congress Control Number: 2023941404

ISBN: 9781638220602 (pbk)
ISBN: 9781003523901 (ebk)

DOI: 10.4324/9781003523901

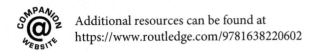

Additional resources can be found at
https://www.routledge.com/9781638220602

DEDICATION

This book is dedicated to all my past, current, and future occupational therapy students
who make teaching a wonderful and rewarding experience
and to my family who makes life worth living.

—*Crystal A. Gateley, PhD, OTR/L*

CONTENTS

ACKNOWLEDGMENTS

First, I would like to thank Sherry Borcherding who taught me how to document 30 years ago and asked me to serve as co-author on this book back in 2009. Beyond the professional collaboration required for three book revisions, she has provided support and encouragement for my transition into a faculty role and incredible patience for my ever-changing life circumstances, which often delayed the book revision process. Although her name is no longer on the cover of this book, it would not exist without her initial vision and efforts, continued guidance and suggestions, and eagle eye for catching my typos.

Thank you to Brien Cummings, former Senior Acquisitions Editor, who guided me through four book publications with SLACK Incorporated. Thank you also to Tony Schiavo, Jenn Cahill, Saige Avery, Doris Zheku, Erin O'Reilly, and all the behind-the-scenes staff at SLACK Incorporated for your guidance and contributions to this edition.

I am grateful for the support of all my departmental colleagues at University of Missouri: Tim Wolf, Stephanie Allen, Bill Janes, Gina Pifer, Tiffany Bolton, Rachel Proffitt, Anna Boone, Katelyn Mwangi, Whitney Henderson, Melanie Tkach, Brittney Stevenson, Lea Ann Lowery, Winnie Dunn, Sam Shea Lemoins, Kristi Peterson, Angie Wolf, Juliana Earwood, Shelly Crawford, Bethany Kendrick, Jean Griffith, and Sheila Marushak. I am blessed to work in a collaborative environment where excellence in occupational therapy practice, education, and research are valued and respected. To Angie Williams, I dearly miss you and our early morning conversations. The department copier would never have survived without your interventions during my fits of frustration! I am thankful for Bailey Baucum who served as a co-instructor for the documentation course and made it better with each suggestion. Thank you also to Megan Kotil and Mikayla Simons for assistance with proofreading and other manuscript preparation tasks.

I am also thankful for my colleagues and friends "down the hall" in the Department of Physical Therapy and across the College of Health Sciences. Your friendship and support make it a joy to come to work. Special thanks to Jamie Hall for following me to three different jobs over the past 25 years, the many lunch dates at Chipotle and Campus Bar & Grill, and all the years of mutual support through graduate school, job transitions, and kid-raising adventures!

I would like to acknowledge Joe Sadewhite and my dozens of occupational therapy, physical therapy, and speech-language pathology colleagues at Boone Health for your friendship, support, and last-minute shift coverage when I needed it over the past few years for family emergencies. I am blessed to have not one but two jobs that I love. Special thanks to Mackenzie Cullifer for providing some new examples for this edition.

I also would like to acknowledge Bruce VanBerkum and Cheryl Harrington of My School Therapy and Karthik Rao and Sanjay Patel of Practice Pro for their assistance in providing screenshots of their electronic documentation software for this textbook. Thank you for your quick responses to my many requests for the last two editions of this book!

Most of this book revision took place at my "second office" at Panera in Jefferson City, Missouri. For the past 2 years, I was greeted each visit with a smile by Margaret Millington at the register. I was inspired by the kindness and enthusiasm of employee Tristian Reynolds, who is a living testimony that you can persevere and have a bright future and a positive impact on others, no matter your past life circumstances. Special thanks to fellow Panera patron Larry Surface, who beat me to the parking lot every day no matter how early I arrived, always saved my favorite booth for me, and asked each day how the book project was going. I truly have enjoyed getting to know each of you!

In 2018, I stumbled upon a small online group of college parents who welcomed me into their private club. This small group of approximately 30 parents spread out across the nation has been a constant source of emotional support and encouragement as our students and families have navigated countless challenges and celebrations over the past 5 years. They are the first ones I turn to when I have good or bad news that I can't share publicly. To my 2018 CC Family, thank you for all the laughs, tears, and virtual hugs. Although the vast majority of us have never met, we have built an incredible community, and I look forward to many more years of friendship and support.

A huge thank you goes out to our circle of friends who always provide the much-needed escape from the stress of work and life and make us laugh. I often feel like we are living our own version of *A Million Little Things*. Thank you to Myles and Lora Hinkel, Mark and Ustena Simenson, Russ and Jamie Drury, James and Whitney Scurlock, Michael Abbott, and Brad Fortson. Here's to many more float trips, backyard fires, relaxed dinners, and impromptu gatherings! Thank you to Erick Taylor for the weekly *Survivor* nights and for always listening to and supporting me through life's ups and downs. Last but not least, huge thank you to my best friend of 30+ years, Michelle Bass, who is simultaneously my best and worst influence. I am thankful for our many adventures, both meticulously planned and ridiculously spontaneous. I am looking forward to making many more memories with you!

Most importantly, I want to thank my husband, Curt, and my two daughters, Katrina and Lauren, for your continued patience, love, and support through all of my educational and professional endeavors. Curt, thank you for the most wonderful 28 years of marriage and for making me laugh every single day. I love you so much! Katrina, over the past few years I watched you graduate from the University of Mississippi in the middle of a pandemic and then had the pleasure of calling you a Boonie colleague for over a year as you worked a very challenging job on the hospital's primary COVID-19 unit. Then I watched you surpass everyone's expectations by earning acceptance to Yale University for graduate school. Lauren, I saw you earn a spot in and complete the Haslam Scholars Program, the most prestigious and selective honors program at the University of Tennessee. Although the pandemic took away so many college experiences, you persevered and made us so proud with all your accomplishments, and we are amazed at the independent young woman you have become. We can't wait to see where life takes both of you over the next several years!

—*Crystal A. Gateley, PhD, OTR/L*

ABOUT THE AUTHOR

Crystal A. Gateley, PhD, OTR/L is Associate Chair and Teaching Professor at the University of Missouri, Department of Occupational Therapy, where she has been a full-time faculty member since 2009. She serves as Program Director for the Entry-Level Occupational Therapy Doctorate (OTD) program, providing oversight of curriculum revision and accreditation compliance. She also assists with new program development and the myriad of issues faced by a growing department. In addition to her administrative responsibilities, she teaches a variety of courses across the curriculum including Clinical Reasoning and Documentation, Foundations and Theory in Occupational Therapy, Conditions in Occupational Therapy, Psychosocial Aspects of Occupational Therapy, Emerging Trends in Occupational Therapy, Professional Seminar, Capstone Mentor Hour I and II, and Leadership, Management, and Policy. She also has taught interdisciplinary courses including Clinical Pathophysiology and Introduction to the Health Professions.

Crystal graduated Summa Cum Laude from the University of Missouri in 1995 with a Bachelor of Health Science in Occupational Therapy. She went on to complete a master's (2003) and doctorate (2015) in Educational Leadership and Policy Analysis with an Emphasis in Higher Education and Administration, also from the University of Missouri. Crystal has worked in a variety of occupational therapy practice settings throughout her career, including acute care, inpatient and outpatient rehabilitation, skilled nursing, home health, early intervention, outpatient pediatrics, public schools, and community programs for adults with developmental disabilities. She still provides occasional occupational therapy coverage at Boone Health in Columbia, Missouri, on weekends and holidays, and her experiences there with patients and interprofessional colleagues inform her teaching as she passes along insights from contemporary occupational therapy practice to her students.

Beyond her love for college teaching and occupational therapy practice, Crystal enjoys spending time with friends and family in outdoor activities including hiking, camping, fishing, canoeing, and rafting along various Missouri rivers. She is an avid football fan, and she is still basking in the glory of the Kansas City Chiefs' Super Bowl victories in 2020 and 2023! She currently lives in rural Holts Summit, Missouri, with her husband Curt, her parents, and her two cats, Cora and Loki. Crystal treasures the occasional phone calls and visits from her two daughters, Katrina and Lauren, who are pursuing their dreams in Connecticut and Tennessee.

Chapter 1

Documenting the Occupational Therapy Process

Welcome to a new style of writing. The first time you see an experienced occupational therapist make an entry in a health record, you may think you will never be able to do it with such ease. The technical language alone can be intimidating. Then there is the amazing attention to detail in the client observation, the insightful assessment, and the plan that just seems to roll off the therapist's fingertips while you are wondering how long it will take you to predict a course of treatment like that.

Professional documentation is a skill, and like any skill, you can learn it and eventually master it. Learning a new skill requires two things: instruction and practice. I have designed this book to provide you with both parts of the process. I introduce information about each part of the documentation process, and I present worksheets to let you practice each step as you learn it.

The material presented here emerged from a course on clinical documentation taught to occupational therapy students at the University of Missouri. With each new edition, I rely on my students for suggestions to ensure the information I present is understandable and effective in helping you learn both documentation and the professional reasoning skills underlying the documentation process.

Occupational therapy practitioners use different formats for documentation depending on their practice settings. This manual introduces specific formats for writing occupation-based problem statements and goals. In addition, the manual presents a systematic approach to one form of documentation: the SOAP note. SOAP is an acronym for the four parts of an entry into a health record. The letters stand for *Subjective, Objective, Assessment,* and *Plan.* Although not all practice settings use the SOAP note format, the professional reasoning skills underlying SOAP note documentation can be adapted to nearly any occupational therapy practice setting. Additionally, although narrative note writing has become much less common with the evolution of electronic health records, many documentation software products still use a SOAP structure to organize information into electronic flowsheets.

OUR EVOLVING PROFESSION

The American Occupational Therapy Association (AOTA) represents the interests and concerns of occupational therapy practitioners and students in all aspects of professional practice, including provision of quality services, improvement of consumer access to services, promotion of professional development, education of the public, and advancement of the profession (AOTA, 2021). AOTA publishes mission and vision statements that help guide the profession (see text box for details). AOTA updates these statements every few years to reflect contemporary practice.

Gateley, C. A. *Documentation Manual for Occupational Therapy, Fifth Edition* (pp. 1-6). © 2024 Taylor & Francis Group.

MISSION AND VISION STATEMENTS OF THE AMERICAN OCCUPATIONAL THERAPY ASSOCIATION

Mission Statement: "To advance occupational therapy practice, education, and research through standard setting and advocacy on behalf of its members, the profession, and the public." (AOTA, 2021, para. 6)

Vision 2025: "As an inclusive profession, occupational therapy maximizes health, well-being, and quality of life for all people, populations, and communities through effective solutions that facilitate participation in everyday living." (AOTA, 2021, para. 7)

These statements serve as a roadmap for all aspects of professional practice, including documentation. Current occupational therapy practice is in many ways determined by which services are reimbursable, and documentation of client care is the vehicle through which we communicate those services. As the profession continues to move toward evidence-based practice in a context where payer sources are rewarding service quality over service quantity, occupational therapy is well poised to be a leader in the health care arena. "There is compelling evidence that occupational therapy provides cost-effective interventions that address many of the U.S. health care system's greatest needs" (Hart & Parsons, 2015, p. 1). In fact, one recent study found that occupational therapy services are associated with a significant reduction in hospital readmissions for particular diagnoses including heart failure, pneumonia, and myocardial infarction (Rogers et al., 2016). Researchers based that study in part on the occupational therapy documentation included in patients' Medicare claims, again highlighting the importance of what and how we communicate about the services we provide to our clients.

Occupational therapy practitioners must combine the ever-changing knowledge base of the profession with its historical foundations and this visionary roadmap for the future. Leaders in the profession have identified four principles to guide contemporary occupational therapy practice (Boyt Schell et al., 2019, p. 64):

1. Client-centered practice
2. Occupation-centered practice
3. Evidence-based practice
4. Culturally relevant practice

OUR EVOLVING PROFESSIONAL LANGUAGE

Although various health care professions share a common language in terms of diagnoses and procedures, each profession has its own specific language that explains its unique role in addressing a client's health care needs, typically found in some sort of official documents. This section will review the most important documents that guide occupational therapy documentation.

Occupational Therapy Practice Framework: Domain and Process, Fourth Edition

Several decades ago, leaders in our profession recognized the need for a system of uniform terminology. The original document, *Occupational Therapy Product Output Reporting System and Uniform Terminology for Reporting Occupational Therapy Services*, was developed in 1979 in response to a change in public laws targeted at reducing fraud and abuse of the Medicare and Medicaid systems (AOTA, 1989). That original document evolved into the *Occupational Therapy Practice Framework: Domain and Process* (AOTA, 2002). AOTA revises the *Occupational Therapy Practice Framework* approximately every 5 to 6 years.

At the time of this writing, the most recent version is the *Occupational Therapy Practice Framework: Domain and Process, Fourth Edition*, hereafter referred to as *OTPF-4* (AOTA, 2020). If you are reading this textbook in 2026 or beyond, I encourage you to explore the AOTA website to determine if an *OTPF-5* has been published and to familiarize yourself with minor changes. The *American Journal of Occupational Therapy* publishes each revision of the document, and this journal is readily available to AOTA members. You also may be able to access the journal online through your academic library. I am writing this section with the assumption that most readers will already be somewhat familiar with the *OTPF-4* before encountering this documentation textbook. Therefore, the summary that follows is very brief.

The *OTPF-4* "describes the central concepts that ground occupational therapy practice and provides a common understanding of the basic tenets and vision of the profession" (AOTA, 2020, p. 4). The authors emphasize that the document builds on values established by the profession's founders back in 1917. The *OTPF-4* is divided into two major sections, which "are linked inextricably in a transactional relationship" (AOTA, 2020, p. 6):

1. *Domain*: This section of the document outlines the purview of occupational therapy practice and identifies the areas in which occupational therapy practitioners have knowledge and expertise.
2. *Process*: This section focuses on the delivery of occupational therapy services, with an emphasis on occupation-based and client-centered practices.

Domain of Occupational Therapy

The aspects of occupational therapy's domain have a dynamic and transactional relationship. "All aspects are of equal value and together interact to affect occupational identity, health, well-being, and participation in life" (AOTA, 2020, p. 6).

- *Occupations*: In the *OTPF-4*, the term *occupation* refers to "personalized and meaningful engagement in daily life events by a specific client" (AOTA, 2020, p. 7). Activities are actions not related to a specific client or context but may be used as interventions to enhance occupational engagement. Occupations include:
  - Activities of daily living (ADLs)
  - Instrumental activities of daily living (IADLs)
  - Health management
  - Rest and sleep
  - Education
  - Work
  - Play
  - Leisure
  - Social participation
- *Contexts*: Context refers to the environmental factors and personal factors that influence occupational performance.
- *Performance Patterns*: "Performance patterns are the acquired habits, routines, roles, and rituals used in the process of engaging consistently in occupations and can support or hinder occupational performance" (AOTA, 2020, p. 12).
- *Performance Skills*: Performance skills include the motor skills, process skills, and social interaction skills that clients use to engage in activities and occupations.
- *Client Factors*: Client factors are the "specific capacities, characteristics, or beliefs that reside within the person, group, or population and influence performance in occupation" and include values, beliefs, and spirituality; body functions; and body structures (AOTA, 2020, p. 15).

Process of Occupational Therapy Service Delivery

The occupational therapy process is "facilitated by the distinct perspective of occupational therapy practitioners engaging in professional reasoning, analyzing occupations and activities, and collaborating with clients" (AOTA, 2020, p. 17). Service delivery does not occur in a linear fashion. It is a dynamic and fluid process that allows occupational therapy practitioners to focus on identified outcomes while continually reflecting on and accommodating new developments and insights throughout the service delivery process. Accurate and effective documentation during all phases of service delivery is essential to communicate the necessity and benefit of occupational therapy to all involved parties. The process of occupational therapy service delivery involves (AOTA, 2020):

- **Evaluation**
  - *Occupational Profile*: The occupational therapist summarizes information related to the client's occupational history, experiences, daily living patterns, interests, values, needs, contexts, and reasons for seeking services.
  - *Analysis of Occupational Performance*: After obtaining a thorough occupational profile, the occupational therapist identifies the client's assets, limitations, and potential problems through observation and assessment of the client's performance.
  - *Synthesis of Evaluation Process*: The occupational therapist interprets the information gathered from the occupational profile and the analysis of occupational performance to determine priorities for intervention and outcomes, working collaboratively with the client to create goals.
- **Intervention**
  - *Intervention Plan*: "The occupational therapy practitioner integrates information from the evaluation with theory, practice models, frames of reference, and research evidence" to develop an action plan for addressing targeted goals and outcomes in collaboration with the client (AOTA, 2020, p. 24).
  - *Intervention Implementation*: The occupational therapy practitioner implements the action plan and continually monitors the client's response to interventions, which may include therapeutic use of occupations and activities, interventions to support occupations, education, training, advocacy, self-advocacy, group intervention, or virtual intervention.
  - *Intervention Review*: The occupational therapy practitioner reviews the effectiveness of the intervention plan and the client's progress toward targeted goals and outcomes.
- **Outcomes**
  - *Selecting Outcome Measures*: The occupational therapist selects valid, reliable methods to measure any of the following targeted outcomes: occupational performance, prevention, health and wellness, quality of life, participation, role competence, well-being, or occupational justice (AOTA, 2020).
  - *Measuring Progress and Adjusting Goals and Interventions*: Throughout the occupational therapy process, the practitioner uses the selected outcome measures to monitor progress, update goals, modify interventions, and plan for transition and/or discontinuation of occupational therapy services.

Other Publications of the American Occupational Therapy Association

The content of this book reflects the domain and process of contemporary occupational therapy practice as described in the *OTPF-4*. The *OTPF-4* is just one of many *Official Documents* published by AOTA that influence occupational therapy practice and therefore documentation. *Official Documents* are divided into the following types (AOTA, 2019):

- *Guidelines*: Guidelines provide descriptions, examples, or recommendations of procedures pertaining to occupational therapy practice or education.
- *Position Papers*: Position papers present AOTA's official stance on a particular issue or subject.
- *Standards*: Standards include a general description of a topic relevant to occupational therapy practice and define the minimum requirements for performance and quality.
- *Statements*: Statements describe and clarify an aspect or issue relevant to occupational therapy practice or education. Although they do not present an official stance like position papers, statements link to fundamental concepts of occupational therapy.
- *Societal Statements*: Societal statements are typically written as a public announcement that identifies a societal issue of concern to individuals, groups, or communities and may offer recommendations of action to be taken.

Each AOTA *Official Document* undergoes review approximately every 5 years (AOTA, 2019). This book incorporates information from the most recent documents available at the time of writing that are relevant to occupational therapy documentation. Practitioners should remain informed about revisions that affect practice and documentation. Updated documents are approved by AOTA's Representative Assembly and published in the *American Journal of Occupational Therapy*. All *Official Documents* are also available on the AOTA website (https://www.aota.org).

The Accreditation Council for Occupational Therapy Education (ACOTE) publishes accreditation standards for educational programs at the levels of associate and baccalaureate degrees for the occupational therapy assistant and master's and doctoral degrees for the occupational therapist. This book is a tool for becoming competent in the documentation skills specified in the accreditation standards. There are minor wording differences between standards for the different educational levels, particularly regarding role differences between occupational therapists and occupational therapy assistants. Like AOTA's routine revision of *Official Documents*, ACOTE updates its standards periodically, and students and educators should ensure they are working toward meeting the most current standards. This book addresses ACOTE standards related to documentation, reporting data, reimbursement, and electronic documentation systems.

In summary, numerous documents and publications affect the occupational therapy profession as a whole and professional documentation in particular. Each occupational therapy practitioner has a responsibility to be familiar with current literature, standards, and state and federal regulations that affect documentation. Leaders in the profession are continually researching and publishing both revised and novel works that affect occupational therapy practice. Staying current with all professional publications allows occupational therapy practitioners to engage in evidence-based practice, and this must be reflected in your documentation.

OVERVIEW

This book arranges information in the order most easily learned by students or new practitioners, with foundational concepts presented first. More complex concepts build on these foundational concepts as professional reasoning is developed. Below is a very brief description of each of the following chapters.

- Chapter 2 provides an overview of the health record including its function, uses, and history.
- Chapter 3 reviews reimbursement, coding, and billing guidelines that impact occupational therapy practice and documentation.
- Chapter 4 reviews legal, regulatory, and ethical considerations that influence occupational therapy practice and documentation.
- Chapter 5 presents the rules and mechanics that guide occupational therapy documentation.
- Chapter 6 discusses the process of developing functional problem statements that can be addressed through occupational therapy intervention.
- Chapter 7 introduces the COAST format for writing occupational therapy goals, a format that has been endorsed by AOTA (Amini, 2016; Sames, 2015).
- Chapter 8 explains the Subjective portion of the SOAP note format.
- Chapter 9 reviews the Objective portion of the SOAP note format.
- Chapter 10 covers the Assessment portion of the SOAP note format.
- Chapter 11 discusses the Plan portion of the SOAP note format.
- Chapter 12 introduces the intervention planning process.
- Chapter 13 discusses documentation requirements in different practice settings.
- Chapter 14 reviews how the professional reasoning underlying SOAP notes can translate into the use of electronic documentation software.
- Chapter 15 discusses requirements specific to various settings and funding sources and provides related examples from numerous practice settings and client populations. This chapter has its own Table of Contents for ease of locating each note.
- The Appendix provides suggestions for completing the worksheets found throughout this book. You will learn the most from attempting the worksheets on your own before comparing them with the suggested responses in the Appendix. Remember also that there are multiple "correct" ways to document, and the suggested responses are simply one example to help you learn.

NEW IN THIS EDITION

This edition of *Documentation Manual for Occupational Therapy* is based on the *OTPF-4* (AOTA, 2020) and on the *Guidelines for Documentation of Occupational Therapy* (AOTA, 2018). Information regarding reimbursement, coding, and billing has been expanded significantly in a separate chapter with an emphasis on recent Medicare changes, specifically the use of Section GG in post-acute practice settings. The use of symbols commonly used in written documentation has been eliminated to reflect the predominant use of electronic documentation in health care. Examples have been updated and added throughout the book to reflect contemporary practice across a variety of occupational therapy practice settings. Several tables have been added throughout the book to improve readability and highlight important concepts.

REFERENCES

Accreditation Council for Occupational Therapy Education. (2020). *2018 Accreditation Council for Occupational Therapy Education (ACOTE) standards and interpretive guide (effective July 31, 2020), December 2020 interpretive guide version.* https://acoteonline.org/

American Occupational Therapy Association. (1989). Uniform terminology for occupation therapy (2nd ed.). *American Journal of Occupational Therapy, 43*(12), 808-815. https://doi.org/10.5014/ajot.43.12.808

American Occupational Therapy Association. (2002). Occupational therapy practice framework: Domain and process. *American Journal of Occupational Therapy, 56*(6), 609-639. https://doi.org/10.5014/ajot.56.6.609

American Occupational Therapy Association. (2018). Guidelines for documentation of occupational therapy. *American Journal of Occupational Therapy, 72*(Suppl. 2), 7212410010p1-7212410010p7. https://doi.org/10.5014/ajot.2018.72S203

American Occupational Therapy Association. (2019). Official Documents available from the American Occupational Therapy Association. *American Journal of Occupational Therapy, 73*(Suppl. 2), 7312410005p1-7312410005p3. https://doi.org/10.5014/ajot.2017.716S2OffDoc

American Occupational Therapy Association. (2020). Occupational therapy practice framework: Domain and process (4th ed.). *American Journal of Occupational Therapy, 74*(Suppl. 2), 7412410010. https://doi.org/10.5014/ajot.2020.74S2001

American Occupational Therapy Association. (2021). *About AOTA.* https://www.aota.org/

Amini, D. (2016). *AOTA documentation series—Module 2: Occupational based goal writing for OT practice* [Online continuing education module]. American Occupational Therapy Association. https://www.aota.org/

Boyt Schell, B. A., Gillen, G., & Coppola, S. (2019). Contemporary occupational therapy practice. In B. A. Boyt Schell & G. Gillen (Eds.), *Willard and Spackman's occupational therapy* (13th ed., pp. 56-71). Wolters Kluwer.

Hart, E. C., & Parsons, H. (2015). *Occupational therapy: Cost-effective solutions for a changing health system.* https://www.aota.org/

Rogers, A. T., Bai, G., Lavin, R. A., & Anderson, G. F. (2016). Higher hospital spending on occupational therapy is associated with lower readmission rates. *Medical Care Research and Review,* 1-19. https://doi.org/10.1177/1077558716666981

Sames, K. (2015). *AOTA documentation series—Module 1: The nuts and bolts of effective documentation* [Online continuing education module]. American Occupational Therapy Association. https://www.aota.org/

The Health Record

The health record, often called the *medical record*, is a compilation of data that includes the client's past and present health information. The purpose of the health record is to serve as the medical and legal document of a client's history, current condition and status, the intervention provided, and the client's response to intervention (Kettenbach & Schlomer, 2016; Quinn & Gordon, 2016; Sullivan, 2019; Sutton, 2015). Like many aspects of health care, the health record is continuously undergoing changes. Before moving on to the specific processes involved in documenting occupational therapy practice, it is important to understand the history of health records in general and the implications for occupational therapy documentation. This chapter provides a brief history of health records in general, a history and overview of SOAP notes, a very brief overview of other documentation formats, and a discussion of the many audiences and functions of the health record.

HISTORY OF HEALTH RECORDS

The recording of patient information can be traced back through antiquity from the cave paintings and stone carvings of prehistoric times to Egyptian surgical case reports documented on papyrus (Gillum, 2013; Synapse Medical, 2019). As civilizations developed, people transitioned to pen and paper for recording events. In the 1700s, businesses in the United States, including banks, stores, and eventually hospitals, used ledgers to record information. Benjamin Franklin, secretary of one of the first incorporated hospitals in Pennsylvania in the mid-1700s, kept records of clients' names, addresses, disorders, and dates of admission and discharge (Gensel, 2005; University of Pennsylvania, 2015). With the establishment of major teaching hospitals across the United States, more formal medical records were developed (Gillum, 2013). As medicine has advanced, so has the complexity and detail of the record. An entire profession, now called *health information management*, emerged to oversee the collection, classification, storage, retrieval, and dissemination of health records (American Health Information Management Association [AHIMA], 2021).

The use of computers to support health records management began in the late 1960s (Gillum, 2013). Over the past several decades, the use of electronic health records (EHRs) or electronic medical records (EMRs) has transitioned from the exception to the rule in many health care settings (Kettenbach & Schlomer, 2016; Quinn & Gordon, 2016; Sullivan, 2019). Garrett and Seidman (2011) explained a critical difference between EMRs and EHRs. **EMRs contain medical and treatment information for a patient at a single location.** In contrast, "EHRs focus on the total health of the patient—going beyond standard clinical data collected in the provider's office and inclusive of a broader

Gateley, C. A. *Documentation Manual for
Occupational Therapy, Fifth Edition* (pp. 7-14).
© 2024 Taylor & Francis Group.

view on a patient's care" (Garrett & Seidman, 2011, para. 6). Rather than being restricted to a single practice, **EHRs are designed to share information across many providers and locations**, including laboratories and specialists, so that all clinicians involved in the patient's care have quick and easy access to the information about the individual's history and current condition. The use of EHRs has the potential to streamline and improve the overall quality of client care, increase efficiency of health practitioners, and reduce health care costs (Office of the National Coordinator for Health Information Technology, 2019).

"Whether paper-based or electronic, the health record is the link connecting all of health care" (Smith, 2016, p. 3). In addition to the clinical information documented by providers, health records also contain an administrative section including demographic information, payment source, account number, patient identification number, referral information, consent to release information, acknowledgment of patient rights and privacy notices, and advance directives (Kettenbach & Schlomer, 2016). Depending on the setting, occupational therapy practitioners may be responsible for gathering some of this information.

HISTORY OF THE SOAP NOTE

EHRs allow members of a client's health care team to access information with a few simple clicks of the mouse. While many health care organizations have moved fully or partially to EHRs, printed health records are still in use in many settings and are the default back-up plan when EHRs experience technological glitches. Printed health records typically are organized in one of the following methods (Clark, 2004):

- *Source-oriented*: Documents are grouped together by the source from which they came (e.g., laboratory results, radiology results, physician notes, nursing notes, therapy notes).
- *Integrated*: Documents from various sources are entered in chronological or reverse chronological order.
- *Problem-oriented*: Documents are organized according to the client's problem list.

Each of these formats has its advantages and disadvantages. However, the problem-oriented medical record (POMR) is the basis for the SOAP note format presented in this manual. Dr. Lawrence Weed introduced the POMR in the late 1960s to standardize physician and nursing documentation (Aronson, 2019; Weed, 1968). Weed believed that the POMR format offered a more client-centered approach by focusing on the client's problems and the progress made toward solving those problems. As part of the more client-centered approach to documentation, Weed recommended organizing the progress note into four sections, including the client's own perception of the situation, which previously had been considered irrelevant. He used the acronym SOAP to define the four sections (Podder et al., 2020; Weed, 1968):

- *S—Subjective*: This section includes the **client's report** of their problems, limitations, and needs as well as the client's perception of treatment and progress. Typically, the Subjective section of the progress note is brief. However, in an initial evaluation report, the "S" might be longer since it will include the information obtained in the initial interview for the client's occupational profile.
- *O—Objective*: This section contains the health professional's **observation** of the client's performance and the treatment provided. In an initial evaluation note, this section also includes all of the measurable, quantifiable, and observable data that were collected.
- *A—Assessment*: This section is the health professional's **analysis and interpretation** of the events reported in the Subjective and Objective sections. This section shows the practitioner's professional reasoning. An initial evaluation contains the functional problem list and the client's rehabilitation potential. Subsequent progress notes will focus on one or more problems from that list as well as the progress made and rehabilitation potential.
- *P—Plan*: This section is the health professional's plan of **what to do next**, and it includes the anticipated frequency and duration of services. An initial evaluation includes a detailed intervention plan. Subsequent progress notes specify the planned focus for future sessions with the client. This section may also include plans to refer the client to other disciplines when appropriate.

SOAP notes help standardize documentation among physicians as well as nurses, pharmacists, psychologists, therapists, and many other health care professionals (Hovey, 2019; Quinn & Gordon, 2016). In fact, SOAP notes have been described as "the most common method of documentation used by providers to input notes into patients' medical records" (CareCloud, 2021, para. 2). Many EHRs are built around the SOAP note concept and contain options for data entry in a SOAP note format. "A major advantage of the SOAP format is its widespread acceptance and the resulting familiarity with the format. ... It emphasizes clear, complete, and well-organized reporting of findings with a natural progression from data collection to assessment to plan" (Quinn & Gordon, 2016, p. 11).

Table 2-1

COMPONENTS OF DIFFERENT NOTE FORMATS

DART		FOCUS	
D	Data observed and reported	Focus of the concern	
A	Action taken	Data	
R	Response of the client	Action	
T	Teaching given	Response	
PIE		**SBAR**	
P	Problem observed and reported	S	Situation observed or reported
I	Interventions taken	B	Background information
E	Evaluation of the client's response	A	Assessment
		R	Recommendation
SOAPIE		**SOAPIER**	
S	Subjective	S	Subjective
O	Objective	O	Objective
A	Assessment	A	Assessment
P	Plan	P	Plan
I	Implementation of interventions	I	Implementation of interventions
E	Evaluation of outcomes	E	Evaluation of outcomes
		R	Revision

Data source: Rebar, 2009.

It is important to remember that SOAP is just a format—an outline for organizing information. Any note can be written in this format, although the SOAP format works better for some types of notes than others. An initial assessment can be quite lengthy when written in the SOAP format because it will contain an occupational profile, prior level of functioning, a summary of functional problems, and the detailed intervention plan including long- and short-term goals. For this reason, many practice settings do not use the SOAP format for the initial evaluation report, but the facility may use the SOAP format for treatment and progress notes.

The SOAP format is an alternative to narrative notes, which tend to be disorganized and subjective. It forces the writer to look at all four aspects of the therapy session and to present the information in an orderly fashion. Learning the SOAP format is an excellent way for students and practitioners to develop the professional reasoning process that underlies therapeutic intervention. Practitioners who learn to use the SOAP format will be able to adapt their documentation skills to nearly any practice setting as well as to EHRs. A more detailed explanation of each section of the SOAP note is provided in Chapters 8 through 11.

OTHER FORMATS FOR NOTES

SOAP notes are only one method for writing notes. Although very common for occupational therapy practitioners, you may encounter other note formats, particularly in inpatient hospital settings. Rebar (2009) described several alternative formats for clinical documentation including DART, FOCUS, PIE, SBAR, SOAPIE, and SOAPIER. Although it is beyond the scope of this textbook to provide in-depth examples of each of these formats, it is important to understand how practitioners organize information in each format. Table 2-1 lists the components of each format.

PURPOSES OF CLIENT CARE DOCUMENTATION

The primary and obvious purpose of the health record is to document a client's health information for future reference. Documentation is the evidence that occupational therapy practitioners create to prove that a client or caregiver interaction occurred (Quinn & Gordon, 2016; Sames, 2015). It is important to consider the many potential audiences and functions of the health record whenever you make an entry into a client's record.

Client Care Management

The health record is one of the ways the treatment team communicates with each other about the day-to-day aspects of the client's care. Other occupational therapy practitioners and members of the interprofessional treatment team will read your notes to coordinate care (Quinn & Gordon, 2016; Sames, 2015). In your notes, you share the results of your evaluation, report the client's progress toward established goals, and advise other members of the team of your plan for continuing care, all of which are important to the treatment team. Good documentation is particularly important in ensuring continuity of care within and between settings as a single client may encounter multiple occupational therapy practitioners during the intervention process.

Reimbursement

The health record is the source for which services were provided and which services may be billed. Third-party payers such as Medicare, Medicaid, and private insurance companies may review documentation, not only for frequency and duration, but also to determine if the services provided to the client are worth paying for. Documentation in the health record is the primary means of justifying reimbursement for intervention (Combs, 2020; Quinn & Gordon, 2016; Sames, 2015). In all settings, but particularly outpatient settings where services typically are billed on a fee-for-service model, occupational therapy practitioners must ensure that their documentation about the treatment session justifies the billing codes that were used for the client's visit (Fusion Web Clinic, 2022). Documentation that is inaccurate or poorly written may be used by reimbursement sources to deny payment for occupational therapy services (Sames, 2015).

Utilization Review and Utilization Management

The health record may be used for determining whether services provided to a client are appropriate, medically necessary, and efficient according to the policies and procedures established by federal and state regulatory agencies. Duchinsky (2016) explained the distinction between *utilization review* and *utilization management*, two terms that often are used interchangeably but have different processes and meanings. Utilization review is a review of the health record that occurs **after** services have been provided to a client and "safeguards against unnecessary and inappropriate medical care" (Duchinsky, 2016, para. 2).

In contrast, utilization management involves the proactive processes that take place **before and during** a client's provision of health services. These processes may include discharge planning or precertification for an acute care or rehabilitation unit stay. For example, in acute care settings, physicians, social workers, and case managers rely heavily on the recommendations of occupational and physical therapy practitioners to determine whether a patient is safe to discharge home or needs continued therapy services via home health, inpatient rehabilitation, or skilled nursing facility. Utilization management "ensures healthcare systems continuously improve and deliver appropriate levels of care, reducing the risk of cases that need review for inappropriate or unnecessary care" (Duchinsky, 2016, para. 3).

The goals of both utilization review and utilization management are to ensure compliance of health care providers and organizations to regulatory standards and to use a client's funds for health care in the most cost-effective manner. In either situation, documentation of occupational therapy services may help determine whether a client's admission and continued treatment are necessary and appropriate.

The Legal System

The health record is a legal document that substantiates what occurred during a client's illness and treatment. Any entries made in the health record, whether in print or electronic format, become a part of that legal document and may be subpoenaed (Kettenbach & Schlomer, 2016; Quinn & Gordon, 2016; Sames, 2015). If you as an occupational therapy practitioner have to appear in court to testify, it will be helpful if your documentation is clear, accurate, and thorough. Court cases often occur years after the event or intervention that is being contested (Sames, 2015). You may not even remember the event or the client. What you have written in the health record will provide you with the information you need to testify. However, Scott (2013) explained that "despite its broad range of variegated uses as a legal instrument, healthcare recordkeeping … should not be carried out with a defensive legal focus. Rather, the creation of patient care records should be guided primarily by patient welfare-oriented healthcare principles" (p. 94).

Quality Improvement

Quality improvement, often referred to as QI, is a framework for improving the quality of health care delivery by measuring and analyzing various processes within a health care system, identifying areas for improvement, and implementing new strategies to address those issues (Agency for Healthcare Research and Quality [AHRQ], 2013). "In the United States there has been an evolution from quality assurance, where the emphasis was on inspection and punishment for medical errors (the 'bad apple' theory) to QI, where we ask, 'How did the system fail to support the worker involved in an error?'" (AHRQ, 2013, para. 2).

The health record is one of the primary sources of information used in the quality improvement process. An example of a quality improvement process is the review of occupational therapy documentation to determine whether practitioners were consistently documenting a client's pain level according to hospital policy, followed by the implementation of measures to increase the compliance with the hospital policy, such as a pop-up reminder in an EHR when a practitioner attempts to sign a note without documenting the patient's pain level. Another example of a quality improvement process is the review of client care records to determine whether specific standardized assessments were performed for particular populations according to departmental or facility policy and subsequent modifications to the electronic documentation flowsheet with more prominent cues as therapists document an evaluation.

Accreditation

Health care settings that bill Medicare and/or Medicaid for services must be accredited by a state survey agency or a national accreditation organization approved by the Centers for Medicare & Medicaid Services (CMS) to ensure compliance with applicable laws and regulations (CMS, 2021). Some health care facilities voluntarily seek accreditation from private entities to improve their professional reputation as a provider of quality health care. For example, The Joint Commission, the oldest and largest health care accreditation entity in the United States, accredits more than 22,000 health care organizations and programs (The Joint Commission, 2022a). The Joint Commission accredits hospitals, nursing care centers, home care agencies, ambulatory care clinics, laboratory services, and behavioral health care programs. The Joint Commission's mission is "to continuously improve health care for the public, in collaboration with other stakeholders, by evaluating health care organizations and inspiring them to excel in providing safe and effective care of the highest quality and value" (The Joint Commission, 2022b, para. 1). The Commission on Accreditation of Rehabilitation Facilities (CARF) is another accrediting agency that occupational therapy practitioners may encounter. Founded in 1966 in the United States, CARF International now accredits more than 62,000 programs and services worldwide in the areas of aging services, behavioral health, child and youth services, employment and community services, and medical rehabilitation (CARF International, 2022). Accreditation surveyors always rely heavily on the review of client health records during the accreditation survey of a facility.

Education and Research

The health record may be used as a teaching tool. Students in various health care professions use the health record to gain information about a client's medical history and current clinical condition. An occupational therapy or occupational therapy assistant student may review the health record to learn about quality occupational therapy interventions or to gain a better understanding of the roles and interventions of other members of the client's health care team.

The health record may also be used to provide data for research by a variety of individuals. Public health entities may use the health record to identify and document the incidence of certain medical conditions. In recent decades, there has been a demand for evidence-based practice in all health care professions, including occupational therapy, to improve client outcomes and reduce health care costs (Cullen, 2018). For example, researchers may collect and analyze data from the health record to improve methods of disease and injury prevention or to analyze client outcomes to determine efficacy of specific therapeutic interventions. Good documentation practices help ensure that credible and valid data are available to clinical researchers (Sames, 2015).

Business Development and Management

Management teams use the information contained in the health record to plan and market services provided by a facility. For example, are there enough referrals for outpatient occupational therapy driving evaluations to warrant the cost of purchasing expensive assessment equipment and providing specialized training for staff? Does the number of referrals for inpatient occupational therapy following total joint replacement justify the need for additional occupational therapy staffing on the orthopedic unit? Are there significant differences in discharge outcomes for clients who received daily occupational therapy sessions as opposed to a frequency of three to five times per week in the acute care setting? If so, a rehabilitation director may be able to justify a new occupational therapist or occupational therapy assistant position.

Health care records can also provide a productivity measure of occupational therapy practitioner workload and performance. Productivity is a measure of the amount of billable time in a practitioner's workday (Braveman, 2022). Although many practitioners cringe at the mention of productivity standards, "workload expectations and productivity measurement are legitimate management tools utilized to ensure appropriate staffing resources for service delivery as well as to maximize reimbursement, with the goal of achieving economic sustainability" (American Occupational Therapy Association [AOTA] Ethics Commission, 2019).

Client Access

Another significant user of the health record is the client. When you are documenting in the health record, always remember that the client owns the information and may choose to exercise the right to review or obtain a copy of the health record (U.S. Department of Health & Human Services [DHHS], 2020). As health care has evolved to a more client-centered, collaborative approach, encouraging and increasing client access to health records can improve clients' sense of control over their health and well-being. Clients who access their own health information "are better able to monitor chronic conditions, adhere to treatment plans, find and fix errors in their health records, track progress in wellness or disease management programs, and directly contribute their information to research" (U.S. DHHS, 2020, para. 1).

A recent trend in the United States is encouraging clients to use a personal health record (PHR), which is a way to organize and manage health information that may be scattered across various health care facilities and providers (Sarwal & Gupta, 2021). Unlike EHRs, PHRs are maintained and controlled by the client rather than the provider and may be kept in either written or electronic form. While providers still maintain a health record on each client, the PHR allows the individual to keep health information in an organized fashion for personal reference and for ease of communication with health care providers. A client may choose to include information in the PHR about occupational therapy services you have provided.

Advocacy

You may be able to use your documentation to advocate for a client. For example, perhaps a client needs a customized power wheelchair to meet positioning and mobility needs. Your documentation helps the payer understand why each feature of the wheelchair is medically necessary. Or perhaps you can use your documentation to convince a local charitable organization to fund home modifications for a client who otherwise would not be able to remain at home. On a larger scale, occupational therapy documentation may serve as a tool for advocating for our profession:

> Good documentation can help educate others, including other healthcare professionals, third party payers, and patients themselves, about the services that physical or occupational therapy can provide. Although the services may seem obvious to us, they are not so obvious to people outside our profession. (Kettenbach & Schlomer, 2016, p. 22)

A team of researchers recently discovered that higher hospital spending on occupational therapy services was associated with lower readmission rates (Rogers et al., 2016), prompting a call by AOTA for occupational therapy services to be utilized more in hospital settings (AOTA, 2017). That research was based in part on documentation by occupational therapy practitioners.

REFERENCES

Agency for Healthcare Research and Quality. (2013). *Module 4: Approaches to quality improvement.* https://www.ahrq.gov/

American Health Information Management Association. (2021). *Who we are.* https://ahima.org/

American Occupational Therapy Association. (2017). *AOTA responds to New York Times article, "The high price of failing America's costliest patients."* https://www.aota.org/

American Occupational Therapy Association Ethics Commission. (2019). *Ethical considerations for productivity, billing, and reimbursement.* https://www.aota.org/

Aronson, M. D. (2019). The purpose of the medical record: Why Lawrence Weed still matters. *American Journal of Medicine, 132*(11), 1256-1257. https://doi.org/10.1016/j.amjmed.2019.03.051

Braveman, B. (2022). Financial planning, management, and budgeting. In B. Braveman (Ed.), *Leading & managing occupational therapy services* (3rd ed., pp. 331-351). F. A. Davis.

CareCloud. (2021). *How SOAP notes paved the way for modern medical documentation.* https://www.carecloud.com/

CARF International. (2022). *Who we are.* http://www.carf.org/

Centers for Medicare & Medicaid Services. (2021). *Become a Medicare provider or supplier.* https://www.cms.gov/

Clark, J. (2004). *Documentation for acute care.* American Health Information Management Association.

Combs, T. (2020). *The importance of high-quality clinical documentation across the healthcare continuum.* Journal of Ahima. https://journal.ahima.org/

Cullen, L. (2018). *Evidence-based practice and the bottom line: An issue of cost.* Healthcare Financial Management Association. https://www.hfma.org/topics/article/58754.html

Duchinsky, E. (2016). *Understanding utilization review versus utilization management.* BHM Healthcare Solutions. https://bhmpc.com/

Fusion Web Clinic. (2022). *A complete guide to occupational therapy billing.* https://fusionwebclinic.com/

Garrett, P., & Seidman, J. (2011). EMR vs EHR—What is the difference? https://www.healthit.gov/

Gensel, L. (2005). The medical world of Benjamin Franklin. *Journal of the Royal Society of Medicine, 98*(12), 534-583. https://doi.org/10.1177/014107680509801209

Gillum, R. F. (2013). From papyrus to the electronic tablet: A brief history of the clinical medical record with lessons for the digital age. *American Journal of Medicine, 126*(10), 853-857. https://doi.org/10.1016/j.amjmed.2013.03.024

Hovey, N. (2019). *The importance of SOAP notes in an EHR.* Best Notes. https://www.bestnotes.com/

Kettenbach, G., & Schlomer, S. L. (2016). *Writing patient/client notes: Ensuring accuracy in documentation* (5th ed.). F. A. Davis Company.

Office of the National Coordinator for Health Information Technology. (2019). What is an electronic health record (EHR)? https://www.healthit.gov/

Podder, V., Lew, V., & Ghassemzadeh, S. (2020). SOAP Notes. In: *StatPearls* [Internet]. StatPearls Publishing. https://www.ncbi.nlm.nih.gov/books/NBK482263/

Quinn, L., & Gordon, J. (2016). *Documentation for rehabilitation: A guide to clinical decision making in physical therapy* (3rd ed.). Elsevier.

Rebar, C. (2009). *DocuNotes: Clinical pocket guide to effective charting.* F. A. Davis.

Rogers, A. T., Bai, G., Lavin, R. A., & Anderson, G. F. (2016, September 2). Higher hospital spending on occupational therapy is associated with lower readmission rates. *Medical Care Research and Review,* 1-19. dx.doi.org/10.1177/1077558716666981

Sames, K. (2015). *AOTA documentation series—Module 1: The nuts and bolts of effective documentation* [Online continuing education module]. American Occupational Therapy Association. https://www.aota.org/

Sarwal, D., & Gupta, V. (2021). *Personal health record.* https://www.ncbi.nlm.nih.gov/books/NBK557757/

Scott, R. W. (2013). *Legal, ethical, and practical aspects of patient care documentation: A guide for rehabilitation professionals* (4th ed.). Jones & Bartlett Learning.

Smith, J. (2016). Overview of the health record. In G. Kettenbach & S. L. Schlomer (Eds.), *Writing patient/client notes: Ensuring accuracy in documentation* (5th ed., pp. 3-8). F. A. Davis.

Sullivan, D. D. (2019). *Guide to clinical documentation* (3rd ed.). F. A. Davis.

Sutton, R. (2015). *The counselor's STEPs for progress notes* (2nd ed.). CreateSpace Independent Publishing Platform.

Synapse Medical. (2019). *A history of medical records in the ancient world.* https://synapsemedical.com.au

The Joint Commission. (2022a). *Facts about The Joint Commission.* https://www.jointcommission.org/

The Joint Commission. (2022b). *Mission statement.* https://www.jointcommission.org/

University of Pennsylvania. (2015). *History of Pennsylvania Hospital.* http://www.uphs.upenn.edu/paharc/timeline/1751/

U.S. Department of Health & Human Services. (2020). *Individuals' right under HIPAA to access their health information.* https://www.hhs.gov/

Weed, L. L. (1968). Medical records that guide and teach. *New England Journal of Medicine, 278*(11), 593-600. https://www.nejm.org/doi/full/10.1056/NEJM196803142781105

Chapter 3

Reimbursement, Coding, and Billing

The previous chapter provided an overview of the various purposes and uses of the health record and the potential impacts on the documentation of occupational therapy practitioners. Some of those issues warrant further explanation and discussion. Because documentation is the primary means of justifying reimbursement for services (Moninger, 2021), it is important for occupational therapy practitioners to understand various reimbursement systems as well as the coding and billing systems that affect reimbursement. Reimbursement, coding, and billing issues vary considerably between practice settings, and occupational therapy practitioners work in diverse health care settings. This chapter will provide a general foundation of information to guide documentation, but practitioners will need to stay up to date on policy changes that affect occupational therapy documentation and reimbursement.

SOURCES OF REIMBURSEMENT

Medicare

Medicare is a federal health insurance program managed by the Centers for Medicare & Medicaid Services (CMS; 2022d). Medicare helps pay the health care costs of people over age 65 years, people under age 65 years with certain disabilities, and people with end-stage renal disease. See Table 3-1 for a brief explanation of the four parts of Medicare benefits.

Some Medicare beneficiaries have a supplemental insurance policy from a previous employer to help cover the portion of costs that Medicare does not. Others choose to purchase Medigap, which is a supplemental policy sold by private insurance companies. Medigap policies may help cover deductibles, copayments, and coinsurance, although "Medigap plans sold to people new to Medicare [since January 1, 2020] can no longer cover the Part B deductible" (CMS, 2022g, para. 2).

People who are eligible for Medicare have a variety of options to consider when selecting their Medicare coverage. Each client you treat will have different benefits, co-pays, and deductibles depending on the coverage options they have selected. In many situations, your clients may have little to no understanding of their Medicare benefits. Occupational therapy services may be billed through Medicare Parts A, B, and C. Occupational therapy services covered under Medicare must be medically necessary and skilled (Kroll & Richman, 2018). *Medically necessary* means that services are consistent with accepted standards of practice for the client's condition. *Skilled* means that

Gateley, C. A. *Documentation Manual for Occupational Therapy, Fifth Edition* (pp. 15-30). © 2024 Taylor & Francis Group.

	Table 3-1
	BENEFITS UNDER DIFFERENT PARTS OF MEDICARE
MEDICARE PART A	Inpatient care in hospitals and critical access hospitals, skilled nursing facilities (SNFs), home health care, and hospice.
MEDICARE PART B	Physicians' services and outpatient care, including occupational therapy; services in long-term care facilities when the client does not qualify for coverage under Part A; durable medical equipment (DME) and preventive services such as vaccines, screening, and wellness visits.
MEDICARE PART C	Private insurance companies contract with Medicare to provide individuals with their Part A, B, and D benefits through Medicare Advantage Plans rather than through Original Medicare. These plans function like health maintenance organizations (HMOs) or preferred provider organizations (PPOs) in which beneficiaries typically may see providers only in a particular network to have services covered. These plans may also include coverage for vision, hearing, and dental services that are not covered under Original Medicare.
MEDICARE PART D	Covers a portion of prescription drug costs.

Data source: Centers for Medicare & Medicaid Services, 2022d.

the services provided require the decision making, clinical judgment, and highly complex competencies of an occupational therapist or occupational therapy assistant with a knowledge base of human functioning and occupational performance. *Nonskilled* services are those that are routine or maintenance types of therapy that could be carried out by nonprofessional personnel or caregivers.

Furthermore, occupational therapy services should result in documentable improvements within a reasonable and predictable time period based on contemporary practice standards. Documentation should "make the correlation between intervention and outcomes as explicit as possible" (Kroll & Richman, 2018, Slide 101). However, in 2013, the *Jimmo v. Sebelius* settlement agreement clarified that Medicare also covers skilled interventions that are intended to maintain function by slowing or preventing decline, so long as these services require the skill of a licensed practitioner (CMS, 2021a). In other words, coverage cannot be denied simply because an individual does not have the potential for improvement.

"The *Jimmo* Settlement Agreement clarified that when a beneficiary needs skilled nursing or therapy services under Medicare's skilled nursing facility (SNF), home health (HH), and outpatient therapy (OPT) benefits in order to maintain the patient's current condition or to prevent or slow decline or deterioration (provided all other coverage criteria are met), the Medicare program covers such services and coverage cannot be denied based on the absence of potential for improvement or restoration. … It does not matter whether such care is expected to improve or maintain the patient's clinical condition. In addition, although such maintenance coverage standards do not apply to services furnished in an inpatient rehabilitation facility (IRF) or a comprehensive outpatient rehabilitation facility (CORF), the *Jimmo* Settlement Agreement clarified that for services performed in the IRF setting, coverage should never be denied because a patient cannot be expected to achieve complete independence in the domain of self-care or because a patient cannot be expected to return to his or her prior level of functioning" (CMS, 2021a, para. 1).

Because Medicare regulations and guidelines are constantly changing, it is important that you stay abreast of current issues related to Medicare reimbursement for occupational therapy services. Several online resources are available to help you understand Medicare reimbursement:

- CMS website: https://www.cms.gov/
- Medicare website: https://www.medicare.gov/
- American Occupational Therapy Association (AOTA) website: https://www.aota.org/

The following sections will provide more detail about Medicare Parts A, B, and C, the three parts of Medicare that may serve as a source of reimbursement for occupational therapy services.

Medicare Part A

Medicare Part A has multiple reimbursement systems for providers and health care facilities. Although you may not be directly involved in billing and reimbursement processes, your occupational therapy documentation provides information about an individual's condition and performance, and you should have a general understanding of the reimbursement systems at your fieldwork site or place of employment (Healthinsurance.org, LLC, 2022). Here is a very brief overview of some of the most common reimbursement systems for Medicare Part A:

- *Fee-for-Service*: In this reimbursement model, health care providers are paid separately for each service provided (CMS, 2021f).
- *Prospective Payment Systems*: Under a Prospective Payment Systems model of reimbursement, Medicare payments are based on a predetermined fixed amount according to a patient's diagnosis-related group (CMS, 2021g).
- *Value-Based Bundled Payments*: Under this payment system, multiple entities and providers work together to manage each episode of care. For example, a hospital may team up with one or more physician groups, and collectively they are paid for the client's overall episode of care based on the client's outcomes. This model shifts incentives away from volume (more services provided = more money) to value (accountable use of resources and better client outcomes = more money; CMS, 2022f).
- *Patient Driven Payment Model (PDPM)*: This payment model for SNFs went into effect in late 2019. Prior to the implementation of PDPM, Medicare SNF payments were based in large part on the number of therapy minutes that each resident received. Thus, there was an incentive to provide high volumes of therapy to maximize payment (Net Health, 2022). Under PDPM, reimbursement is based on resident classifications and anticipated resource needs. "SNFs who over-deliver therapy won't get paid for services provided beyond the reimbursement level for each resident classification. But under-delivering therapy will lead to poor patient outcomes and potential Medicare audits and take-backs" (Net Health, 2022, para. 3).
- *Patient Driven Groupings Model (PDGM)*: Like PDPM, the PDGM model for home health services emphasizes "value over volume, eliminating therapy services thresholds as a reimbursement factor" (CareCentrix, Inc., 2020). Under PDGM, patients are classified into one of more than 400 case-mix groups based on the following factors (CMS, 2021c; Vontran & Gehne, 2019):
  - **Source of admission**: This is determined by whether the referral came from an institution (e.g., hospital, SNF, long-term care hospital, inpatient rehabilitation, inpatient psychiatric facility) or from the community (e.g., primary care physician).
  - **Clinical groupings**: The client's primary diagnosis is assigned to one of 12 clinical groups as the main reason for needing home health services. A few examples are neurorehabilitation, surgical aftercare, behavioral health, infectious disease, wound care, and respiratory conditions.
  - **Timing of episode of care**: Each 30-day period is classified as early or late. The first 30-day period of home health services is considered early. All subsequent 30-day periods are classified as late.
  - **Functional impairment level**: This level is classified as low, medium, or high based on client ability to complete grooming, dressing, bathing, toileting, transfers, and ambulation/locomotion and the risk for hospitalization.
  - **Comorbidities**: The comorbidity adjustment level of none, low, or high is based on the presence of secondary diagnoses. Multiple comorbidities are tied to more complex medical needs, poorer health outcomes, and higher costs.

Table 3-2

TOOLS FOR DOCUMENTING PATIENT STATUS IN POST-ACUTE CARE SETTINGS

INPATIENT REHABILITATION FACILITY—PATIENT ASSESSMENT INSTRUMENT (IRF-PAI)	The IRF-PAI collects "patient assessment data for quality measure calculation and payment determination in accordance with the IRF Quality Reporting Program (QRP)" (CMS, 2022a, para. 4). The IRF-PAI is required for all patients in an IRF who have Medicare Part A or Part C.
LONG-TERM CARE HOSPITAL (LTCH) CONTINUITY ASSESSMENT RECORD AND EVALUATION (CARE) DATA SET	For simplification, CMS refers to this document as the LCDS. The LCDS is the instrument used to collect patient assessment information in LTCHs (CMS, 2022b).
LONG-TERM CARE MINIMUM DATA SET (MDS)	The MDS is the electronic document used for "clinical assessment of all residents in Medicare and Medicaid certified nursing homes," regardless of individual payment source for each resident, and "provides a comprehensive assessment of each resident's functional capabilities" (CMS, 2021e, para. 1; CMS, 2022b).
OUTCOME AND ASSESSMENT INFORMATION SET (OASIS)	This tool is used to collect information about Medicare beneficiaries receiving home health services. Home health providers use the OASIS to collect information about a client's health conditions, living arrangements, and level of functional performance (CMS, 2022e).

By now you probably have realized that Medicare has a lot of acronyms to describe various aspects of health care delivery, documentation, and reimbursement. See Table 3-2 for a list of other terms and acronyms that you may encounter if you work with Medicare Part A beneficiaries in post-acute settings, in other words, after the individual is discharged from an acute care hospital. Each of the documentation tools listed in Table 3-2 has a Section GG that assigns a numerical score to the client's performance on several specific tasks related to self-care and mobility (Strunk, 2019). See Tables 3-3 and 3-4 for a brief overview of these scores and the self-care categories that occupational therapy practitioners most often score. Please note that occupational therapy practitioners may also be involved in scoring the mobility items on Section GG and/or the cognitive items in other portions of the post-acute care documentation tools. It is beyond the scope of this book to provide an extensive overview for all these items. If you work or have fieldwork in a post-acute setting, you likely will be required to complete training and an annual certification examination.

Scores are collected at admission, a discharge goal is set, and then scores are collected again at the time of the client's discharge from the respective setting. At the time of this writing, all post-acute care settings are experiencing or anticipating payment reforms. Data from Section GG, which may be completed in whole or part by occupational therapy practitioners, may be used to determine reimbursement levels and incentives for quality care (Grote, 2022). Prior to the creation of Section GG, the various post-acute care settings

… were collecting their own data with their own definitions and rating scales, which created a challenge in caring for patients when they were transferred from one setting to another. Section GG, which provides a universal language relative to functional ability, is expected to decrease variability, standardize communication and care across settings, and provide the basis for comparing patient types, outcomes, and costs. (Strunk, 2019, para. 5)

Table 3-3

SELF-CARE AND MOBILITY SECTION GG SCORES

ACTIVITY WAS PERFORMED, WITH OR WITHOUT ASSISTIVE DEVICES	
6—Independent	Activity is completed with **no assistance** from a helper, with or without adaptive equipment.
5—Set-Up or Clean-Up Assistance	Helper provides set-up **before** the activity and/or clean-up **after** the activity. The individual completes the activity without helper assistance **during** the activity. In other words, the helper can leave the room during the activity.
4—Supervision or Touching Assistance	Helper provides **verbal cues** and/or **touching/steadying** and/or **contact guard assist** as the individual completes the activity. Assistance may be intermittent or provided throughout the activity.
3—Partial/Moderate Assistance	Helper assists by lifting, holding, or supporting the trunk or limbs during the activity, but overall provides **less than half** of the total effort to complete the activity.
2—Substantial/Maximal Assistance	Helper assists by lifting, holding, or supporting the trunk or limbs during the activity, but overall provides **more than half** of the total effort to complete the activity.
1—Dependent	Helper performs **all** of the effort to complete the activity, and the individual exhibits **none** of the effort, or the assistance of **two or more helpers** is required for the individual to complete the activity.
ACTIVITY WAS NOT ATTEMPTED	
07—Individual Refused	Every effort should be made to encourage the individual to complete the activity during the assessment period, but if the **individual completely refuses**, this score would be entered for the activity.
09—Not Applicable	Activity is not something the client was able to complete before the current injury, illness, or exacerbation and is **not relevant for the client now**. Example: Client has bilateral lower extremity above the knee amputations and does not have prostheses, so putting on and taking off footwear would be not applicable. In another example, if a client did not eat or drink by mouth prior to this admission (i.e., received tube feedings or total parenteral nutrition), then eating by mouth would be not applicable.
10—Not Attempted Due to Environmental Limitations	Activity is something relevant for the client, but **contextual circumstances prevent assessment** of the client's performance. May include lack of equipment or weather conditions. Example: If a facility does not have a car simulator indoors, and it is too cold or icy to take the individual outdoors to assess performance of a car transfer, then the activity would not be attempted due to environmental limitations.

(continued)

Table 3-3 (continued)

SELF-CARE AND MOBILITY SECTION GG SCORES

ACTIVITY WAS PERFORMED, WITH OR WITHOUT ASSISTIVE DEVICES	
88—Not Attempted Due to Medical Condition or Safety Concerns	Activity is something relevant for the client, but assessing this activity is **not possible due to current medical status or would put the patient at risk**. Example: If the client currently does not eat or drink by mouth due to aspiration risk, but did eat and drink by mouth prior to the illness or event leading to this admission, then eating by mouth would be unsafe to attempt for this assessment.

Data source: American Occupational Therapy Association, 2022d.

Table 3-4

SELF-CARE SECTION GG ITEMS AND DEFINITIONS

Eating	Bring food and/or liquid to the mouth using suitable utensils and swallowing, after meal is placed in front of person.
Oral Hygiene	Use of suitable utensils to clean teeth. If the individual has dentures, this item includes removal and insertion of dentures as well as the ability to manage materials required for soaking and rinsing.
Toilet Hygiene	Perineal hygiene and the adjustment of clothing before and after voiding or having a bowel movement. If the individual has an ostomy, this item includes wiping the opening, but **not** applying or removing the ostomy equipment.
Wash Upper Body	Wash, rinse, and dry the face, hands, chest, and arms while sitting in a chair or bed. (As of 2023, this item is reported only in LTCH setting.)
Shower/Bathe Self	Wash, rinse, and dry self. Does not include washing back or hair; also does not include tub or shower transfer. (As of 2023, this item is only reported in IRF, SNF, and home health settings.)
Upper Body Dressing	Dress and undress self above the waist, including applicable fasteners. May include bra, shirt, neck or back brace, abdominal binder, and any applicable upper extremity orthotic or prosthetic items.
Lower Body Dressing	Dress and undress self below the waist, including applicable fasteners. May include underwear, incontinence brief, shorts or pants, skirts, knee brace, stump shrinker or sock, and any applicable lower extremity prosthetic. This item does **not** include footwear.
Putting On/Taking Off Footwear	Put on and take off socks, shoes, or other footwear needed for safe mobility. This includes compression stockings, an ankle foot orthosis (AFO), orthopedic walking boot, or other foot orthotic.

Data sources: American Occupational Therapy Association, 2022d; Deutsch & Dass, 2019.

Medicare Part B

Medicare Part B covers occupational therapy services in outpatient clinics and long-term care settings when an individual is not eligible for SNF level of care. "Medicare Part B (Medical Insurance) helps pay for medically necessary outpatient occupational therapy if your doctor or other health care provider certifies you need it" (CMS, 2022d, para. 1). Original Medicare beneficiaries typically have a monthly premium for this medical coverage and pay 20% of the Medicare-approved amount for occupational therapy services after meeting the Part B deductible. If the individual has an additional insurance supplement, that supplemental policy may cover the 20% that Medicare Part B does not cover. Medicare Advantage plans set their own rules regarding deductibles and coinsurance.

An important change since the last edition of this book is that Medicare no longer sets a "therapy cap" or monetary limit on the amount of outpatient occupational therapy services a patient can receive in one calendar year. However, if billed occupational therapy services exceed a particular threshold (e.g., $2230 for 2023), services must be billed with a particular code called a KX modifier (CMS, 2021d, 2023). Once a client's billed occupational therapy services exceed a targeted medical review threshold, currently set at $3000 through 2028, the claim may be selected for review (American Physical Therapy Association [APTA], 2022). "Factors used to select claims for review may include any of the following:

- The provider has had a high claims denial percentage for therapy services or is less compliant with applicable requirements.
- The provider has a pattern of billing for therapy services that is aberrant compared with peers, or otherwise has questionable billing practices for services, such as billing medically unlikely units of services within a single day.
- The provider is newly enrolled or has not previously furnished therapy services.
- The services are furnished to treat targeted types of medical conditions.
- The provider is part of a group that includes another provider identified by the above factors" (APTA, 2022, para. 9).

If future therapy services are not reasonable and necessary, or if the client is not expected to demonstrate significant functional improvement within a reasonable amount of time, the occupational therapist must provide the Medicare beneficiary with an Advanced Beneficiary Notice of Noncoverage (ABN). The ABN informs clients that services are not likely to be paid by Medicare so they can make decisions about whether they want to receive those services and pay for them out of pocket (AOTA, 2020a). Many clients think that just because a physician has ordered occupational therapy, Medicare will automatically cover those services. However, the responsibility lies with the occupational therapy practitioner to document the functional status and improvement of the client to prove medical necessity.

Medicare Part C

Medicare Part C plans, also known as *Medicare Advantage plans*, are offered by private Medicare-approved insurance companies, which administer the client's Parts A, B, and D benefits (CMS, 2022c). Although these private insurance companies must follow general rules set by Medicare, they establish their own rules about how clients access various health care services, including occupational therapy. For example, a Medicare Advantage plan can limit which facilities and providers are covered under the plan. In acute care settings, occupational therapy practitioners often are involved in making recommendations for a patient to go to a SNF or an inpatient rehabilitation facility (IRF). Under Original Medicare, patients can choose any SNF or IRF that will accept them. However, a Medicare Advantage plan may require additional preauthorization and may limit which facilities the patient goes to. People who enroll in Medicare Advantage plans "often give up the freedoms that come along with Original Medicare in exchange for the additional benefits" like dental and vision coverage (Elite Insurance Partners LLC, 2022, para. 9). Furthermore, insurance companies administering Medicare Advantage plans can set their own out-of-pocket costs such as deductibles and copayments.

Medicaid and Children's Health Insurance Plan

Medicaid is a health insurance program jointly funded by the federal government and each individual state (Benefits.gov, 2021). It covers individuals who have limited income and meet certain eligibility requirements. Medicaid is administered by each individual state. While all states must follow general federal guidelines, there is considerable variance between states in terms of which individuals are eligible for Medicaid and which services are covered. There may also be differences within a single state between services that are covered by Medicaid for adults versus children.

> While Medicaid serves both children and adults in low-income families, CHIP [Children's Health Insurance Plan] was created to help build upon Medicaid coverage for low-income children and does not provide additional coverage for adults. Medicaid programs are required to provide certain coverage by federal standards, while CHIP's coverage requirements are established by the individual states. (Benefits.gov, 2021, para. 3)

Occupational therapy practitioners must become familiar with Medicaid and CHIP documentation and reimbursement guidelines for the state in which they are practicing if these serve as sources for reimbursement in their practice settings.

Private Insurance

Private insurance coverage may be offered through an individual's employer or the employer of the individual's spouse, partner, or significant other. Individuals may also be covered through an insurance policy offered by a parent's employer, up through age 26 (U.S. Department of Health & Human Services, 2017). The cost of such plans often is subsidized by the employer. Individuals may also sign up for private health insurance coverage via the Health Insurance Marketplace at www.healthcare.gov. All insurance plans in the Marketplace must cover 10 essential health benefits (CMS, 2022h, para. 1):

1. Ambulatory patient services (outpatient care)
2. Emergency services
3. Hospitalization
4. Pregnancy, maternity, and newborn care
5. Mental health and substance use disorder services
6. Prescription drugs
7. Rehabilitative and habilitative services and devices
8. Laboratory services
9. Preventive and wellness services and chronic disease management
10. Pediatric services, including oral and vision care (however, adult dental and vision care are **not** classified as essential health benefits)

There are many different private insurance plans with varying coverage, and there may be specific requirements that must be followed for the insurance company to pay for health care services, including occupational therapy. These requirements may include seeking health care from only particular providers considered in-network, getting preauthorization or prior approval before seeing a health care provider, and limiting the number of visits per year to a particular type of provider. Many health care settings have individuals whose primary role is to deal with these insurance issues, but occupational therapy practitioners may have more direct involvement in the process in some settings. Documentation must meet the requirements of the individual practice setting, and there may be additional documentation required for a client's specific insurance plan. AOTA (2022a, para. 2) explained:

> For practitioners in the private practice/outpatient setting, private insurance reimbursement can be a significant portion of their practice revenue. Any change in benefit, coverage, or reimbursement policy for occupational therapy services by a commercial insurance company can have a profound impact on private practitioners and their clients.

Workers' Compensation

Workers' Compensation is a type of business insurance that covers "loss of income, medical expenses, and other related expenses when an employee is injured or develops a health condition related to their work environment" (AOTA, 2022c, para. 1). Each state has different requirements for its Workers' Compensation program. Occupational therapy may be a service covered under the medical expenses of the program. When a client has Workers' Compensation as the funding source, therapeutic interventions and documentation should focus on improving the individual's capacity to return to work. In some cases, occupational therapists may be called upon to conduct an Ergonomic Worksite Analysis to determine if a client's injury, disease, or condition is work related (Heller-Ono, 2021). The U.S. Department of Labor (2022) has a webpage that provides contact information for state Workers' Compensation officials and links to each state's website.

Schools

Reauthorized in 2004, and later amended in 2015 through the Every Student Succeeds Act, "the Individuals with Disabilities Education Act (IDEA) is a law that makes available a free appropriate public education [FAPE] to eligible children with disabilities throughout the nation and ensures special education and related services to those children" (U.S. Department of Education, 2022, para. 1). Part B of IDEA requires schools to provide students with disabilities a FAPE in the least restrictive environment (LRE). The law applies to students ages 3 through 21 years. Children who qualify for special education services under Part B may be eligible for occupational therapy services if those services are necessary to benefit from education.

Section 504 of the Rehabilitation Act of 1973 and Title II of the Americans with Disabilities Act (ADA) of 1990 prohibit schools from excluding a student with a disability from participating in educational activities (U.S. Department of Education, 2020). In other words, Section 504 ensures that children receive necessary accommodations and modifications for equal access to education:

> A student on a 504 plan may require related services such as occupational therapy. This may take the form of an OT helping develop accommodations, consultative services, and in rare cases, direct services. … It's important to note that IDEA is a function of **special** education and Section 504 is a facet of **general** education. (Breithart, 2021, para. 12-13)

Schools use an Individualized Education Program to document the student's educational needs, goals, and services (Hanft & Shepherd, 2016). Documentation requirements vary from school to school, but the services provided must be relevant to the educational setting. In some cases, school-based services may be covered by Medicaid. In such cases, services must meet requirements of both educational relevance and medical necessity (Laverdure & LeCompte, 2021).

Early Intervention Programs

The Early Intervention Program for Infants and Toddlers with Disabilities (Part C of IDEA) is a federal grant program that assists states in operating a program of early intervention services for infants and toddlers from birth through a child's third birthday, along with their families (U.S. Department of Education, 2022). The program targets children who have a diagnosis associated with developmental delay and children who are deemed at risk for developmental delay. A major provision of Part C is that services are to be provided in a child's *natural environment*. These include the child's home and community settings that are typical for children without disabilities, such as preschools, day care centers, and other community settings. Eligibility requirements vary among states based on each state's definition of developmental delay, the degree to which a child must exhibit such a delay, and the physical or mental diagnoses that are identified as placing a child at risk for developmental delay (Early Childhood Technical Assistance Center, 2021).

Just as some school-based services are covered by Medicaid, occupational therapy services provided through early intervention programs may also be covered by Medicaid (Stuart, 2022). Each child served in an early intervention program will have an Individualized Family Service Plan (IFSP) that includes (U.S. Department of Education, 2017):

- The child's present physical, cognitive, communication, adaptive, and social or emotional developmental level
- The family's resources, concerns, and priorities for the child
- Expected results or outcomes of intervention
- Early intervention services needed to meet the identified needs of the child and family
- Medical or other services provided through other sources
- Projected dates and duration of services
- Identification of a service coordinator
- A transition plan out of Part C services

Occupational therapy is one of the many services that may be provided as part of the IFSP, and specific documentation requirements vary across states.

BILLING CODES

Occupational therapy practitioners will encounter multiple coding systems as part of their documentation and billing processes. These coding systems are intended to provide a standard language between health care providers and reimbursement sources for describing a client's diagnosis and the services provided (American Medical Association [AMA], 2022a; Centers for Disease Control and Prevention [CDC], 2022). It should be noted that the coding systems described in this section are updated frequently, and practitioners must keep track of changes that may affect their documentation.

ICD-10 Codes

Originally designed in the 1800s by the International Statistical Institute to track causes of death (mortality), the *International Classification of Diseases* (ICD) currently is maintained by the World Health Organization (WHO) and now includes codes for illness and disease while a person is still alive (morbidity; American Association of Professional Coders [AAPC], 2021). Countries use variations of the ICD coding system, "each modified to align with their unique healthcare infrastructure. The US version of ICD-10, created by the Centers for Medicare & Medicaid Services (CMS) and the National Center for Health Statistics (NCHS)," consists of two sets of codes (AAPC, 2021, para. 2):

1. *ICD-10-CM (Clinical Modification)*: These are alphanumeric **diagnosis codes used in all health care settings**. These codes allow a high degree of specificity about a client's condition. "ICD-10-CM is a standardized classification system of diagnosis codes that represent conditions and diseases, related health problems, abnormal findings, signs and symptoms, injuries, external causes of injuries and diseases, and social circumstances" (AAPC, 2021, para. 5).
   - Example: I69.351—Hemiplegia and hemiparesis following cerebral infarction affecting right dominant side
2. *ICD-10-PCS (Procedure Classification System)*: These are the codes used to classify and bill for the **procedures in inpatient hospital settings only**. Like the diagnosis codes, the procedure codes allow for a high degree of specificity.
   - Example: F0FZ1FZ—Caregiver training in dressing using assistive, adaptive, supportive, or protective equipment

In most hospital and clinic settings, there are individuals or entire departments whose responsibility it is to review documentation and ensure that applicable codes were included in a client's health record and related billing documentation. However, those individuals rely on the detailed documentation of health professionals, including occupational therapy practitioners, to assign the appropriate codes. As mentioned previously, coding systems are updated frequently. At the time of this writing, WHO had already published ICD-11 (2022), but it is unclear when the U.S. health care system will transition from the current ICD-10 coding system.

Current Procedural Terminology Codes

Current Procedural Terminology (CPT) codes are owned and copyrighted by the AMA (2022a, 2022b). The codes are a standardized listing of descriptive and identifying terms for reporting medical services and procedures. CMS adopted the use of CPT codes in 1983 as the mandatory system of coding for **outpatient services** under Medicare Part B. CPT codes, also known as *HCPCS Level I codes*, comprise one of the subsystems of the Healthcare Common Procedure Coding System used by Medicare and other health insurance programs to process health care claims. Most managed care and private insurance companies also base their reimbursements on the CPT relative value units (RVUs) established by CMS. The RVU of each code is based on three factors (Jordan et al., 2022):

1. *Work*: The technical skill and physical effort, mental effort and judgment, time to perform the service, and the psychological stress incurred by the provider.
2. *Practice expense*: The clinical staff, medical equipment, and medical supplies needed to perform the service or procedure.
3. *Professional liability*: The insurance premiums for specialists that perform a service based on risk of performing the service.

CPT codes are continuously reviewed, and new and revised CPT codes are published yearly. Some codes are deleted, and new codes are added. This annual review process "ensures clinically valid codes are issued, updated, and maintained on a regular basis to accurately reflect current clinical practice and innovation in medicine" (AMA, 2022a, para. 4). Furthermore, the AMA collaborates with AOTA and other organizations to modify existing codes and create new codes when needed. For example, following years of advocacy by AOTA and other professional organizations, the AMA established new CPT codes in 2017 to distinguish different levels of occupational therapy evaluation (Table 3-5). Occupational therapy evaluations are categorized as Low Complexity, Moderate Complexity, or High Complexity based on the complexity of three primary factors:

1. **Occupational profile and client history**, including both medical and therapy history
2. **Assessment of occupational performance** with identification of performance deficits that result in activity or participation restrictions
3. **Clinical decision making** in analyzing the occupational profile, the assessment data, and the number of treatment options

To bill for a High Complexity evaluation, the complexity of each of the three factors **must meet** the High Complexity criteria in Table 3-5. To bill for a Moderate Complexity evaluation, the complexity of each of the three criteria must be **no lower than** the Moderate Complexity criteria. In other words, you must bill an evaluation at the lowest complexity of any of the three individual factors. For example, if two factors meet Moderate Complexity criteria but one factor only meets Low Complexity criteria, you must bill the entire evaluation as Low Complexity. AOTA has a training video to better understand the use of these evaluation codes (AOTA, 2019).

It is the responsibility of each occupational therapy practitioner and employer to understand the current codes that may be assigned for services provided. Each year, AOTA provides members with a list of CPT codes from the AMA of the most frequently used codes by occupational therapy practitioners to classify and bill for services. The following are just a few of those common codes. Please note that this list is not all-inclusive (AOTA, 2022f):

- 97165   Occupational therapy evaluation, low complexity
- 97166   Occupational therapy evaluation, moderate complexity
- 97167   Occupational therapy evaluation, high complexity
- 97168   Occupational therapy re-evaluation
- 97110   Therapeutic procedure (exercises for strength, endurance, ROM)
- 97112   Neuromuscular reeducation
- 97129   Therapeutic interventions focused on cognitive function (first 15 minutes)
- 97130   Each additional 15 minutes of cognitive therapeutic interventions
- 97140   Manual therapy (mobilization, lymphatic drainage, traction)
- 97530   Therapeutic activities (dynamic activities to improve function)
- 97533   Sensory integrative techniques
- 97535   Self-care/home management training
- 97537   Community/work reintegration training
- 97545   Work hardening/conditioning (initial 2 hours)

Table 3-5

OCCUPATIONAL THERAPY EVALUATION CODES

CPT CODE AND EVALUATION CATEGORY	OCCUPATIONAL PROFILE AND CLIENT HISTORY	ASSESSMENT OF OCCUPATIONAL PERFORMANCE	CLINICAL DECISION MAKING IN THE COLLECTION AND ANALYSIS OF DATA
97165 OT Evaluation: Low Complexity	Occupational profile and history with **brief** review of medical/therapy records related to presenting problem and functional performance	**1 to 3 performance deficits** relating to physical, cognitive, or psychosocial skills limiting activity or participation	Data collection and analysis from **problem-focused** assessment/s
97166 OT Evaluation: Moderate Complexity	Occupational profile and history with **expanded** review of medical/therapy records related to presenting problem and functional performance	**3 to 5 performance deficits** relating to physical, cognitive, or psychosocial skills limiting activity or participation	Data collection and analysis from **detailed** assessment/s
97167 OT Evaluation: High Complexity	Occupational profile and history with **extensive** review of medical/therapy records related to presenting problem and functional performance	**5 or more performance deficits** relating to physical, cognitive, or psychosocial skills limiting activity or participation	Data collection and analysis from **comprehensive** assessment/s

Data source: American Occupational Therapy Association, 2016.

- 97546   Each additional hour of work hardening/conditioning
- 97755   Assistive technology assessment
- 97760   Orthotic management and training—Initial encounter
- 97761   Prosthetic training—Initial encounter
- 97763   Orthotic or prosthetic management and training, subsequent encounters
- 92526   Treatment of swallowing dysfunction and/or oral function for feeding
- 96110   Developmental screening
- 96112   Developmental test administration
- 98977   Remote therapeutic monitoring

Each of the codes above has specific guidelines for use. Each year the AMA publishes a new CPT code book with thorough descriptions and details of how to use each code correctly (AMA, 2022b). Some CPT codes are billed as a single unit regardless of time spent on the activity described by the code. For example, the three codes for occupational therapy evaluation are billed as a single unit, regardless of time spent on the evaluation. Other codes are billed in 15-minute units and follow the 8-minute rule, which differs by payment source.

Table 3-6

BILLING CURRENT PROCEDURAL TERMINOLOGY CODES USING THE CENTERS FOR MEDICARE & MEDICAID SERVICES 8-MINUTE RULE

NUMBER OF 15-MINUTE UNITS THAT CAN BE BILLED	TOTAL BILLABLE INTERVENTION TIME IN MINUTES
0	1 to 7
1	8 to 22
2	23 to 37
3	38 to 52
4	53 to 67
5	68 to 82
6	83 to 97

Data source: American Occupational Therapy Association, 2021.

Centers for Medicare & Medicaid Services 8-Minute Rule

The CMS 8-minute rule stipulates that a service must have been provided for at least 8 minutes to bill one 15-minute CPT code. A second billable unit cannot be billed "until you have at least 8 minutes past the 15-minute mark. If more than one timed CPT code is billed during a calendar day, then the total treatment time determines the number of units billed" (AOTA, 2021, para. 2). See Table 3-6 for a quick reference of how many units you can bill based on the number of intervention minutes when you are working with a Medicare beneficiary or another payer source that follows CMS guidelines. **Under the CMS 8-minute rule, you cannot bill more than 4 units in an hour.**

Substantial Portion Methodology or the American Medical Association 8-Minute Rule

Some private insurance companies do not follow the CMS 8-minute rule. Instead, they follow the Substantial Portion Methodology or the AMA 8-minute rule (AOTA, 2021). This method follows CPT coding conventions. **If you have performed a substantial portion of the timed service, you can bill the code, even if the total number of 15-minute codes exceeds 1 hour.** For example, suppose that in a single 1-hour session, you perform 10 minutes each of 97110—Therapeutic procedure, 97112—Neuromuscular reeducation, 97140—Manual therapy, 97530—Therapeutic activities, and 97535—Self-care/home management training. In this case, you could bill one 15-minute unit for each of the five codes. The total number of timed codes is 75 minutes, although you only saw the patient for 60 minutes. You must be certain that you are using the correct method of billing for your client's payer source. Check with your fieldwork educator or employer for further guidance.

Modifiers for Current Procedural Terminology Codes

"A modifier is an addition to a CPT code that provides additional information that can be used for payment or tracking purposes" (AOTA, 2020c, Slide 2). Use of modifiers depends on the requirements of each payment source. Here are some of the most common modifiers used for occupational therapy services:

- *Modifier 59*: Indicates that two codes that typically would not be billed during the same therapy session were in fact distinct and different procedures with no overlap.
- *Modifier GO*: Indicates that the service was performed under an occupational therapy plan of care; required by Medicare and some private insurance companies.

- *Modifier CO*: Indicates that an occupational therapy assistant performed at least 10% of the service independently. As of 2022, services coded with the CO modifier will be reimbursed at a 15% reduced rate by Medicare and other private insurances that follow this reimbursement policy. At the time of this writing, this controversial change was the focus of considerable advocacy by AOTA to reverse the policy (AOTA, 2022b).
- *Modifier KX*: Indicates that the service is still considered medically necessary despite having exceeded a particular annual monetary threshold established each year by Medicare. For example, in 2023, the annual threshold amount for outpatient occupational therapy services was $2230 (CMS, 2023).
- *Modifiers 96 and 97*: Modifier 96 indicates habilitative services to help clients develop skills or function they did not previously have. Modifier 97 indicates rehabilitative services to help clients regain previous function or skills that have been lost.
- *Modifier 95*: Indicates that services were provided via telehealth.
- *Modifier GA*: Indicates that an ABN is on file because the occupational therapy practitioner believes that the service will not be covered by Medicare.

Healthcare Common Procedure Coding System Level II Codes

Whereas CPT codes identify **services and procedures** provided by health care professionals, including occupational therapists, HCPCS Level II codes identify **products and supplies** such as durable medical equipment, orthotics, and prosthetics (CMS, 2021b). Like the use of CPT codes, occupational therapy practitioners may encounter certain limitations from payer sources and state regulatory agencies for specific HCPCS Level II codes. Furthermore, you should be aware that not all codes are accepted by Medicare and other payers.

Providing a product and bill does not guarantee that the client's funding source will pay for that product, particularly if a same or similar product has been billed to that patient in the past 5 years (AOTA, 2020b). Each year, AOTA provides members with a list of selected HCPCS Level II codes that are frequently used codes by occupational therapy practitioners to report fabrication and fitting of upper extremity orthoses.

Not all codes are accepted by all payers, including Medicare. State regulations and/or payer policies may establish limitations on the use of one or more of these codes. Always review state rules and the official HCPCS book, and request information from specific insurers concerning the use of codes and payment policy. (AOTA, 2022e, para. 1)

Here are examples of HCPCS Level II codes that occupational therapy practitioners may use in various settings:

- L3764—Elbow Wrist Hand Orthosis, includes one or more nontorsion joints, elastic bands, turnbuckles; may include soft interface, straps, custom fabricated; includes fitting and adjustment
- L3923—Hand Finger Orthosis, without joints, may include soft interface, straps, prefabricated item that has been trimmed, bent, molded, assembled, or otherwise customized to fit a specific patient by an individual with expertise

REFERENCES

American Association of Professional Coders. (2021). *What is ICD-10?* https://www.aapc.com/icd-10/
American Medical Association. (2022a). *CPT overview and code approval.* https://www.ama-assn.org/
American Medical Association. (2022b). *CPT 2022: Professional edition.* American Medical Association.
American Occupational Therapy Association. (2016). *New occupational therapy evaluation coding overview.* https://www.aota.org/
American Occupational Therapy Association. (2019). *Coding a new occupational therapy evaluation* [Video]. https://www.aota.org/
American Occupational Therapy Association. (2020a). *Am I required to bill Medicare? Understanding the Medicare Advanced Beneficiary Notice.* https://www.aota.org/
American Occupational Therapy Association. (2020b). *DMEPOS training* [Video]. https://www.aota.org/practice/practice-essentials/coding
American Occupational Therapy Association. (2020c). *Modifiers training* [Video]. https://www.aota.org/
American Occupational Therapy Association. (2021). *Timed codes: The 8-minute rule.* https://www.aota.org/
American Occupational Therapy Association. (2022a). *Advocacy issues.* https://www.aota.org/

American Occupational Therapy Association. (2022b). *OTA payment advocacy.* https://www.aota.org/

American Occupational Therapy Association. (2022c). *Payment policy: Worker's compensation.* https://www.aota.org/

American Occupational Therapy Association. (2022d). *Section GG self-care (activities of daily living) and mobility items.* https://www.aota.org/

American Occupational Therapy Association. (2022e). *Selected 2022 HCPCS Level II codes.* https://www.aota.org/

American Occupational Therapy Association. (2022f). *2022 CPT® codes for occupational therapy.* https://www.aota.org/

American Physical Therapy Association. (2022). *Medicare payment thresholds for outpatient therapy services.* https://www.apta.org/

Benefits.gov. (2021, February 3). *What to know about applying for Medicaid and CHIP in your state.* https://www.benefits.gov/news/article/417

Breithart, D. (2021, May 10). *IEPs, 504s, and school-based OT—Oh my!* https://devonbreithart.com/ieps-504s-school-based-ot

CareCentrix, Inc. (2020). *PDGM/PDPM payment models: The impact on home health.* https://www.carecentrix.com/blog/pdgm-pdpm-payment-models-the-impact-on-home-health/

Centers for Disease Control and Prevention. (2022). *International Classification of Diseases (ICD-10-CM/PCS) transition—Frequently asked questions.* https://www.cdc.gov/

Centers for Medicare & Medicaid Services. (2021a). *Frequently asked questions (FAQs) about Jimmo settlement agreement.* https://www.cms.gov/

Centers for Medicare & Medicaid Services. (2021b). *Healthcare Common Procedure Coding System (HCPCS) Level II coding procedures.* https://www.cms.gov/

Centers for Medicare & Medicaid Services. (2021c). *Home Health Patient Driven Groupings Model.* https://www.cms.gov/

Centers for Medicare & Medicaid Services. (2021d). *Implementation of the Bipartisan Budget Act of 2018.* https://www.cms.gov/

Centers for Medicare & Medicaid Services. (2021e). *MDS 2.0—Public quality indicator and resident reports.* https://www.cms.gov/

Centers for Medicare & Medicaid Services. (2021f). *Medicare fee-for-service payment regulations.* https://www.cms.gov/

Centers for Medicare & Medicaid Services. (2021g). *Prospective payment systems—General information.* https://www.cms.gov/

Centers for Medicare & Medicaid Services. (2022a). *Inpatient Rehabilitation Facility Patient Assessment Instrument (IRF-PAI) and IRF-PAI manual.* https://www.medicaid.gov/

Centers for Medicare & Medicaid Services. (2022b). *Long-Term Care Hospital (LTCH) Quality Reporting Program (QRP).* https://www.medicaid.gov/

Centers for Medicare & Medicaid Services. (2022c). *Medicare Advantage plans.* https://www.medicare.gov

Centers for Medicare & Medicaid Services. (2022d). *Medicare basics.* https://www.medicare.gov/

Centers for Medicare & Medicaid Services. (2022e). *OASIS data sets.* https://www.medicare.gov/

Centers for Medicare & Medicaid Services. (2022f). *Value-based programs.* https://www.cms.gov/

Centers for Medicare & Medicaid Services. (2022g). *What's Medicare supplement insurance (Medigap)?* https://www.medicare.gov/

Centers for Medicare & Medicaid Services. (2022h). *What Marketplace health insurance plans cover.* https://www.healthcare.gov/

Centers for Medicare & Medicaid Services. (2023). *Therapy services: CY 2023 therapy services update.* https://www.cms.gov/

Deutsch, A., & Dass, M. (2019). *Section GG: Functional abilities and goals.* Centers for Medicare & Medicaid Services. https://www.cms.gov/

Early Childhood Technical Assistance Center. (2021). *Summary of state and jurisdictional eligibility definitions for infants and toddlers with disabilities under IDEA Part C.* https://ectacenter.org/topics/earlyid/state-info-summary.asp

Elite Insurance Partners LLC. (2022). *Top 3 reasons why people leave Medicare Advantage plans.* https://www.medicarefaq.com/

Grote, C. (2022). *Everything you need to know about Section GG.* Amplify OT. https://amplifyot.com/

Hanft, B., & Shepherd, J. (2016). *Collaborating for student success A guide for school-based occupational therapy* (2nd ed.). AOTA Press.

Healthinsurance.org, LLC. (2022). *Frequently asked questions about health insurance.* healthinsurance.org/faqs/

Heller-Ono, A. (2021, July 6). *Disability management & ergonomic worksite analysis: A critical link in stay-at-work and return-to-work.* Medbridge. https://www.medbridgeeducation.com/

Jordan, K., Sandhu, S., Walsh-Sterup, M, & Silva, Z. (2022, March 31—April 3). *Understanding payment: A deep dive into the process of occupational therapy coding and reimbursement* [Conference session]. 2022 AOTA Annual Conference & Expo, San Antonio, TX.

Kroll, C., & Richman, N. (2018). *Skilled nursing facilities 101: Documentation, reimbursement, and ethics in practice* (2nd ed.). AOTA Continuing Education.

Laverdure, P., & LeCompte, B. (2021). *Continuing education article: Medicaid in education during times of COVID-19.* American Occupational Therapy Association. https://www.aota.org/

Moninger, S. (2021, July 7). *Skilled service documentation tips for reimbursement.* BTE. https://www.btetechnologies.com/

Net Health. (2022). *Understanding the Patient-Driven Payment Model (PDPM).* https://www.nethealth.com/

Strunk, E. (2019, January 7). *Section GG changes: What do they mean for your organization?* Medbridge. https://www.medbridg-eeducation.com/blog/2019/01/section-gg-changes-what-do-they-mean-for-your-organization/

Stuart, A. (2022). *Early intervention services: Who pays for what?* Understood. https://www.understood.org/articles/en/early-intervention-services-who-pays-for-what

U.S. Department of Education. (2017). *Sec. 303.344—Content of an IFSP.* https://sites.ed.gov/idea/regs/c/d/303.344

U.S. Department of Education. (2020). *Protecting students with disabilities: Frequently asked questions about Section 504 and the education of children with disabilities.* https://www2.ed.gov/about/offices/list/ocr/504faq

U.S. Department of Education. (2022). *About IDEA.* https://sites.ed.gov/idea/about-idea/

U.S. Department of Health & Human Services. (2017). *Young adult coverage.* https://www.hhs.gov/healthcare/about-the-aca/young-adult-coverage/index.html

U.S. Department of Labor. (2022). *State worker's compensation officials.* https://www.dol.gov/agencies/owcp/wc

Vontran, K., & Gehne, W. (2019). *Overview of the patient-driven groupings model (PDGM).* Centers for Medicare & Medicaid Services. https://www.cms.gov/

World Health Organization. (2022). *International Classification of Diseases, 11th edition: The global standard for diagnostic health information.* https://icd.who.int/en

Chapter 4

Legal, Regulatory, and Ethical Considerations

Practitioners must be aware of federal and state laws and regulations that affect reimbursement and documentation. It is also necessary to understand the impact of *Official Documents* of the American Occupational Therapy Association (AOTA) on documentation. In addition, it is important to consider the ethical implications that practitioners may encounter regarding the documentation of occupational therapy services. This chapter will provide a general overview of the legal, regulatory, and ethical considerations that guide documentation. However, policies, statutes, and guidelines change frequently and vary greatly among occupational therapy practice settings. Occupational therapy practitioners must remain current with legal, regulatory, and ethical issues that affect their current practice setting.

HEALTH CARE POLICY AND LEGISLATION

Health care policy and legislation have a direct impact on how occupational therapy services are provided, documented, billed, and reimbursed. In recent years, new legislation and policies have improved the ability of occupational therapy practitioners to be reimbursed for mental health services, to open home health cases, and to provide telehealth services (AOTA, 2022). Unfortunately, some policies and legislation have led to cuts for services provided by occupational therapy assistants and pressure by some post-acute facilities to provide group and concurrent therapy sessions to cut labor costs under new payment models. As our health care system is continually evolving, you should stay abreast of current issues that may impact your practice. AOTA's website has a section dedicated to advocacy issues.

HEALTH INSURANCE PORTABILITY AND ACCOUNTABILITY ACT

If you have been to any health care provider in the past 2 decades, you or your legal guardian likely had to sign a form indicating you have been made aware of your patient rights and the privacy guidelines of the facility. Originally passed by Congress in 1996 to ensure that employees could maintain health benefits when changing jobs, the Health Insurance Portability and Accountability Act (HIPAA) also established federal standards for the security, use, and disclosure of a client's protected health information (PHI; U.S. Department of Health & Human Services [DHHS],

Gateley, C. A. *Documentation Manual for Occupational Therapy, Fifth Edition* (pp. 31-41).
© 2024 Taylor & Francis Group.

2022a). A major goal of the HIPAA Privacy Rule "is to assure that individuals' health information is properly protected while allowing the flow of health information needed to provide and promote high quality health care and to protect the public's health and well being" (U.S. DHHS, 2022b, para. 3). Clients are also accorded several rights under HIPAA:

- The right to view and obtain a copy of the health record
- The right to request revision or omission of information in the health record that is incorrect
- The right to know how health information is used and shared with others
- The right to decide if PHI can be used for purposes of marketing and research
- The right to authorize the release of health information to selected individuals
- The right to file a complaint if it is believed that health information has been used in a way that violates the law

"The Privacy Rule protects all individually identifiable health information held or transmitted by a covered entity or its business associate, in any form of media, whether electronic, paper, or oral. … Individually identifiable health information is information, including demographic data, that relates to:
- the individual's past, present, or future physical or mental health condition,
- the provision of health care to the individual, or
- the past, present, or future payment for the provision of health care to the individual,

and that identifies the individual or for which there is a reasonable basis to believe it can be used to identify the individual. Individually identifiable health information includes many common identifiers (e.g., name, address, birth date, Social Security Number)" (U.S. DHHS, 2022a, para. 14).

HIPAA has several implications for occupational therapy practitioners, particularly as many health care settings have transitioned to electronic health records (EHRs). In 2013, the HIPAA Security Rule implemented new requirements to address technological advances (Collmer, 2015). The new rule "not only strengthened privacy and security safeguards for PHI, but it also created steeper civil and criminal penalties for violation" (Collmer, 2015, p. 13). In recent years, numerous health care providers, from individual practitioners to entire health care systems, have incurred penalties ranging from a few thousand dollars to several million dollars for HIPAA violations (Alder, 2022). Some of the most common compliance issues involve (Jannenga, 2019, para. 5):

- Impermissible uses and disclosures of PHI
- Lack of safeguards of hard copy and electronic PHI
- Inability for patients to access their PHI
- Use or disclosure of more than the minimum necessary PHI

In any fieldwork or practice setting, you should have a clear understanding of the site's strategies for HIPAA compliance and your role in maintaining client confidentiality. Although not all-inclusive, the following is a list of strategies that will help maintain compliance with HIPAA guidelines (Alder, 2021; CareCloud, 2022; Collmer, 2015):

- Do not discuss client PHI with anyone who does not have a need to know the information, including coworkers or personal acquaintances.
- Do not discuss client PHI in an area where it may be overheard by others.
- Do not leave paper charts out on a desk for easy access by unauthorized users.
- Do not leave client records open on a computer screen or other electronic device.
- Do not access a health record unless needed for work.
- Do not share your password with other staff.
- Always log off from electronic devices containing health records.
- When working on electronic devices, position yourself and the device in a manner to prevent others from viewing the screen.
- Make sure electronic devices containing PHI are locked up to prevent physical access by unauthorized users.
- Make sure that you are using encrypted emails or encrypted cloud-based software programs to share electronic PHI with other authorized users.

- Complete required HIPAA training offered by the site.
- Avoid documenting in public areas with unsecured wireless access.
- Never share any client information on social media.

I want to draw particular attention to three of the points above, particularly for students and new practitioners. First is the issue of not accessing health records unless needed for work purposes. This includes your own health record, those of family or friends, and those of well-known individuals. It can be very tempting when you see a name you recognize on the patient census for your facility to want to do a little exploring about the patient's situation. It is human nature to think, "Hmm … I wonder what's going on with that person?" **Your curiosity can get you fired and sued if you access the health record of someone who is not your client.** You leave an electronic "fingerprint" on every record that you access, and your facility can determine every individual that has accessed any given EHR.

Another important issue for further discussion is to **make sure that others cannot see your screen when you are documenting outside of designated staff areas.** For example, the hospital where I do some weekend work has a computer in every patient room, so it is common for me to document while I am with the patient, particularly as I gather information about the client's occupational profile, prior level of function, and home environment. It is not concerning for the client to see you documenting the information that they are reporting to you. However, clients and families are curious too, and they might ask you to check on other aspects of the health record. Be very careful with the information that you share. A patient may have just had a test that revealed a serious new medical condition, such as cancer, and it is not your role to be the first one to deliver that information. In that situation, you can simply say, "Your doctor or provider will be reviewing all your test results the next time they make rounds" or "I'll let your nurse know that you have questions about your tests." You should also be cautious about documenting on a patient while in a different patient's room. The patient, or more likely a visitor, may unexpectedly walk by your screen and see the PHI of another individual before you can close out of the chart.

A final issue that warrants further discussion is social media and HIPAA. Many of us use social media on a frequent basis to share moments of our day with others in our social network, but what you consider to be an innocent post may result in criminal charges and disciplinary action, including termination of your job. **No matter how tempted you are to share information about one of your clients, just don't do it!** Alder (2021, para. 12) listed the following common social media HIPAA violations:

- Posting of images and videos of patients without written consent
- Posting of gossip about patients
- Posting of any information that could allow an individual to be identified
- Sharing of photographs or images taken inside a health care facility in which patients or PHI are visible
- Sharing of photos, videos, or text on social media platforms within a private group

> "HIPAA was enacted several years before social media networks such as Facebook and Instagram were launched, so there are no specific HIPAA social media rules. However, as with all healthcare-related communications, the HIPAA Privacy Rule still applies whenever covered entities or business associates—or employees of either—use social media networks" (Alder, 2021, para. 1).

"Compliance with the HIPAA Security Rule means more than following the law. Occupational therapy practitioners who comply with the requirements protect their organization and themselves from hefty penalties and reputational damage" (Collmer, 2015, p. 16). Furthermore, occupational therapy practitioners must follow the AOTA *Code of Ethics* (2020). Principle 3 of the *Code of Ethics* states "occupational therapy personnel shall respect the right of the person to self-determination, privacy, confidentiality, and consent" (AOTA, 2020a, p. 3). The related standard of conduct specifies that occupational therapy personnel shall maintain high standards of confidentiality in all written, verbal, electronic, or virtual communication.

In summary, you should have a clear understanding of the privacy safeguards that exist at your place of fieldwork or employment and your role in ensuring compliance with HIPAA laws. For example, which procedure should you follow if a client asks for a copy of the health record? Which form must be signed to allow you to discuss health information with a client's relative or friend? What should your response be if another client innocently asks, "What's wrong with that person over there?"

FAMILY EDUCATIONAL RIGHTS AND PRIVACY ACT

The Family Educational Rights and Privacy Act (FERPA) is a federal law enacted in 1974 that protects the privacy of educational records (U.S. Department of Education, 2021). FERPA applies to educational institutions that receive government funding through the U.S. Department of Education. School occupational therapy practitioners have access to student educational records and must comply with FERPA regulations. In some instances, school practitioners may also be subject to HIPAA guidelines. For example, if a practitioner is providing occupational therapy services as outlined in the child's Individualized Education Program (IEP) but Medicaid is billed for the services, the billing procedures must comply with HIPAA guidelines, while the documentation for the services becomes part of the educational record and therefore falls under FERPA guidelines (Barboza et al., 2008). When in doubt about whether you can share information about school-based occupational therapy services, you should consult with school administrators and your employer if you are providing contract services and are employed by another entity.

REGULATORY AND ETHICAL GUIDELINES

Occupational therapy practitioners must be aware of legal, regulatory, and ethical standards that affect documentation. The AOTA publishes several *Official Documents* that guide occupational therapy practice and have direct implications on documentation. In addition, each state has a practice act that further regulates occupational therapy practice. This section will highlight the key points of several documents that affect the documentation of occupational therapy practitioners. Keep in mind that AOTA *Official Documents* are revised approximately every 5 years, and state practice acts may be updated annually. Occupational therapy practitioners must be familiar with the most current documents available. The most recent *Official Documents* described below are located on the AOTA website, and state practice acts can be located on the website of the occupational therapy regulatory board for each state.

Scope of Practice

This document delineates the domain and process of occupational therapy practice and describes the educational and certification requirements for occupational therapy practitioners. The *Scope of Practice* document is based on the *Occupational Therapy Practice Framework: Domain and Process, Fourth Edition* (OTPF-4; AOTA, 2020c). Occupational therapy is defined as "the therapeutic use of everyday life occupations with person, groups, or populations (i.e., clients) for the purpose of enhancing or enabling participation" (AOTA, 2021b, p. 2). Documentation should demonstrate that the services provided to a client fall within the scope of practice for the occupational therapy profession. Furthermore, practitioners must abide by state laws for licensure, continuing education, and supervision. Such laws may affect the credentials included in a practitioner's signature on documentation and the type of documentation required to reflect that appropriate supervision has been provided to occupational therapy assistants during the delivery of services.

Standards of Practice for Occupational Therapy

This document defines the standards that must be met to practice as an occupational therapist or occupational therapy assistant (AOTA, 2021d). It outlines the education, examination, and licensure requirements for occupational therapy practitioners. The document goes on to outline specific expectations of occupational therapy practitioners related to the following standards:

- Standard I—Professional Standing and Responsibility
- Standard II—Service Delivery
- Standard III—Screening, Evaluation, and Reevaluation
- Standard IV—Intervention Process
- Standard V—Outcomes, Transition, and Discontinuation

The *Standards of Practice* document explains that occupational therapy documentation must abide "by the time frames, formats, and standards established by practice settings, federal and state laws, other regulatory and payer requirements, external accreditation programs, and AOTA *Official Documents*" (AOTA, 2021d, p. 4).

Guidelines for Supervision, Roles, and Responsibilities During the Delivery of Occupational Therapy Services

This document outlines the roles, responsibilities, and supervision requirements of occupational therapists, occupational therapy assistants, and occupational therapy aides in the provision of occupational therapy services, including documentation practice (AOTA, 2020b). The document explains that "supervision is based on mutual understanding between the supervisor and supervisee about each other's education, experience, credentials, and competence" (AOTA, 2020b, p. 1).

Occupational Therapists

Occupational therapists are considered autonomous practitioners, meaning they are independent in all aspects of service delivery, including documentation of the evaluation, intervention plan, intervention implementation, and outcomes (AOTA, 2020b). Occupational therapists initiate and direct the evaluation, interpret the data, develop and direct the intervention plan, modify or discontinue the intervention plan when appropriate, and interpret outcomes of a client's occupational performance. They collaborate with occupational therapy assistants by delegating selected assessments and interventions and exchanging information throughout the evaluation and intervention process. Documentation should reflect an occupational therapist's involvement throughout the delivery of occupational therapy services.

Occupational Therapy Assistants

Occupational therapy assistants must deliver occupational therapy services under the supervision of an occupational therapist (AOTA, 2020b). The amount of supervision that must be provided will vary depending on the state of practice and funding source. Occupational therapy assistants may contribute to the evaluation process by implementing assessments that have been delegated by the occupational therapist and providing verbal and written reports of the client's performance to the occupational therapist. They may collaborate with the occupational therapist during the development of the intervention plan.

Occupational therapy assistants are responsible for knowing the client's occupational therapy goals and targeted outcomes, and they provide written documentation and verbal reports to the occupational therapist about the client's progress toward those goals and outcomes. Finally, in collaboration with the supervising occupational therapist, occupational therapy assistants select, implement, and modify "occupational therapy interventions consistent with demonstrated competence levels, client goals, and the requirements of the practice setting, including payment source requirements" (AOTA, 2020b, p. 4). Their accompanying documentation should reflect that all guidelines have been followed throughout the delivery of occupational therapy services.

In some situations, occupational therapy practitioners may use their education and expertise to work in settings that are not related to the delivery of occupational therapy. "In these other arenas, supervision of the occupational therapy assistant may be provided by non–occupational therapy professionals, or supervisory relationships may not be applicable when the occupational therapy assistant is a sole proprietor" (AOTA, 2020b, p. 4).

Occupational Therapy Aides

Occupational therapy aides provide supportive nonskilled services specifically delegated by the occupational therapist or occupational therapy assistant (AOTA, 2020b). Ultimately, the occupational therapist is responsible for the use and actions of the aide, but aides may be supervised by the occupational therapy assistant. Aides may provide non–client-related tasks such as clerical, maintenance, and work area or equipment preparation. They may also perform routine client-related tasks under stable, predictable circumstances if they have previously demonstrated competence in the task. Occupational therapy practitioners must adhere to state and payer regulations when using aides and documenting the services provided by an aide.

Occupational Therapy Students and Occupational Therapy Assistant Students

Although not addressed in an *Official Document*, AOTA issues periodic updates to clarify supervision requirements for students when occupational therapy services are billed under Medicare. AOTA works "with a coalition of organizations to advocate for additional government support for educating allied health providers and to develop long-term solutions to the problems caused by Medicare's limitations on reimbursement when students participate in service delivery" (AOTA, 2021c, para. 17). Other payer sources may have different guidelines, and state laws and facility guidelines may be even more restrictive. The Medicare supervision requirements summarized by AOTA (2021c) are as follows:

- *Medicare Part A—Hospital and Inpatient Rehabilitation*: State and local laws and practice standards should be considered when determining supervision of students in these settings. "Services provided by therapy students may count toward the IRF three-hour rule/intensity of therapy services requirement" (AOTA, 2021c, para. 4).

- *Medicare Part A—SNF*: Services of an occupational therapy student or occupational therapy assistant student may be recorded on the MDS as minutes of therapy received by the client if the supervising occupational therapy practitioner provides skilled direction to the student. CMS does not require that services be provided within the line-of-sight of an occupational therapy practitioner. "Within individual facilities, supervising therapists/assistants must make the determination as to whether or not a student is ready to treat patients without line-of-sight supervision. Additionally, all state and professional practice guidelines for student supervision must be followed" (AOTA, 2021c, para. 6). Supervising occupational therapy practitioners should be physically present in the facility and immediately available for guidance as needed by the student.

- *Medicare Part A—Hospice*: CMS has not issued specific rules regarding student supervision in hospice. AOTA recommends that the approach for Part A inpatient settings be followed and that practitioners consult state practice acts for additional guidance (AOTA, 2021c).

- *Medicare Part A—Home Health*: CMS regulations define "qualified personnel" who may provide and bill for home health services. Students are not included in the definition of qualified personnel. AOTA offers the following clarification:

    CMS has not issued specific restrictions regarding students providing services in conjunction with a qualified OT or OTA. Services by students can be provided (as allowed by state law) as part of a home health visit, when the student is supervised by an OT or OTA in the home. (AOTA, 2021c, para. 9)

    AOTA recommends that the approach for Part A inpatient settings be followed and that practitioners consult state practice acts for additional guidance.

- *Medicare Part B—Outpatient/SNF/Home Health/Private Practice*: There are very specific rules regarding the use of occupational therapy students in the provision of services under Part B reimbursement. "Only the services of the therapist can be billed and paid under Medicare Part B. The services performed by a student are not reimbursed, even if provided under 'line of sight' supervision of the therapist" (AOTA, 2021c, para. 13). However, the presence of an occupational therapy or occupational therapy assistant student in the room does not make the services unbillable. AOTA further explains that students can assist a qualified practitioner in the provision of occupational therapy services:

    Students can participate in the delivery of services when the qualified practitioner (OT) is directing the service, making the skilled judgment, responsible for the assessment and treatment in the same room as the student, and not simultaneously treating another patient. The qualified practitioner is solely responsible and must sign all documentation. (AOTA, 2021c, para. 11)

Guidelines for Documentation of Occupational Therapy

This document articulates the purposes of documentation, explains different types of documentation, and lists the fundamental elements that should be present in all occupational therapy documentation (AOTA, 2018). There should be documentation any time occupational therapy services are provided to a client. The term *client* may be used to describe a person, group, or population as defined in the *OTPF-4* (AOTA, 2020c). According to the *Guidelines for Documentation of Occupational Therapy*, "the purpose of documentation is to:

- Communicate information about the client's occupational history and experiences, interests, values, and needs
- Articulate the rationale for provision of occupational therapy services and the relationship of those services to client outcomes
- Provide a clear, chronological record of client status, the nature of the occupational therapy services provided, client response to occupational therapy intervention, and client outcomes
- Provide an accurate justification for skilled occupational therapy necessity and reimbursement" (AOTA, 2018, p. 1)

Different types of documentation may be required throughout the occupational therapy process. Types of documentation include:

- *Screening report*: Documents need, or lack thereof, for occupational therapy evaluation
- *Evaluation report*: Includes thorough occupational profile, types of assessments used and results, analysis of occupational performance, summary and analysis, and recommendations
- *Re-evaluation report*: Completed "when, in the professional judgment of the occupational therapist, new clinical findings emerge, a significant change in the patient's condition requiring further tests and measures is observed, the client demonstrates a lack of response as expected in the plan of care, additional information is required for discharge, or when required by practice guidelines and payer, facility, and state and federal guidelines and requirements" (AOTA, 2018, pp. 2-3)
- *Intervention plan/plan of care*: Based on evaluation or re-evaluation results; may include goals, intervention approaches, types of approaches, service delivery mechanisms (e.g., location, frequency, duration), plan for discharge, and outcome measures
- *Contact report*: Daily treatment notes to document any contact or missed visit; includes client report, interventions and responses, devices used or fabricated, education or consultation provided, and present level of performance
- *Progress report*: Includes summary of client sessions/contacts, services provided, current client performance, and recommendations about changes or continuation of services
- *Transition plan*: Documents plan for a formal transition between service settings including expected time frame, outline of transition activities, and recommendations for occupational therapy services, accommodations, assistive technology, and/or environmental modifications
- *Discharge or discontinuation report*: Summarizes the intervention process, progress toward goals, outcomes, and recommendations for follow-up and/or referral to other professionals or agencies

Each type of documentation listed above will be discussed in more detail in Chapter 15 with examples provided. There are several fundamental elements that are essential to all documentation types (AOTA, 2018):

- Name, date of birth, gender, and case or health record number (if applicable)
- Date and type of occupational therapy contact
- Terminology, acronyms, and abbreviations acceptable to the setting
- Clear rationale for provision of skilled occupational therapy services
- Professional signature including name and credentials
- Co-signature and credentials if required by supervision guidelines, payer policy, state or federal laws, or facility standards
- Errors noted and initialed or signed
- Adherence to state and federal regulations, payer and facility requirements, practice guidelines, and confidentiality requirements for documentation storage and disposal

Occupational Therapy Code of Ethics

This document outlines the principles to promote and maintain ethical standards of conduct and is based on the core values of the occupational therapy profession: altruism, equality, freedom, justice, dignity, truth, and prudence (AOTA, 2020a). It is intended to guide decision making when ethical issues arise. In simple terms, practitioners must always consider the implications of their decisions and actions on occupational therapy clients. The six ethical principles and standards of conduct are summarized as follows (AOTA, 1993, 2020a):

1. *Beneficence*: Occupational therapy practitioners will demonstrate concern for the safety and well-being of their clients.
2. *Nonmaleficence*: Occupational therapy practitioners will not engage in actions that pose harm to their clients.
3. *Autonomy*: Practitioners will collaborate with clients to determine goals, obtain informed consent for services, respect the client's right to refuse services, and protect all confidential information.
4. *Justice*: Practitioners will provide fair, respectful, inclusive, and equitable services to their clients.
5. *Veracity*: Practitioners will provide comprehensive, objective, and accurate information in all forms of communication and avoid communication that is false, fraudulent, or deceptive.
6. *Fidelity*: Practitioners will demonstrate respect, fairness, discretion, and integrity in relationships with clients, colleagues, and other professionals.

These ethical principles have many direct implications for documentation of occupational therapy services. An individualized evaluation and plan of care should be documented for each client, and the collaborative process between practitioner and client must be well documented. Documentation and accompanying billing must accurately reflect the services that were provided and must comply with applicable laws, guidelines, and regulations. Documentation must include accurate credentials of the practitioner providing service and a description of appropriate levels of supervision during service delivery when applicable to comply with legal and facility guidelines. Documentation should not contain false information or fabricated data, and practitioners must always maintain client confidentiality.

Students and practitioners are highly encouraged to read the *Code of Ethics* (AOTA, 2020a) in its entirety. However, I would like to highlight two key points from the document directly related to documentation and other forms of communication that are particularly salient for students and early career practitioners:

- "Do not follow arbitrary directives that compromise the rights or well-being of others, including unrealistic productivity expectations, fabrication, falsification, plagiarism of documentation, or inaccurate coding" (AOTA, 2020a, p. 6).
- "Demonstrate responsible conduct, respect, and discretion when engaging in digital media and social networking, including but not limited to refraining from posting protected health or other identifying information" (AOTA, 2020a, p. 8).

Violations of the standards above, or any other standards in the *Code of Ethics*, not only endanger your clients but also place your professional licensure and certification at risk for probation, suspension, revocation, or other disciplinary action (AOTA, 2021a; National Board for Certification in Occupational Therapy, 2020).

State Practice Acts

Each state regulates the practice of occupational therapy. State practice acts address issues such as scope of occupational therapy practice, qualification and licensure requirements, continuing competence, supervision of students and occupational therapy personnel, referral requirements, documentation requirements, and disciplinary actions for violations of any state requirements. Each of these issues may have either direct or indirect implications on a practitioner's documentation, and it is the responsibility of each practitioner to know and abide by statutes that govern occupational therapy practice. You should be able to locate your state practice act on the website of your state regulatory board or via a link on the AOTA website.

REIMBURSEMENT, LEGAL, AND ETHICAL ISSUES

When practitioners do not abide by all of the guidelines presented in this chapter that affect practice and documentation, they may encounter unfortunate reimbursement, legal, and ethical situations. In some cases, even those practitioners who consistently meet all guidelines still find themselves in unfortunate situations. Some of the common situations involving occupational therapy documentation will be discussed in this section.

Reimbursement Denials

Medicare and other reimbursement sources look at health care documentation with increasing scrutiny when determining whether billed services will be reimbursed. Appealing a reimbursement denial requires valuable time and resources. Denials often can be avoided by consistently providing thorough documentation that meets all necessary requirements. Reavis (2022), Griswold (2019), and Fusion Web Clinic (2022) listed several reasons for reimbursement denials by Medicare and other payers related to occupational therapy documentation:

- Use of abbreviations unknown to the claim reviewer
- Illegible documentation
- Incomplete documentation (patient name, signatures, dates, minutes of treatment)
- Missing physician order or signed plan of care
- Lack of support for billing codes
- Incorrect diagnosis codes
- Failure to document progress within reasonable time frame
- Skilled care not justified
- Lack of support for medical necessity
- Standardized scores reported without interpretation of functional impact for client
- Repetitive documentation between sessions with no evidence of significant improvement
- Excessive duration of sessions and/or duration of care
- Excessive use of KX modifiers to override therapy limits
- Lack of required co-signatures for students and/or therapy assistants
- Lack of thorough explanation of client's comorbidities and prior/current functional status
- Failure to document rationale for changing intervention plan or frequency/duration of treatment
- Too much emphasis on client factors (e.g., strength, range of motion) without relation to function
- Documentation suggests duplication of service with another discipline
- No authorization on date of session
- Yearly session limit exceeded

Billing Fraud and Abuse

CMS (2021, p. 6) defined fraud as "knowingly submitting, or causing to be submitted, false claims or making misrepresentations of fact" to obtain health care payments. Examples of billing practices that may constitute fraud include knowingly filing claims for services that were not rendered and knowingly billing for services at a higher complexity level than what was provided, such as billing for individual occupational therapy services when multiple clients were treated simultaneously. CMS (2021, p. 7) defines abuse as "practices that may directly or indirectly result in unnecessary costs to the Medicare program. Abuse includes any practice that does not provide patients with medically necessary services or meet professionally recognized standards of care." Examples include billing for services that were not medically necessary, charging excessively for services or supplies, and misuse of codes to maximize reimbursement. CMS describes abuse as **bending the rules**, whereas fraud involves **intentional deception**. In either case, providers may be subject to administrative, civil, or criminal liability. Occupational therapy practitioners must be diligent in documenting and billing for their services appropriately to avoid claims of fraud and abuse. You can lose your job and your license if you are found to be involved in fraud or abuse. Most employers will require you to complete an annual training to remind you about acceptable practices and how to report concerns.

Malpractice and Other Legal Claims

Health care malpractice claims may result from professional negligence, breach of client–professional contractual promise, liability for defective equipment or abnormally dangerous care-related activities that cause injury, or intentional misconduct. From a legal perspective, the documentation that appears in a client's health record is often considered the best evidence of what transpired between the client and health care provider. It is essential that occupational therapy practitioners document client interactions accurately and completely. If an occupational therapy practitioner is found guilty of malpractice, they may face serious consequences, including monetary loss, loss of reputation, and state and/or federal punitive action including loss of license to practice (Omnisure, 2021).

> "The medical record is viewed as 'the witness that never dies and never lies.' Often the first analysis of medical negligence begins with a review of the medical record. The record is a legal document that provides the most valuable evidence as to what transpired between the patient and the healthcare provider. The medical record can be entered into evidence as proof that what it says is true" (Omnisure, 2021, p. 17).

Ethical Dilemmas

Many occupational therapy practitioners will encounter ethical dilemmas involving their documentation at some point in their careers. For example, suppose it is time to provide a progress note to a client's insurance company to request authorization for additional outpatient visits. In your opinion, the client has made great progress and really does not need any additional services, but the client tells you that they hope they can keep seeing you for a few more weeks so they can get even stronger. While you always have the client's best interests in mind, you should never falsify or withhold information about a client's performance in your documentation.

The issue of productivity expectations can also lead to ethical dilemmas. Productivity is measured by comparing the number of units or minutes billed to the number of hours worked (Bermudez, 2022). "Workload expectations and productivity measurement are legitimate management tools used to ensure appropriate staffing resources for service delivery as well as to maximize reimbursement, with the goal of achieving economic sustainability" (AOTA, 2019, p. 1). Many settings have stringent productivity targets with the expectation that clients will be treated concurrently or in groups. While treating multiple clients simultaneously is not unethical, as long as the intervention is beneficial for each client and does not pose a safety risk, the services must be documented and billed appropriately.

Occupational therapy practitioners may find themselves torn between meeting the productivity expectations of their employer and providing quality, individualized care to their clients. AOTA explained that "the financial interests of the institutional provider and the individual practitioner should not supersede concerns for the client's own health-related benefit in the planning or provision of occupational therapy" (AOTA, 2019, p. 1). Examples of ethical issues related to occupational therapy practice and documentation include the following:

- Placing or keeping clients on caseload who do not need skilled services or meet payer coverage criteria
- Administrative mandates regarding treatment frequency, duration, or intensity
- Providing treatment without client consent
- Counting nonbillable time as treatment time
- Inappropriate coding or changes to coding without approval of the treating therapist
- Falsifying or changing documentation to misrepresent services delivered or time spent with client

Occupational therapy practitioners who find themselves faced with ethical dilemmas can take any of the following steps (AOTA et al., 2014):

- Stop the questionable practice
- Contact an administrator or corporate compliance officer for the facility
- Contact state and national professional associations for guidance (AOTA)
- Consider seeking legal counsel
- If appropriate, consider reporting information to CMS or the Office of the Inspector General

REFERENCES

Alder, S. (2021, December 12). *HIPAA social media rules.* The HIPAA Journal. https://www.hipaajournal.com/

Alder, S. (2022, January 2). *The most common HIPAA violations you should be aware of.* The HIPAA Journal. https://www. hipaajournal.com/

American Occupational Therapy Association. (1993). Core values and attitudes of occupational therapy practice. *American Journal of Occupational Therapy, 47,* 1085-1086. https://doi.org/10.5014/ajot.47.12.1085

American Occupational Therapy Association. (2018). Guidelines for documentation of occupational therapy. *American Journal of Occupational Therapy, 72*(Suppl. 2), 7212410010. https://doi.org/10.5014/ajot.2018.72S203

American Occupational Therapy Association. (2019). *Ethical considerations for productivity, billing, and reimbursement.* https:// www.aota.org/

American Occupational Therapy Association. (2020a). AOTA 2020 occupational therapy code of ethics. *American Journal of Occupational Therapy, 74*(Suppl. 3), 741341005. https://doi.org/10.5014/ajot.2020.74S3006

American Occupational Therapy Association. (2020b). Guidelines for supervision, roles, and responsibilities during the delivery of occupational therapy services. *American Journal of Occupational Therapy, 74*(Suppl. 3), 7413410020. https://doi. org/10.5014/ajot.2020.74S3004

American Occupational Therapy Association. (2020c). Occupational therapy practice framework: Domain and process (4th ed.). *American Journal of Occupational Therapy, 74*(Suppl. 2), 7412410010. https://doi.org/10.5014.ajot.2020.74S2001

American Occupational Therapy Association. (2021a). Enforcement procedures for the AOTA occupational therapy code of ethics. *American Journal of Occupational Therapy, 75*(Suppl. 3), https://doi.org/10.5014/ajot.2021.75S3006

American Occupational Therapy Association. (2021b). Occupational therapy scope of practice. *American Journal of Occupational Therapy, 75*(Suppl. 3), 7513410030. https://doi.10.5014/ajot.2021.75S3005

American Occupational Therapy Association. (2021c). *OT/OTA student supervision & Medicare requirements.* https://www.aota. org/

American Occupational Therapy Association. (2021d). Standards of practice for occupational therapy. *American Journal of Occupational Therapy, 75*(Suppl. 3), 7513410030. https://doi.org/10.5014/ajot.2021.75S3004

American Occupational Therapy Association. (2022). *Advocacy issues in focus.* https://www.aota.org/

American Occupational Therapy Association, American Physical Therapy Association, & American Speech-Language-Hearing Association. (2014). *Consensus statement on clinical judgment in health care settings.* https://www.aota.org/

Barboza, S., Epps, S., Byington, R., & Keene, S. (2008). HIPAA goes to school: Clarifying privacy laws in the education environment. *Internet Journal of Law, Healthcare and Ethics, 6*(2), 1-5.

Bermudez, M. (2022). Surviving and thriving in high-demand settings. In B. Braveman (Ed.), *Leading & managing occupational therapy services: An evidence-based approach* (3rd ed., pp. 353-377). F. A. Davis.

CareCloud. (2022). *14 best practices to keep your staff HIPAA compliant.* https://www.carecloud.com/

Centers for Medicare & Medicaid Services. (2021). *Medicare fraud & abuse: Prevent, detect, report.* https://www.cms.gov/

Collmer, V. (2015). Navigating the HIPAA security rule: Practical strategies for the occupational therapy practitioner. *OT Practice, 20*(14), 13-16.

Fusion Web Clinic. (2022). *Common mistakes occupational therapists make when billing.* https://fusionwebclinic.com/

Griswold, B. (2019, May 27). *The top 10 (mostly preventable) reasons your claim could be denied.* https://theinsurancemaze.com/ articles/denials/

Jannenga, H. (2019). *What is HIPAA?* WebPT. https://www.webpt.com/

National Board for Certification in Occupational Therapy. (2020). *Procedures for the enforcement of the NBCOT candidate/certificant code of conduct.* https://nbcot.org

Omnisure. (2021). *Key areas of risk for occupational therapy practitioners: Reducing risks and enhancing patient safety.* Proliability. https://www.proliability.com/

Reavis, M. (2022). *Top 10 reasons for costly rehab denials.* PESI Rehab. https://rehab.pesi.com/blog/details/2015/top-10-reasons-for-costly-rehab-denials

U.S. Department of Education. (2021). *Family Educational Rights and Privacy Act (FERPA).* https://www2.ed.gov/

U.S. Department of Health & Human Services. (2022a). *Summary of the HIPAA privacy rule.* https://www.hhs.gov/

U.S. Department of Health & Human Services. (2022b). *Your rights under HIPAA.* https://www.hhs.gov/

Chapter 5

General Guidelines for Documentation

The first four chapters of this book have detailed the importance of good documentation skills. The health record is a communication tool while the client is receiving services, but it is also the source for financial, legal, and clinical accountability. Occupational therapy documentation should always contain the following:

- Which services were provided and when they were provided
- What was said and what happened
- Why the skill of an occupational therapy practitioner was required rather than the services of an aide, a family member, or another professional

Before you write or type anything in the health record, make these assumptions:

- Someone else will have to read and understand what I write because I may be sick or out of town the next time this client needs to be treated.
- This entry I am about to make will be scrutinized by a third-party payer. If I were a Medicare or insurance reviewer, would I want to pay for the services I am about to record?
- My client will exercise their right to read this record.

Some payers are looking for different outcomes than others. With a Medicare client, you will discuss activities of daily living (ADLs) and instrumental activities of daily living (IADLs), and you will write goals for self-care and home management. With a Workers' Compensation client, you will write goals that are oriented toward returning to work. In home health care, you may need to document that your client is unable to leave home to receive services or that education on safety issues was provided to the caregiver. With a child, you will need to focus on educationally relevant services identified in the Individualized Education Program (IEP) for school-based services or family-centered goals identified in the Individualized Family Service Plan (IFSP) for early intervention services.

It is essential to remember that your documentation is a reflection of your professional identity and abilities. It is also a reflection of your academic institution, your department, and occupational therapy as a profession. Unless they have witnessed you treating a client, your documentation may be the primary way that others form an impression about your skills and professionalism. This chapter will review general rules for documenting in the health record, guidelines for documenting special situations, considerations in electronic documentation, abbreviations and symbols for documentation, and common documentation errors.

Gateley, C. A. *Documentation Manual for Occupational Therapy, Fifth Edition* (pp. 43-61). © 2024 Taylor & Francis Group.

"Other readers will assume, rightly or wrongly, that you practice … much in the same way that you document. If your documentation is sloppy, full of errors, or incomplete, others will assume that is the way you practice. Conversely, thorough, legible, and complete documentation will infer that you provide care in the same way, thus establishing your credibility" (Sullivan, 2019, p. 2).

GENERAL RULES FOR DOCUMENTING IN THE HEALTH RECORD

There are several rules that should always be followed when documenting in the health record:

- *Always use waterproof, nonerasable black or blue ink in written records* (American Health Information Management Association [AHIMA], 2014a, 2014b): This prevents smearing, erasing, or otherwise changing the health record. Black and blue ink show up best when part of the health record needs to be photocopied or electronically scanned.
- *Correct errors*: Never use correction tape or black marker to cover up the inaccurate information. It is considered an illegal alteration of the record. If you make a mistake in a written health record, draw a single line through it, write your correction, and initial the change:

CG

Pt. able to dress lower body with ~~*verbal cues*~~ *min A using a reacher.*

  ◦ If you inadvertently write your note in the wrong client's chart, draw a single line through the entire entry and write "wrong chart" beside it with your signature.
  ◦ If you need to add something after you have written and signed your note, write an addendum with the current date and time.
  ◦ If you are correcting an error in an electronic health record (EHR), the same basic principles apply: "The original entry should be viewable, the current date and time should be entered, the person making the change should be identified, and the reason should be noted" (AHIMA, 2014b, para. 4).
- *Be sure all required data are present*: The *Guidelines for Documentation in Occupational Therapy* (American Occupational Therapy Association [AOTA], 2018) specify the content for each type of note you may be writing. This information will be covered in Chapter 13.
- *Be as concise as possible without leaving out pertinent data*: You will have limited time for documentation under today's productivity standards, and other busy professionals appreciate being able to read what you have written in the shortest time possible (Syed, 2017).
- *Sign and date every entry*: Some facilities and funding sources also require you to document the time of day or number of minutes that the client received services. The standard format is first name, middle initial, last name, and credentials (Kettenbach & Schlomer, 2016). Some facilities may require only first initial and last name (AHIMA, 2014a). Required credentials may vary by state. In written health records, if your signature is not legible, be sure to print your name below your signature. In EHRs, you will be able to sign your name electronically with your electronic user identification and password. Notes by students must be co-signed by a supervising therapist, and in some settings, notes by occupational therapy assistants must be co-signed by the supervising occupational therapist.
  ◦ Signature Example for Students: *Truman Tiger, OTS*
  ◦ Signature Example for Therapists: *Crystal Gateley, OTR/L*

The second example above shows that the therapist is **registered** with the National Board for Certification in Occupational Therapy (NBCOT) and **licensed** in a particular state. Some therapists choose not to maintain their certification with NBCOT after initially passing the national certification exam. Maintaining certification and the use of the "R" in a signature requires proof of continuing education and a fee every 3 years (Lyon, 2022; NBCOT, 2022). In that case the signature would end with "OT/L." Many therapists also include their degree and/or other specialty credentials relevant to occupational therapy practice in their signatures (Lyon, 2022). For example:
  ◦ Signature Examples With Degrees:
    ▪ *Stephanie Allen, MOT, OTR/L*
    ▪ *Whitney Henderson, MOT, OTD, OT/L*
    ▪ *Crystal Gateley, PhD, OTR/L*

- ° Signature Examples With Specialty or Board Certifications:
  - *Mark Simenson, OTR/L, CHT* (Certified Hand Therapist)
  - *Gina Pifer, OTR/L, BCPR* (AOTA Board Certification in Physical Rehabilitation)
  - *Monica Holmes, OTR/L, CLT* (Certified Lymphedema Therapist)

Please note: Your state's practice act may dictate how you must sign your name. For example, some states do not require or even allow practitioners to use OTR/L or OT/L. Instead, they must include their state license number. For example:

Crystal Gateley, OT, #003434

It is your responsibility to be familiar with your state practice act and follow all requirements related to documentation.

- *Identify the client on every page of documentation*: In a written health record, every page must include the client's full name and other identifying information as required by the facility in indelible ink or in the form of a stamp (AHIMA, 2014a).

- *Document in a timely manner*: It is best to document as soon after a session as possible. This allows for the best communication between team members. It also ensures that your recollection of events will be accurate. As many facilities move toward the use of EHRs, occupational therapy practitioners are being asked to complete point-of-service documentation, in which the therapist electronically documents the occupational therapy services during the session (Waite, 2012). However, Sames (2015) cautioned practitioners to maintain communication and periodic eye contact when completing point-of-service documentation.
  - ° If you encounter a situation in which you need to document a session that occurred on another date, you should document "Late entry for [date]" at the beginning of the note.

- *Use appropriate terminology for the recipient of services*: When referring to the persons who receive occupational therapy services, the terms *client, patient, consumer, resident, veteran, participant, individual, student, teacher, child, caregiver, employer,* or *family* may be used (Costa et al., 2019). You may also simply use the individual's preferred name. Use the term that is considered most respectful for your practice setting. You will see a variety of terms used throughout this textbook.

- *Be prudent in using abbreviations*: Although abbreviations save time and help with writing concise notes, "using too many or incorrect abbreviations can also cause denial of payment if the reviewer at the reimbursement agency cannot understand what happened in physical or occupational therapy" (Kettenbach & Schlomer, 2016, p. 37). Your facility should provide you with an accepted list of abbreviations.

- *Focus on the client's experience and leave yourself out*: "Notes discuss the patient, not the therapist" (Kettenbach & Schlomer, 2016, p. 25). Unless it is absolutely relevant, do not mention yourself in the note. It is not necessary to say, "Therapist provided caregiver with skilled instruction in assisting client with self-care." Simply say, "Caregiver received skilled instruction in assisting client with self-care." In the rare cases when it is necessary to mention yourself in the note, refer to yourself in the third person. Do not use "I" or "me." Instead, use "the therapist," "the clinician," or "the occupational therapist." For example: "Client cursed and pushed therapist's hand away when physical assistance was provided for grooming task." Chapter 8 will provide additional examples about how to write from the client's point of view while simultaneously showing the skilled therapy that was provided.

- *Always adhere to legal and ethical guidelines*: Be familiar with laws, regulatory guidelines, facility policies, and AOTA *Official Documents* that affect documentation (AOTA, 2018; Sames, 2015; Sullivan, 2019).

- *Always be accurate and objective*: Report what was actually observed and avoid judging or interpreting the observations other than in the Assessment portion of your note. "Criticism of other staff members, colleagues, or the patient, or complaints about working conditions are not to be included in the patient care note. The note is about the patient's condition, not about the healthcare provider or the healthcare provider's reactions to other people" (Kettenbach & Schlomer, 2016, p. 23).

- *In terms of fiscal and legal accountability, "If it's not documented, it didn't happen"*: No activity or contact is ever considered a service that has been provided until a clinical entry has been made in the health record. "Documentation that happens today is future evidence of the quality of care of the intervention the client received. If any portion is left unsaid, it leaves the door open for doubt about the entire care of the client and could be a potential liability" (McCann, as cited in AOTA, 2021, para. 10). In the current era of health care reimbursement scrutiny, you should also think to yourself, "If it's not documented well, my company might not get reimbursed."

- *Avoid spelling, grammar, and punctuation errors*: As previously stated, your documentation is a reflection of your skills and professionalism. Errors in documentation can also present safety concerns for your client if another professional misinterprets your documentation due to such errors. Although some software programs for EHRs offer a spellcheck option, many do not (Lai et al., 2015). Occupational therapy practitioners should carefully review what they have entered into an EHR prior to providing an electronic signature.

- *Be aware of "red-flag" words*: Words such as *continued* and *maintained* suggest that progress is not occurring, and funding sources may not reimburse for those services. However, in 2013, the U.S. Supreme Court ruling in the *Jimmo v Sebelius* case clarified that the potential for improvement is not required for Medicare reimbursement. Rather, "Skilled therapy services are covered when an individualized assessment of the patient's clinical condition demonstrates that the specialized judgment, knowledge, and skills of a qualified therapist ('skilled care') are necessary for the performance of a safe and effective maintenance program" (Centers for Medicare & Medicaid Services, 2021). In such cases, be very clear in your documentation that the skills of an occupational therapy practitioner were required due to the nature of the client's condition or the complexity of the intervention.

DOCUMENTING SPECIAL SITUATIONS
Change in Client Status

Any unusual situations regarding the client should be documented (AOTA, 2018). In many cases, therapy personnel may be the first to recognize a change in patient status indicative of a significant underlying medical issue. For example, suppose during your morning ADL session with a client that you observe pain and swelling of the lower leg (symptoms of a blood clot) or a decrease in cognition from previous sessions. Those symptoms should be documented in the health record. It is also important to communicate any status change to the client's nurse and/or physician and to document that you have passed the information on to the appropriate person. Example:

During lower body dressing, client observed to have redness, pitting edema, and pain in L LE. Skin also noted to be warm to touch. Discontinued ADL session. Notified nurse and physician of patient status.

In another example, suppose you are working with a toddler diagnosed with hydrocephalus. When you arrive to the child's home for a scheduled early intervention session, you note that the child is more irritable and lethargic than you have observed in previous sessions, and the parent reports that the child has been hitting her head repeatedly, all of which are signs of shunt malfunction (Cincinnati Children's Hospital Medical Center, 2018). You should document your follow-up actions. Example:

Upon arrival to child's home for occupational therapy session, Chloe noted to be significantly more irritable and lethargic than previous sessions. Parent reports Chloe has been crying and hitting right side of her head all morning. Redness noted at shunt site. Recommended parent seek immediate medical attention for Chloe to rule out shunt malfunction. Family transported Chloe to emergency department at Children's Hospital. Notified Chloe's pediatrician and early intervention case manager. No other occupational therapy intervention provided on this date.

Missed Visits

Any scheduled or attempted visits that are missed should be documented with an explanation for the missed visit and any other pertinent information regarding follow-up (Kettenbach & Schlomer, 2016):

- *Client cancelled scheduled outpatient visit due to inclement weather. Confirmed next appointment on 12-15-2023.*
- *Attempted twice this date to see pt. for initial OT eval. Pt. off unit to diagnostic testing (TEE) in am, then on bed rest this pm following sedation from test. Will reattempt tomorrow.*
- *Resident declined participation in therapeutic exercise this am, citing fatigue. Rescheduled for this pm.*
- *Child missed two scheduled OT sessions on 11/14 and 11/16 due to being absent from school 11/13–11/17/2023 with illness. Will resume 30-minute sessions 2x/wk next week.*
- *Attempted scheduled home visit for early intervention. Child and family not home at scheduled time/date. Attempted twice to contact by phone, no answer, left message on voicemail. Notified service coordinator of situation.*

Lack of Compliance

A client's lack of compliance with medical and therapy recommendations is another situation that should be documented. For example, if a client is not following safety recommendations, such as hip precautions or the use of an assistive device for ambulation during ADLs, it is important to document these observations along with any reasons that the client may provide for choosing not to follow the recommendations. It is, however, necessary to distinguish between voluntary lack of compliance and cognitive deficits that limit the client's ability to remember to comply with recommendations. Examples:

- *Client does not consistently adhere to post-surgical hip precautions during ADL performance. Reviewed hip precautions. Client able to articulate 3 of 3 precautions but reports difficulty remembering to follow them during functional activities.*
- *During home health visit, client reported she had not been using shower chair for bathing as recommended to reduce fall risk. "I just don't like having all that stuff cluttering up my bathroom."*
- *Child has missed 4 of 8 scheduled therapy visits this month. Caregiver reports difficulty balancing therapy schedule with numerous other medical and school-related appointments. After discussion with caregiver, frequency of sessions reduced to 1x/wk with a plan for increased emphasis on home program activities. Insurance case manager notified.*

Incident Reports

Another special situation that requires documentation is an incident report. An incident report should be completed for events such as client falls, skin tears, inadvertent removal of IV or catheter, and other unplanned events that led to injury or had the potential to lead to the injury of a client, visitor, or staff person. Scott (2013) and Rebar (2009) reiterated that **the incident report should not be contained in the health record**, as it contains administrative information about follow-up of the incident. The health record should contain only the objective clinical information related to the event, and no mention of the incident report. Example:

Client experienced ½-inch skin tear to dorsal aspect of L hand when reaching into kitchen cabinet during cooking activity. Pressure and gauze bandage applied; nursing notified. Client stated, "I'm fine" and continued with cooking activity.

Health care settings have special forms and procedures for documenting incident reports, which serve the following purposes (Hooiveld, 2022; Rebar, 2009; Scott, 2013):

- Ensuring that optimal care was provided to the injured party
- Protecting the staff member and facility from unwarranted liability exposure
- Identifying the need for further staff training to prevent similar incidents and enhance patient care and safety

Each facility will have a particular form (written or electronic) for documenting adverse incidents. The following information is typically included in an incident report (Hooiveld, 2022; Rebar, 2009; Scott, 2013):

- Patient name, address, date of birth, and health record identification number
- Incident date, time, and location
- Patient diagnosis and summary of care received following the incident
- Type of incident (e.g., fall, skin tear, modality-related, equipment malfunction)
- Condition of person affected by incident
- Course of action (e.g., notifying nurse or physician)
- Witness names and contact information
- Concise yet thorough explanation of event in objective terms, without speculation of cause

An incident involving injury to you will require additional documentation because it is considered a Workers' Compensation issue. Examples include injuring your back while transferring a client, slipping on a wet floor in a client's room, or being struck or bitten by a client. When any event occurs that would require an incident report, it is essential that you notify your supervisor immediately so that appropriate responses can be carried out and documented.

Remember that incident reports should NOT be included in the health record. "Instead of being filed in the client's chart, an incident report is circulated to an appropriate committee that reviews the report and attempts to enact positive change so that similar episodes do not happen again" (Rebar, 2009, p. 44).

PERSON-FIRST AND IDENTITY-FIRST LANGUAGE

Quinn and Gordon (2016) suggested that professionals should always make an intentional effort to refer to the individual first rather than the diagnosis. "Patients should be thought of as people first, not their disability. Labeling patients according to their disability (e.g., stroke victim, amputee) suggests that their disability defines them" (Quinn & Gordon, 2016, p. 15). For example, rather than "the Down baby," we should say "the infant with Down syndrome." Rather than "the stroke in Room 203," we should say "the person in Room 203 who had a stroke."

This concept of person-first language fits well within our profession. One of the guiding principles for the occupational therapy profession is client-centered practice (AOTA, 2020). One way to demonstrate client-centered practice is by using person-first language not just in our verbal interactions but also in our documentation. We should write our notes in terms of what the client needs rather than stating that the client is a particular assist level. Our clients are much more than their assist levels.

Please say: *"Veteran needs max assist ..."* or *"Veteran requires max assist ..."*

Rather than: *"Veteran is max assist ..."*

Although there has been a push for person-first language for decades, in recent years, some groups, particularly the blind, deaf, and autism communities, have pushed back and called for identity-first language that recognizes that disability is intertwined with a person's identity (Employer Assistance and Resource Network on Disability Inclusion, 2022; Jankowski, 2021; Paraquad, 2022). "In the autism community, many self-advocates and their allies prefer terminology such as 'Autistic,' 'Autistic person,' or 'Autistic individual' because we understand autism as an inherent part of an individual's identity, the same way one refers to 'Muslims,' 'African-Americans,' 'Lesbian/Gay/Bisexual/Transgender/Queer,' 'Chinese,' 'gifted,' 'athletic,' or 'Jewish'" (Brown, 2022, para. 3). When in doubt, simply ask the individuals you are working with if they have a preference and use their preferred terminology.

"One certainty we can derive from the ongoing conversation about person-first language and identity-first language is that we share a common goal: to recognize, affirm, and validate all individuals' identities and personhood. It is incumbent ... to endeavor toward centering the voice of disabled people and strive to acknowledge the varied perspectives of self-advocates through thoughtful use of language" (Simonsen & Mruczek, 2022, para. 13).

CONSIDERATIONS IN ELECTRONIC DOCUMENTATION

While EHRs provide many advantages in terms of efficiency, connectivity, and legibility, they also present unique concerns, particularly regarding confidentiality. The Health Insurance Portability and Accountability Act Security Rule established federal standards for the security of EHRs. All employees who have access to EHRs must take precautions to prevent unauthorized access, alteration, or disclosure of a client's health information (Office for Civil Rights, 2022). Occupational therapy practitioners who have access to EHRs will generally have a username and/or password to access client records and to sign documentation that has been entered about occupational therapy services. The following precautions should be taken to adhere to the HIPAA Security Rule (Kettenbach & Schlomer, 2016; Sames, 2015):

- Do not share your username or password with anyone.
- Log out when you are leaving an electronic workstation.
- Do not access any EHRs that you do not have a direct need to see. This includes your own EHR or those of family, friends, etc. Access to unauthorized EHRs can be traced back to your username and may be grounds for disciplinary action, termination of employment, and legal action.
- Be aware of your surroundings and make sure that unauthorized individuals cannot read the screen. Electronic workstations are often located in high traffic areas, such as nurses' stations, patient rooms, hallways, therapy gyms, and shared offices.
- Be familiar and compliant with your employer's EHR safeguards, including the transmission of personal health information via facsimile or electronic mail.

Chapter 14 will provide a more comprehensive overview of considerations in the use of electronic documentation, after you have learned the basics of the SOAP note approach to documentation.

AVOIDING COMMON DOCUMENTATION ERRORS

As previously stated, your documentation is a reflection of you and the profession of occupational therapy. Mistakes in spelling, grammar, and punctuation may give others a negative impression of your knowledge, skills, and professionalism (Sullivan, 2019). Such errors can also lead to serious consequences for you or your client. This section will review several rules to help you avoid common documentation errors:

- Use quotation marks when documenting the exact words that a client or another person said.
  - Incorrect: *Client stated I can't feel my right arm.*
  - Correct: *Client stated, "I can't feel my right arm."*
- Do not use quotation marks when paraphrasing what a client or another person said.
  - Incorrect: *Client reports she "can't feel her right arm."*
  - Correct: *Client reports she cannot feel her right arm.*
- Be consistent in the use of verb tense.
  - Incorrect: *Client demonstrated upper body dressing with min A. Client threads R UE into sleeve first. Client transfers to toilet with SBA. Client completed grooming tasks independently.*
  - Correct: *Client demonstrated upper body dressing with min A. Client threaded R UE into sleeve first. Client transferred to toilet with SBA. Client completed grooming tasks independently.*
- Indicate plurals by adding an "s" to the end of a word without an apostrophe.
  - Incorrect: *The client's participated in a group discussion about time management and ADL's. The OT's then provided additional suggestion's.*
  - Correct: *The clients participated in a group discussion about time management and ADLs. The OTs then provided additional suggestions.*
- Indicate possession of a single person or object by using an apostrophe before the "s."
  - Incorrect: *The clients' spouse was present during the session.*
  - Correct: *The client's spouse was present during the session.*

- Indicate possession of more than one person or object by using an apostrophe after the "s."
  - ○ Incorrect: *The three clients group discussion focused on coping skills.*
  - ○ Correct: *The three clients' group discussion focused on coping skills.*
- Follow the general rules for capitalization (Table 5-1).
- Know the appropriate spelling of commonly misspelled words (Table 5-2).

Previous editions of this textbook included reminders to use singular pronouns for one person and plural pronouns for more than one person. However, "issues of equality and acceptance of transgender and nonbinary people—along with challenges to their rights—have become a major topic in the headlines" in recent years (Wamsley, 2021). Many advocacy groups and publishers now endorse the use of the word "they" to refer to one person. "The singular 'they' is a generic third-person singular pronoun in English. Use of the singular 'they' is endorsed as part of APA style because it is inclusive of all people and helps writers avoid making assumptions about gender" (American Psychological Association, 2019, para. 1).

Table 5-1

GENERAL RULES FOR CAPITALIZATION

CAPITALIZE	DO NOT CAPITALIZE
Proper names in medical terminology (e.g., Alzheimer's disease)	Common nouns in medical terminology (e.g., virus, appendectomy, scapula)
Trade names of products and medications (e.g., Jobst stocking, Advil)	Generic drugs and products (e.g., compression glove, pain reliever)
Specific organizations (e.g., The Joint Commission)	Generic organizations (e.g., accrediting agency)
Academic degrees and professional designations after the person's name (e.g., Crystal Gateley, PhD, OTR/L)	General degrees or generic professional designations (e.g., an associate's degree, an occupational therapist)
Exact test titles (e.g., Peabody Developmental Motor Scales)	Generic test (e.g., sensory test, cognitive test)
Specific department proper names (e.g., Midwest Hospital Occupational Therapy Department)	Generic department names (e.g., an occupational therapy department, the rehab department)
Official titles as part of a name (e.g., Dr. Wolf, Father O'Malley)	Generic or descriptive titles (e.g., the doctor, the clergyperson)

Data source: GrammarBook.com, 2022.

Table 5-2

COMMONLY MISSPELLED WORDS

WORDS THAT SOUND ALIKE	"I" BEFORE "E" EXCEPT AFTER "C" WORDS	MISCELLANEOUS WORDS
• accept (*She wouldn't accept it.*) • except (*all except that one*) • affect (*He had a flat affect. That didn't affect his participation.*) • effect (*That has no effect on me.*) • aid (verb—*to help;* noun—*a helping device, such as a visual aid*) • aide (*person, such as the occupational therapy aide*) • aloud (*She said it aloud.*) • allowed (*Children aren't allowed in there.*) • brake (*Lock the wheelchair brake.*) • break (*Take a break. He will break his arm.*) • gait (*ambulation*) • gate (*an entrance*) • lay (*Lay it on the desk.*) • lie (*He wants to lie on the bed.*) • loose (*not tight*) • lose (*I want to lose weight.*) • patience (*Have some patience!*) • patients (*The patients were in their rooms.*) • peace (*I want some peace and quiet.*) • piece (*piece of the puzzle*) • principal (*the school principal*) • principle (*principles of NDT*) • stationary (*not moving*) • stationery (*writing paper*) • than (*I have more than you.*) • then (*Then he went to bed.*) • their (*It was their house.*) • there (*Put it there.*) • they're (*they are*) • wait (*Wait here.*) • weight (*Her weight has declined.*) • you're (*you are*) • your (*It's your turn.*)	• achieve (after "ch" is still "ie") • believe • brief • hygiene • piece • receive • relieve • retrieve	• activity • Alzheimer's • asymmetry • catheterization • clavicle • current • deferred • definitely • developmentally • dining • doctor • doff • doffed • doffing • dominant • don • donned • donning • equilibrium • exercise • immobilize • independent • input • intention • interest • judgment • paraffin • perform • putty • recommendations • remember • rotator cuff • schizophrenia • stabilization • strength • symmetry • technique • toilet • tolerate • transferring • writing

Data source: Merriam-Webster, 2022.

ABBREVIATIONS AND SYMBOLS

Using abbreviations and symbols when documenting in the client's health record saves valuable time, but these should be used with discretion (Kettenbach & Schlomer, 2016). Remember that your notes may be read by someone who knows little about occupational therapy, and that individual may determine whether to pay for your services. You should be sure that the individual will be able to understand the information you are trying to convey. Health care settings typically have a list of approved abbreviations. You should be familiar with that list and use only abbreviations that are approved for your setting. Do not make up abbreviations. Many people commonly use acronyms or shorthand when chatting online or texting, but those abbreviations are not appropriate for the health record. Also remember that while it is permissible to use abbreviations, it is not required. You may write out any word instead of shortening it.

In this manual, you will find that some notes use more abbreviations and symbols than others. Table 5-3 lists commonly used abbreviations. Please note that this list is not all-inclusive. The Joint Commission, which accredits many hospitals and other health care facilities, does not maintain a list of acceptable abbreviations and symbols for use in documentation. However, The Joint Commission has published an *Official "Do Not Use" List* for abbreviations (The Joint Commission, 2022). The list contains abbreviations and symbols prohibited on all orders, along with handwritten, pre-printed, and electronic forms regarding medications. A few examples of prohibited abbreviations are qd (every day) and qod (every other day) because they can be mistaken for each other. While occupational therapy practitioners would rarely be involved with documentation regarding medications, some facilities prohibit the use of the abbreviations and symbols on the *Official "Do Not Use" List* by any health care provider in any type of documentation. You must be familiar with the list of acceptable and prohibited abbreviations and symbols for your facility.

Table 5-3

ABBREVIATIONS AND SYMBOLS

ABBREVIATIONS FOR DIAGNOSES AND SURGICAL PROCEDURES

AAA	abdominal aortic aneurysm	CA	cancer; carcinoma	DJD	degenerative joint disease
ADD	attention deficit disorder	CABG	coronary artery bypass grafting	DM	diabetes mellitus
ADHD	attention-deficit/hyperactivity disorder	CAD	coronary artery disease	DVT	deep vein thrombosis
		c-diff	*Clostridioides difficile* (bacteria)	ESRD	end-stage renal disease
a-fib	atrial fibrillation	CF	cystic fibrosis	EtOH	alcohol (use/abuse)
AIDS	acquired immune deficiency syndrome	CHF	congestive heart failure	FTT	failure to thrive
		CHI	closed head injury	fx	fracture
AKA	above knee amputation	COPD	chronic obstructive pulmonary disorder	GBS	Guillain-Barré syndrome
AKI	acute kidney injury			GERD	gastroesophageal reflux disease
ALS	amyotrophic lateral sclerosis	CP	cerebral palsy	GSW	gunshot wound
		CRF	chronic renal failure	H/A/HA	headache
ARF	acute renal failure	CRPS	complex regional pain syndrome	HIV	human immunodeficiency virus
ASCVD	atherosclerotic cardiovascular disease	CTR	carpal tunnel release	HTN	hypertension
AVM	arteriovenous malformation	CVA	cerebrovascular accident	ICH	intracerebral hemorrhage
BKA	below knee amputation	DDD	degenerative disc disease		
BPH	benign prostatic hypertrophy				

(continued)

Table 5-3 (continued)

ABBREVIATIONS AND SYMBOLS

ABBREVIATIONS FOR DIAGNOSES AND SURGICAL PROCEDURES

IDDM	insulin dependent diabetes mellitus	NPH	normal pressure hydrocephalus	SDH	subdermal hematoma
LBP	low back pain	N/V	nausea and vomiting	SLE	systemic lupus erythematosus
LOC	loss of consciousness	OA	osteoarthritis	SOB	shortness of breath
MD	muscular dystrophy	ORIF	open reduction and internal fixation	Sz	seizure
mets	metastasis			TBI	traumatic brain injury
MI	myocardial infarction	PD	Parkinson's disease	THA	total hip arthroplasty
MRSA	Methicillin-resistant *Staphylococcus aureus* (bacteria)	PDD	pervasive developmental disorder	THR	total hip replacement
		PVD	peripheral vascular disease	TIA	transient ischemic attack
MS	multiple sclerosis			TKA	total knee arthroplasty
MVA	motor vehicle accident	RA	rheumatoid arthritis	TKR	total knee replacement
NIDDM	non–insulin-dependent diabetes mellitus	RSD	reflex sympathetic dystrophy	URI	upper respiratory infection
NKA	no known allergies	SAH	subarachnoid hemorrhage	UTI	urinary tract infection
NKDA	no known drug allergies	SCD	sickle cell disease	VRE	Vancomycin-resistant *Enterococci* (bacteria)
NOS	not otherwise specified	SCI	spinal cord injury		

ABBREVIATIONS FOR BODY PARTS, FUNCTIONS, AND OTHER CLIENT DESCRIPTORS

A&Ox4	alert and oriented to person, place, time, situation	ENT	ear, nose, throat	PIP	proximal interphalangeal joint
		GI	gastrointestinal		
		HEENT	head, eyes, ears, nose, throat	PNS	peripheral nervous system
abd	abduction				
add	adduction	HR	heart rate	PO	by mouth
ant.	anterior	ht.	height	post.	posterior
A/P	anterior/posterior	IM	intramuscular	PSIS	posterior superior iliac spine
ASIS	anterior superior iliac spine	Ⓛ/L	left		
		LE	lower extremity	Ⓡ/R	right
Ⓑ/B	bilateral	LLQ	left lower quadrant	RLQ	right lower quadrant
BM	bowel movement	LMN	lower motor neuron	RUQ	right upper quadrant
bpm	beats per minute	LUQ	left upper quadrant	UE	upper extremity
CMC	carpometacarpal	MCP	metacarpophalangeal	UMN	upper motor neuron
CNS	central nervous system	NPO	nothing by mouth	wt.	weight
C/O	complains of	peri	perineal	y.o.	years old
CSF	cerebrospinal fluid	PERRLA	pupils equal, round, reactive to light and accommodation	yr	year
DIP	distal interphalangeal joint				
DOB	date of birth				

(continued)

Table 5-3 (continued)

ABBREVIATIONS AND SYMBOLS

ABBREVIATIONS FOR MEDICAL EQUIPMENT, TESTS, AND INTERVENTIONS

ABG	arterial blood gas	EEG	electroencephalogram	PET	positron emission tomography
AE	adaptive equipment	EKG	electrocardiogram		
AFO	ankle foot orthosis	EMG	electromyogram	PMH	past medical history
AMA	against medical advice	e-stim	electrical stimulation	post-op	postoperatively
appt.	appointment	FBS	fasting blood sugar	pre-op	preoperatively
Bi-PAP	bi-level positive airway pressure	F/U	follow up	RBC	red blood cell (count)
		HFNC	high-flow nasal canula	R/O	rule out
BP	blood pressure	H&H	hemoglobin and hematocrit	Rx	prescription
BSC	bedside commode			SCD	sequential compression devices
BUN	blood urea nitrogen (blood test)	H&P	history and physical		
		Hx	history	S/P	status post
CAT	computed axial tomography	I&D	incision and drainage	S/S	signs and symptoms
		I&O	intake and output	Sx	symptoms
cath.	catheter; catheterization	IV	intravenous	TEDS	thromboembolic disease stockings
		KAFO	knee ankle foot orthosis		
CBC	complete blood count	LP	lumbar puncture	TEE	transesophageal echocardiogram
chemo	chemotherapy	LSO	lumbar sacral orthosis		
CO_2	carbon dioxide	meds	medications	TENS	transcutaneous electrical nerve stimulation
CPAP	continuous positive airway pressure	MRA	magnetic resonance angiography		
				TLSO	thoracic lumbar sacral orthosis
CPM	continuous passive motion	MRI	magnetic resonance imaging		
				tPA	tissue plasminogen activator
CPR	cardiopulmonary resuscitation	NC	nasal canula		
		NG	nasogastric	TPN	total parenteral nutrition
CT	computed tomography	NMES	neuromuscular electric stimulation		
CXR	chest x-ray			tx	treatment
DME	durable medical equipment	O_2	oxygen	UA	urinalysis
		PCA	patient-controlled analgesia	US	ultrasound
DNR	do not resuscitate			VC	vital capacity
dx	diagnosis	PEG	percutaneous endoscopic gastrostomy	VS	vital signs
ECG	electrocardiogram			WBC	white blood cell (count)
ECHO	echocardiogram				

ABBREVIATIONS FOR FREQUENCY AND TIME

$\bar{a}$	before	$\bar{p}$	after	tid	three times per day
ad lib	as desired (up on own)	PM/pm	afternoon	1x/wk	one time per week
AM/am	morning	prn	as needed	2x/wk	two times per week
ASAP	as soon as possible	PTA	prior to admission	3x/wk	three times per week
bid	twice per day	qd	every day	1x/mo	one time per month
min	minute	qod	every other day	2x/mo	two times per month
noc	night; bedtime	STAT	immediately/urgently	3x/mo	three times per month

(continued)

Table 5-3 (continued)

ABBREVIATIONS AND SYMBOLS

ABBREVIATIONS FOR LOCATION AND SETTINGS

CCU	coronary (cardiac) care unit	LTC	long-term care	PACU	post-anesthesia care unit
ECF	extended care facility	MICU	medical intensive care unit	PICU	pediatric intensive care unit
ED	emergency department	NICU	neonatal intensive care unit	RCF	residential care facility
ER	emergency room			SICU	surgical intensive care unit
HH	home health	NSICU	neuroscience intensive care unit		
ICU	intensive care unit	OP	outpatient	SNF	skilled nursing facility
IP	inpatient	OR	operating room	SNU	skilled nursing unit
LTCH/ LTACH	long-term acute care hospital				

ABBREVIATIONS FOR LEVELS OF ASSISTANCE

Ⓐ/A	assistance; assist	CGA	contact guard assistance	Ⓓ/D	dependent; dependence
Ⓘ/I	independent; independence	min A	minimal assistance (~25%)	x1	assistance of one person
mod I	modified independence	mod A	moderate assistance (~50%)	x2	assistance of two people
SBA	standby assistance	max A	maximal assistance (~75%)		

MISCELLANEOUS COMMON THERAPY AND HEALTH CARE ABBREVIATIONS

AAROM	active assistive range of motion	DO	doctor of osteopathy	LPN	licensed practical nurse
		ELOS	expected length of stay	LTG	long-term goal
ADLs	activities of daily living	EOB	edge of bed; explanation of benefits	MD	medical doctor
amb	ambulation; ambulated			MMT	manual muscle test
		eval	evaluation	N	normal (muscle grade)
AROM	active range of motion	ext	extension	NDT	neurodevelopmental treatment
ATNR	asymmetrical tonic neck reflex	F	fair (muscle grade)		
		flex	flexion	NP	nurse practitioner
BADLs	basic activities of daily living	ft	foot; feet	NWB	non–weight bearing
		FWB	full weight bearing	OOB	out of bed
BOS	base of support	G	good (muscle grade)	OT	occupational therapist; occupational therapy
CHT	Certified Hand Therapist	HEP	home exercise program		
CLT	Certified Lymphedema Therapist	HOB	head of bed	OTR/L	Occupational Therapist Registered/Licensed
		HOH	hard of hearing		
COTA	Certified Occupational Therapy Assistant	IADLs	instrumental activities of daily living	OTS	occupational therapy student
COTA/L	Certified Occupational Therapy Assistant/ Licensed	IFSP	Individualized Family Service Plan	P	poor (muscle grade)
				PA	physician assistant
CST	craniosacral therapist	IEP	Individualized Education Program	PAM	physical agent modalities
D/C	discharge; discontinue	LOS	length of stay	PLOF	prior level of function

(continued)

Table 5-3 (continued)

ABBREVIATIONS AND SYMBOLS

PNF	proprioceptive neuro-muscular facilitation	rehab	rehabilitation	STM	short-term memory
POC	plan of care	reps	repetitions	STNR	symmetrical tonic neck reflex
PROM	passive range of motion	RN	registered nurse	TDWB	touch down weight bearing
PT	physical therapist; physical therapy	ROM	range of motion		
		SI	sensory integration	TTWB	toe touch weight bearing
pt.	patient	SLP	speech-language pathologist	WBAT	weight bearing as tolerated
PTA	prior to admission	SOAP	Subjective, Objective, Assessment, Plan		
PWB	partial weight bearing			w/c	wheelchair
QI	quality indicator (section GG score)	SOC	start of care	WFL	within functional limits
		STG	short-term goal	WNL	within normal limits

MISCELLANEOUS SYMBOLS

♀	female	°	degree	~	approximately
♂	male	+	plus; positive	%	percent
↓	decrease	-	minus; negative	&	and
↑	increase	#	number; pounds	@	at
c̄	with	/	per	↔	to/from
s̄	without	<	less than	→	to; progressing toward
"	inches	>	greater than	1°	primary
'	feet	=	equals	2°	secondary; due to

Data sources: Kettenbach & Schlomer, 2016; National Library of Medicine, 2022.

CHANGES IN USE OF ABBREVIATIONS IN THIS TEXTBOOK EDITION

- One change in this manual from previous editions is that I will not be using abbreviations in the sample notes that involve circles around letters, such as Ⓐ, Ⓡ, Ⓛ, Ⓑ, Ⓘ, and Ⓓ. Although those abbreviations were often used in **written** documentation, it is common practice in **electronic** documentation to just type the corresponding letter.
- I will not be using abbreviations in the sample notes that involve a line over a letter, such as c̄, s̄, ā, or p̄. Although you occasionally may encounter these abbreviations in written documentation, it is standard practice in electronic documentation to just type out the corresponding word.
- I also will not be using the term *modified independence* or its abbreviation (mod I) in sample notes in this textbook. This terminology is from the Functional Independence Measure (FIM), which previously was used by Medicare and other insurance companies as an indicator of client performance and outcomes (Kindred Health Care, 2018). Modified independence meant that a person could complete a task independently but required adaptive equipment/strategies, extra time, or there was a safety concern. The new Section GG Quality Indicator (QI) scores (explained in detail in Chapter 3) replaced FIM scores in post-acute settings effective October 2019. QI scores do not include a separate category for modified independence. A person is considered **independent** (score of 6) whether adaptive equipment/strategies, extra time, or safety are factors (AOTA, 2022). However, you may still encounter the term *modified independence* in fieldwork or practice because there are therapists who have used FIM terminology for years or even decades, and old habits die hard. The term *modified independence* may also still be embedded in some electronic documentation systems that you encounter in fieldwork or practice.

The abbreviations and symbols discussed above are included in Table 5-3 for your reference since you may still encounter them in practice.

REFERENCES

American Health Information Management Association. (2014a). *Legal documentation standards that apply to medical records.* https://bok.ahima.org/

American Health Information Management Association. (2014b). *Legal guidelines for handling corrections, errors, omissions, and other documentation problems.* https://bok.ahima.org/

American Occupational Therapy Association. (2018). Guidelines for documentation of occupational therapy. *American Journal of Occupational Therapy, 72*(Suppl. 2), 7212410010. https://doi.org/10.5014/ajot.2018.72S203

American Occupational Therapy Association. (2020). Occupational therapy practice framework: Domain and process (4th ed.). *American Journal of Occupational Therapy, 74*(Suppl. 2), 7412410010. https://doi.org/10.5014/ajot.2020.74S2001

American Occupational Therapy Association. (2021). *Do's and don'ts of documentation: Tips from OT managers.* https://www.aota.org/

American Occupational Therapy Association. (2022). *Section GG self-care (activities of daily living) and mobility items.* https://www.aota.org/

American Psychological Association. (2019). *Singular "they."* https://apastyle.apa.org/

Brown, L. (2022). *Identity-first language.* Autistic Self-Advocacy Network. https://autisticadvocacy.org/

Centers for Medicare & Medicaid Services. (2021). *Jimmo Settlement.* https://www.cms.gov/

Cincinnati Children's Hospital Medical Center. (2018). *Shunt malfunction signs.* https://www.cincinnatichildrens.org/health/s/shunt-malfunction

Costa, D., Merceica-Bebber, R., Tesson, S., Siedler, Z., & Lopez, A. (2019). Patient, client, consumer, survivor, or other alternatives? A scoping review of preferred terms for labelling individuals who access healthcare across settings. *BMJ Open, 2019*(9), 1-16. http://dx.doi.org/10.1136/bmjopen-2018-025166

Employer Assistance and Resource Network on Disability Inclusion. (2022). *Person first and identity first language.* https://www.patientsafety.com/

GrammarBook.com. (2022). *Capitalization rules.* https://www.grammarbook.com/punctuation/capital.asp

Hooiveld, J. (2022, April 4). *Why is incident reporting important for healthcare organizations?* The Patient Safety Company. https://www.patientsafety.com/

Jankowski, M. (2021, February 26). *Language matters: Identity-first vs. person-first language.* Simple Practice. https://www.simplepractice.com/

Kettenbach, G., & Schlomer, S. L. (2016). *Writing patient/client notes: Ensuring accuracy in documentation* (5th ed.). F. A. Davis.

Kindred Health Care. (2018). *IRF Final Rule raises important concerns.* https://www.kindredhealthcare.com/our-services/kindred-rehabilitation-services/

Lai, K. H., Topaz, M., Goss, F. R., & Zhou, L. (2015). Automated misspelling detection and correction in clinical free-text records. *Journal of Biomedical Informatics, 55*(6), 188-195. https://doi.org/10.1016/j.jbi.2015.04.008

Lyon, S. (2022). *The ABC's of OT specialty certifications and credentials.* Very Well Health. https://www.verywellhealth.com/

Merriam-Webster. (2022). *Merriam-Webster's online dictionary.* https://www.merriam-webster.com/

National Board for Certification in Occupational Therapy. (2022). *Certification renewal.* https://www.nbcot.org/

National Library of Medicine. (2022). *Appendix B: Some common abbreviations.* https://medlineplus.gov/

Office for Civil Rights. (2022). *Privacy, security, and electronic health records.* https://www.hhs.gov/ocr/

Paraquad. (2022). *People-first language or identity-first language?* https://www.paraquad.org/

Quinn, L., & Gordon, J. (2016). *Documentation for rehabilitation: A guide to clinical decision making in physical therapy* (3rd ed.). Elsevier.

Rebar, C. (2009). *Docunotes: Clinical pocket guide for effective charting.* F. A. Davis.

Sames, K. (2015). *AOTA documentation series—Module 1: The nuts and bolts of effective documentation* [Online continuing education module]. American Occupational Therapy Association. https://www.aota.org/

Scott, R. W. (2013). *Legal, ethical, and practical aspects of patient care documentation: A guide for rehabilitation professionals* (4th ed.). Jones & Bartlett Learning.

Simonsen, M., & Mruczek, C. (2022). *Person-first vs. identity-first language.* The University of Kansas. https://educationonline.ku.edu/community/person-first-vs-identity-first-language

Sullivan, D. D. (2019). *Guide to clinical documentation* (3rd ed.). F. A. Davis.

Syed, S. (2017). *How to document well.* On the Wards. https://onthewards.org/how-to-document-well/

The Joint Commission. (2022). *Managing health information: Use of abbreviations, acronyms, symbols, and dose designations: Understanding the requirements.* https://www.jointcommission.org/

Waite, A. (2012). Record time: Point-of-service documentation strategies help practitioners beat the time crunch. *OT Practice, 17*(1), 9-12.

Wamsley, L. (2021, June 2). *A guide to gender identity terms.* NPR. https://www.npr.org/

WORKSHEET 5-1

Avoiding Common Documentation Errors

Identify and correct the errors in the following statements.

1. *Pt. stated my head really hurts this morning.*

2. *Resident reported "her right hand is working better today."*

3. *Student used right hand to cut with scissors. Student then switches to left hand for coloring tasks. Student did not demonstrate consistent hand preference.*

4. *The client's expressed excitement about the upcoming visit to the mall.*

5. *An occupational therapy referral was recieved from the childs' teacher.*

6. *The resident's were all in the dinning room weighting for there meal.*

7. *Client demonstrated appropriate social interaction by responding your welcome to another group member.*

8. *Pt. required moderate assistance to use dominate right hand in hygeine tasks.*

9. *Client does not demonstrate awareness of the affect of his mood on other member's of the group.*

10. *Pt. expressed intrest in getting dressed. Pt. required verbal cues when doning pullover shirt to utilize adaptive teckniques due to right rotary cup injury.*

WORKSHEET 5-1 (CONTINUED)
Avoiding Common Documentation Errors

11. *The ot noticed assymetry in the childs sitting posture. Parents reports that the client is unable to sit independantly.*

12. *The OTR preformed a Cognitive Test on the client.*

13. *The Doctor called to check on the Patients status.*

14. *Pt. had right arm imobilized due to a clavical fracture.*

15. *Client required several breif rest brakes during ADL's.*

16. *The clinic employs three otr's and two ota's.*

17. *The students principle stated Jimmy is disruptive at school.*

18. *The childrens' mother has difficulty keeping all they're appointment's.*

19. *Client needed a visual aide to help him learn how to preform self-catherization.*

WORKSHEET 5-2

Using Abbreviations

Translate each sentence written with abbreviations into full English-language phrases or sentences.

1. *Client C/O pain in R MCP joint after ~15 min PROM.*

2. *Pt. A&Ox4.*

3. *Client transferred w/c → mat with sliding board & max A x2.*

4. *1° dx L BKA, 2° dx COPD, CHF, DM, & PVD.*

5. *Pt. is S/P R THR. Orders received for OT 2x/day for ADLs & IADLs, WBAT R LE.*

WORKSHEET 5-2 (CONTINUED)

Using Abbreviations

Shorten these sentences using only the standard abbreviations in this chapter.

6. *Client has thirty degrees of passive range of motion in the left distal interphalangeal joint, which is within functional limits.*

7. *Client is able to put on her socks with standby assistance but requires moderate assistance with putting on and taking off left shoe.*

8. *The client requires contact guard assistance for balance during her morning dressing, which she performs while sitting on the edge of her bed.*

9. *The patient participated in a bedside evaluation of activities of daily living. She was able to perform bed mobility with moderate assistance, but she needed maximum assistance to put on her adult undergarment. She was able to go from a supine position to a sitting position with minimum assistance and from a sitting position to a standing position with moderate assistance.*

10. *The resident came to the occupational therapy clinic via wheelchair escort. The resident was observed to lean toward his left. The resident needed verbal cues and minimum assistance in positioning his body in the wheelchair to maintain midline orientation and symmetrical posture. The resident transferred from his wheelchair to the toilet with moderate assistance of one person to help him keep his balance using a standing pivot transfer. He needed verbal cues and visual feedback from a mirror to maintain upright posture.*

11. *The veteran participated in an evaluation in his room to determine relevant client factors. The veteran's short-term memory was three out of three for immediate recall, one out of three after 1 minute, and zero out of three with verbal cues after 5 minutes. The left upper extremity shoulder flexion was a grade of 4, shoulder extension was a grade of 4, elbow flexion was a grade of 4, elbow extension was a grade of 4, wrist flexion was a grade of 4 minus, wrist extension was a grade of 4 minus, and grip strength was 8 pounds. The left upper extremity light touch was intact. The right upper extremity muscle grades and sensation were within functional limits.*

Chapter 6

Writing Occupation-Based Problem Statements

As a part of the initial assessment, the occupational therapist develops a "problem list" identifying the major areas of occupation that have been affected by the client's condition. The contributing factors that affect the client's occupational performance are also identified. Priorities are then set with the client and caregivers so the problems that are most important to them will be addressed. Some clients and caregivers may need clarification of occupational therapy's role to identify problem areas that fall within the scope of occupational therapy practice.

Educating the client about the purpose and potential benefits of occupational therapy is an important part of establishing a therapeutic relationship (Rose, 2021). For example, when you ask clients in the hospital what their goals are, a common response is, "I want to walk." However, ambulation alone is a physical therapy goal. You can probe deeper by asking, "What things do you need to walk for?" Ask about activities such as meal preparation, gathering clothes to wear, and carrying items from place to place at home, school, or work. Clients who take an active role in goal setting often have improved functional outcomes and report greater satisfaction with the occupational therapy process (Cahill, 2021; Moll et al., 2018; Saito et al., 2019; Suc et al., 2020).

There are two parts to a functional problem statement: the **area of occupation** that is a concern and the **contributing factors** that are interfering with the client's engagement in that area of occupation. Let's take a closer look at information that was presented in Chapter 1 about occupational therapy's domain.

AREAS OF OCCUPATION

Occupational therapy practitioners provide interventions for people who have difficulty engaging in one or more areas of occupation. The focus on ability to engage in occupation is what distinguishes the occupational therapy profession from other health care disciplines, and occupation should be the focus of the problem statements we write for our clients (Amini, 2016). The *Occupational Therapy Practice Framework: Domain and Process, Fourth Edition* (*OTPF-4*; American Occupational Therapy Association [AOTA], 2020) categorizes the areas of occupation (Table 6-1) that may be addressed by occupational therapy practitioners. Please refer to the *OTPF-4* for expanded definitions and examples of each area of occupation.

It is essential to remember that the entities and agencies that provide reimbursement for occupational therapy services have different priorities. You should have a good understanding of funding source regulations, and your documentation should target areas of occupation that the funding source considers necessary and reimbursable (Amini, 2016; Finni & Karr, 2022). For example, Medicare is likely to be most concerned with problems and goals that target

Gateley, C. A. *Documentation Manual for Occupational Therapy, Fifth Edition* (pp. 63-76). © 2024 Taylor & Francis Group.

Table 6-1

AREAS OF OCCUPATION

AREA OF OCCUPATION	DESCRIPTION	EXAMPLES
Activities of Daily Living (ADLs)	Activities necessary for care of one's own body and personal independence. May also be referred to as basic activities of daily living (BADLs).	• Bathing/showering (including transfers) • Toileting and toilet hygiene (including transfers, menstrual needs, incontinence products, and any devices needed for bowel and bladder management) • Dressing (including planning and obtaining clothes) • Eating and swallowing • Feeding (self or others) • Functional mobility (while engaged in functional activities) • Personal hygiene and grooming • Sexual activity
Instrumental Activities of Daily Living (IADLs)	Activities involving participation in the home or community that often require more complex problem-solving and social skills than ADLs.	• Care of others • Care of pets and animals • Child rearing • Communication management • Driving and community mobility • Financial management • Home establishment and management • Meal preparation and cleanup • Religious and spiritual expression • Safety and emergency maintenance • Shopping
Health Management	Activities related to improving or maintaining personal health and wellness to support participation in other desired occupations.	• Social and emotional health promotion and maintenance • Symptom and condition management • Communication with the health care system • Medication management • Physical activity • Nutrition management • Personal care device management
Rest and Sleep	Activities related to obtaining the rest and sleep necessary for successful engagement in other areas of occupation.	• Rest • Sleep preparation • Sleep participation
Education	Activities necessary for learning and participating in an educational environment.	• Formal educational participation • Exploration of personal educational needs or interests • Informal educational participation

(continued)

Table 6-1 (continued)

AREAS OF OCCUPATION

AREA OF OCCUPATION	DESCRIPTION	EXAMPLES
Work	Activities related to seeking and carrying out paid employment or volunteer activities.	• Employment interests and pursuits • Employment seeking and acquisition • Job performance and maintenance • Retirement preparation and adjustment • Volunteer exploration • Volunteer participation
Play	Activities that are intrinsically motivated and provide enjoyment, entertainment, humor, or suspension of reality; may be spontaneous or organized; shaped by sociocultural context.	• Play exploration (includes identifying and selecting games with rules as well as exploratory, constructive, pretend, and symbolic play) • Participation in desired play activities
Leisure	Intrinsically rewarding activities that are engaged in when an individual is not obligated to perform other occupations.	• Leisure exploration (including identification of interests, opportunities, and required skills) • Leisure participation (including maintaining an appropriate balance with other occupations)
Social Participation	Interactions that support social interdependence with others in home, community, and virtual settings.	• Community participation • Family participation • Friendships • Intimate partner relationships • Peer group participation

Data source: American Occupational Therapy Association, 2020.

activities of daily living (ADLs) and instrumental activities of daily living (IADLs) to help get the client back to living as independently as possible (AOTA, 2015; Finni & Karr, 2022). What does the client need to be able to do to return home, with or without caregiver assistance, depending on the specific situation? For Workers' Compensation cases, problem statements and goals should focus on work (Stephenson, 2021). Which requirements or work tasks must the client demonstrate to return to work safely at partial or full capacity? In school-based therapy, occupational therapy problems and goals need to be educationally relevant (AOTA, 2016; Gerber, 2019; Millacci, 2021). Which skills and behaviors does the student need to demonstrate in the classroom and other school contexts to be successful?

CONTRIBUTING FACTORS

The second part of the problem statement identifies the contributing factors that limit engagement in the desired occupation. Table 6-2, although not all inclusive, lists several potential contributing factors. The *OTPF-4* (AOTA, 2020) is an excellent resource for identifying contributing factors relevant to occupational performance. The various aspects that comprise occupational therapy's domain are all viewed as having equal value and "together interact to affect occupational identity, health, well-being, and participation in life" (AOTA, 2020, p. 6). While there may be multiple contributing factors to a limitation in occupational performance, **your documentation should focus on those factors that can be addressed through occupational therapy intervention.**

Table 6-2

POTENTIAL CONTRIBUTING FACTORS

POTENTIAL CONTRIBUTING FACTORS	DESCRIPTION	EXAMPLES

Contexts	Environmental and personal factors that influence how individuals, groups, and populations live and perform occupations.	• *Environmental Factors*:
		  ◦ Natural environment and human-made changes to environments
		  ◦ Products and technology used in areas of occupation
		  ◦ Support and relationships (including people and animals)
		  ◦ Attitudes of individuals and society
		  ◦ Services, systems, and policies that affect persons, groups, and populations
		• *Personal Factors*:
		  ◦ Age
		  ◦ Sexual orientation
		  ◦ Gender identity
		  ◦ Race and ethnicity
		  ◦ Cultural identification and attitudes
		  ◦ Social background, social status, and socioeconomic status
		  ◦ Upbringing and life experiences
		  ◦ Habits and behavioral patterns (past and present)
		  ◦ Individual psychological aspects
		  ◦ Education
		  ◦ Profession and professional identity
		  ◦ Lifestyle
		  ◦ Other health conditions and fitness

Performance Patterns	"… the acquired habits, routines, roles, and rituals used in the process of engaging consistently in occupations and can support or hinder occupational performance …" (AOTA, 2020, p. 12)	• *Habits*: Smoking, frequency of exercise, repetitive rocking in response to stress • *Routines*: Established sequences such as morning routine for dressing and grooming or workers attending weekly meetings • *Roles*: Occupational identity of a person, group, or population such as parent, student, community volunteer, retired or disabled veteran, civic or humanitarian group member, or member of the deaf community • *Rituals*: Symbolic actions related to spiritual, cultural, or social meaning such as holiday meal preparation, groups singing a national anthem at events, or populations observing national holidays

(continued)

Table 6-2 (continued)

POTENTIAL CONTRIBUTING FACTORS

POTENTIAL CONTRIBUTING FACTORS	DESCRIPTION	EXAMPLES
Performance Skills	"… observable goal-directed actions that result in a client's quality of performing desired occupations. Skills are supported by the context in which the performance occurs …" (AOTA, 2020, p. 43)	• *Motor Skills*: Positioning, bending, reaching, grasping, manipulating, coordinating, moving, lifting, or transporting • *Process Skills*: Pacing (appropriate tempo), attending, choosing, using, initiating, sequencing, gathering, locating, organizing, navigating, noticing, adjusting • *Social Interaction Skills*: Initiating interaction, gesturing, speaking fluently, looking, transitioning, expressing emotion, acknowledging, taking turns, touching

Client Factors	"… specific capacities, characteristics, or beliefs that reside within a person, group, or population … Client factors are affected by the presence or absence of illness, disease, deprivation, and disability, as well as by life stages and experiences" (AOTA, 2020, p. 15)	• Values, Beliefs, and Spirituality: What is considered good and important, opinions, what is considered to be true, experiences of meaning and reflection
		• Body Functions:
		  ◦ *Mental*: Attention, memory, emotion, sequencing, orientation, temperament, personality, energy
		  ◦ *Sensory*: Visual, hearing, vestibular, taste, smell, proprioceptive, tactile, interoception, pain, sensitivity to pressure and temperature
		  ◦ *Neuromusculoskeletal and movement related*: Joint mobility and stability, range of motion, strength, muscle tone, reflexes, postural reactions, control of voluntary movement, mobility patterns
		  ◦ *Cardiovascular, hematological, immune, and respiratory*: Blood pressure, heart rate, immune response to infection, respiration rate, endurance, fatigability
		  ◦ *Voice and speech, digestive, metabolic, endocrine, genitourinary, and reproductive*: Speech fluency and rhythm, constipation or diarrhea, bowel or bladder incontinence, impotence
		  ◦ *Skin and related structures*: Presence or absence of hair, presence or absence of cuts, presence or absence of wounds and ability of the body to heal them
		• Body Structures:
		  ◦ Nervous system
		  ◦ Eyes and ears
		  ◦ Structures for voice and speech
		  ◦ Structures for cardiovascular, immunological, respiratory, digestive, metabolic, endocrine, genitourinary, and reproductive systems
		  ◦ Structures related to movement

Data source: American Occupational Therapy Association, 2020.

WRITING PROBLEM STATEMENTS

> Note: In this manual, the terms *client, patient, student, child, infant, consumer, resident, individual, veteran,* and first names or initials have been used to reflect the terms used in various practice settings. Names have been fabricated to protect the confidentiality of those people who receive our services. If a note says, "Mr. P participated in an occupational therapy evaluation in his home …," please understand that he is being called "Mr. P" for purposes of confidentiality. In your documentation, please use the term or format that is considered most respectful in your setting.

As occupational therapy practitioners, we recognize that a client's sense of well-being depends partly on the ability to participate in the life roles desired in home, work, school, community, and other settings. To gather information about the client, we develop an occupational profile of the client and conduct an analysis of occupational performance (AOTA, 2020). Through these various evaluation procedures, we identify the areas of occupation affected by a client's condition and the factors contributing to the functional limitation. Whenever possible, we also specify the extent to which occupational performance is limited. **It is important to note that the client's diagnosis is <u>not</u> the contributing factor.** The contributing factors may be a result of the diagnosis, which is listed in other parts of your evaluation or the client's chart, but it is our responsibility to identify the specific factors that contribute to occupational limitations. To summarize, you need to identify the following when writing an occupation-based problem statement:

- **Area of occupation** that is affected, with level of assist if it is known
- **Contributing factor/s** to be addressed in occupational therapy, with measurement if applicable

---

Here is a simple formula for writing an occupation-based problem statement:

_____ results in (or limits) _____ .
      Contributing factor/s   **area of occupation affected**

You will encounter other formats for problem statements in various settings. In this textbook, only this format will be presented because it flows easily into writing the "A" (Assessment) portion of a SOAP note.

Let's take a look at an example of an occupation-based problem statement using this formula:

<u>Decreased B UE AROM</u> limits independence in <u>upper body dressing</u>.
Contributing Factor   **Area of Occupation**

This statement has the two essential elements of the **area of occupation** and a **contributing factor**, but more specific measurable information would be helpful in documenting progress toward goals. Based on the problem statement listed previously, you will not be able to show any increase in function until the client demonstrates full active range of motion (AROM) and is independent in dressing. Rather than saying that the client is **unable to perform** a given activity independently, it is better to state the assist level needed, if it is known. It is also helpful to provide more detailed information about which joint is limited and to what extent. For example:

<u>Limited B shoulder flexion AROM to ½ range results</u> in need for <u>max A with upper body dressing</u>.
Measurable Contributing Factor   **Area of Occupation (with assist level)**

Now we have more information to help us write measurable goals and document progress. Ideally, we can document a decrease in the assist level needed for the area of occupation. However, we may also be documenting measurable changes to contributing factors resulting from occupational therapy intervention. For example:

<u>Limited B shoulder flexion AROM to ¾ range results</u> in need for <u>min A with upper body dressing</u>.
Measurable Contributing Factor   **Area of Occupation (with assist level)**

In this case the client still has a functional limitation, but an insurance reviewer who is examining this client's case would be able to see a change both in the contributing factor and in the assist level needed for occupational performance when comparing the baseline problem statement to the second problem statement several sessions later.

> If you are unfamiliar with the terminology used to describe levels of assistance in occupational therapy documentation, please refer to Table 7-2 in Chapter 7.

In some cases, rather than an assist level, you can make the area of occupation in your problem statement measurable by specifying an amount of time needed for the performance of a specific occupation. For example:

> *Pain level of 5/10 with finger flexion* limits child's *ability to hold a pencil for more than 3 minutes*.
> **Measurable Contributing Factor**   **Area of Occupation (with time factor)**

In other cases, the contributing factor does not have a specific measurement, but we can still provide information about the assist level or time frame needed for occupational performance. Here are some examples:

- *High tone in R UE results in child's need for mod A to cut with scissors during art activities.*
- *Trunk instability results in veteran's need for min A to complete toilet transfer.*
- *Decreased sequencing and motor planning results in need for max verbal cues for consumer to complete a 3-step lunch preparation.*
- *Lack of stress management skills results in client's inability to sustain employment more than 2 weeks.*

In rare situations, an assist level or time frame is not applicable to the occupational performance. Rather, it is simply a "can" or "cannot" activity. For example:

> *Motor planning deficits result in child's inability to complete jumping jacks during gym class.*

She is not dependent for jumping jacks, and she does not need extra time to do jumping jacks. She just cannot do them with any level of assistance or amount of time.

Although we want to provide as much information about the occupational performance deficit as possible, **we can only provide a specific assist level if we have observed it**. Suppose you are on a fieldwork rotation, and you complete an initial evaluation of a client in ICU who has had a stroke. During the evaluation session, you assist the client from the bed to the bedside commode with max A. You identify L side hemiparesis and L side neglect as contributing factors. You can write the following problem statement:

> *L side hemiparesis and L side neglect result in need for max A for BSC transfer.*

Now, assume your fieldwork educator asks you to write two more functional problem statements based on the contributing factors you identified in your first session. You can use your clinical judgment to make some assumptions about limited occupational performance in other areas, but **you cannot specify a level of assist in the problem statement if you did not observe the client performing that area of occupation yet**. Instead, you can use phrases such as "results in decreased independence with" or "limits safety with." Here are some examples for this scenario:

- *L side neglect limits patient's ability to locate dressing items placed in the left visual field.*
- *L side hemiparesis results in decreased independence with lower body dressing.*

Using our clinical judgment, we know that if the client had difficulty locating the commode in his left visual field, then he will have difficulty locating items in his left visual field in other areas of occupation, but **we do not know exactly how much assistance he will need for those other activities because we have not yet observed them**. We also know that if the patient's L side weakness was severe enough that he needed max A for a commode transfer, then he will need assistance with other areas of occupation requiring similar performance skills, but **we cannot state exactly how much assistance he needs because we have not yet observed those activities**.

You may combine multiple contributing factors into one problem statement if they are all related to the same area of occupation. For example:

- *Trunk ataxia and diplopia limit client's ability to perform grooming tasks while standing at the sink.*
- *Post-surgical shoulder precautions, immobilization brace, and pain 8/10 result in need for maximal caregiver assistance for upper body dressing.*
- *Poor trunk control and limited R UE grasp patterns limit child's ability to feed self with utensils.*
- *Sensory seeking behaviors and inability to maintain attention for more than 3 minutes limit child's success in classroom circle time participation.*

EXAMPLES OF FUNCTIONAL PROBLEM STATEMENTS

When formulating problem statements, be sure that the problem identified is one that will respond to occupational therapy intervention. There is no need to identify problems that you do not intend to address. As previously stated, you also need to focus on problems for which treatment is considered necessary and reimbursable by the funding source.

Activities of Daily Living (ADLs)

- *Poor task initiation and sequencing result in client's need for max verbal cues during dressing activity.*
- *3+ B UE strength results in need for mod A to don pants.*
- *Post-surgical back precautions limit client's ability to perform posterior hygiene after toileting.*
- *Attention span of < 3 minutes results in need for mod verbal and tactile cues during grooming tasks.*
- *Halo brace and limited B UE AROM following SCI limit Abby's ability to drink from a standard cup.*
- *Severe shortness of breath limits David's ability to perform more than 10 minutes of ADL participation.*
- *Low toilet, B LE weakness, and decreased balance result in need for 2-person assist with toileting.*
- *5 out of 10 R elbow pain results in veteran needing max A to comb hair.*
- *Poor motor planning results in need for hand-over-hand assist to keep food on fork during feeding.*
- *Oral tactile defensiveness results in limited variety of food intake during snacks and meals.*
- *Low vision results in need for min A for dressing activities.*
- *Poor balance and lack of adaptive equipment results in decreased safety and independence while bathing.*
- *Pronator spasticity limiting R forearm supination to ½ range results in Tamaya's need for mod A for upper body hygiene.*
- *Decreased strength in trunk and UEs results in resident needing max A for dressing EOB.*
- *Asymmetrical positioning in w/c limits child's ability to feed self.*

Instrumental Activities of Daily Living (IADLs)

- *Impaired short-term memory results in safety concerns with client's care of her two young children.*
- *Decreased B grasp strength and hand sensation limit Ashlyn's ability to manipulate infant's clothing during diaper tasks.*
- *Inability to recognize fatigue when standing results in decreased safety with laundry tasks.*
- *Decreased balance results in client being unable to carry 20-lb buckets to feed his outdoor hobby farm animals.*
- *Inability to count money limits client's ability to make independent purchases in the community.*
- *Limited grasp following C6 SCI results in need for another person to apply collar and vest to client's service dog.*
- *Decreased dominant R hand strength and decreased bilateral coordination result in Macy's inability to answer cell phone calls in a timely manner.*
- *Impaired judgment and sequencing result in need for max verbal cues during meal preparation.*
- *Focused attention on auditory hallucinations makes consumer unsafe to live alone.*
- *Impaired R UE sensation results in need for mod verbal cues for safety during cooking tasks.*
- *Cluttered kitchen, decreased balance, and visual perceptual deficits limit client's ability to safely locate and transport items during snack preparation.*
- *Impaired organizational skills and impulsive behaviors limit Alayna's independence with monthly budgeting.*
- *Lifting and bending restrictions due to post-surgical back precautions result in client being unable to complete laundry tasks.*
- *Decreased finger isolation inhibits client's ability to use a computer for online bill paying.*
- *Decreased memory and problem solving result in resident being unable to locate emergency fire exit.*
- *Impaired sequencing and problem solving result in need for max verbal cues to navigate city bus route to doctor's office.*

- *Decreased balance results in safety concerns getting up and down from prayer rug.*
- *Decreased memory and safety awareness results in Malik frequently forgetting to lock apartment when leaving for work or other community outings.*
- *Decreased fine motor skills limit client's ability to retrieve money or credit cards from wallet when making purchases.*
- *Impaired cognitive and visual perceptual skills limit client's ability to use cell phone to arrange ride share service for community outings.*

Health Management

- *Limited B UE function from C5 SCI results in dependence on caregiver to empty catheter bag.*
- *Decreased task initiation and memory deficits result in client inconsistently taking daily medications.*
- *Pain and post-surgical back precautions limit Felipe's ability to complete established home workout routine.*
- *Decreased dominant L hand coordination limits client's ability to manage glucometer.*
- *Decreased problem solving skills from TBI result in parent's inability to determine correct dose of insulin to manage child's type 1 diabetes.*
- *Impulsive behaviors and limited organization skills limit consumer's ability to make healthy food selections when grocery shopping.*
- *Decreased sensation of dominant R hand limits teen's ability to place contact lenses in eyes.*
- *Decreased executive function skills limit client's ability to manage health care appointments.*
- *Impaired memory skills limit client's understanding of purpose of medications.*
- *Decreased B hand strength limits client's ability to don and doff L LE prosthesis.*

Rest and Sleep

- *Auditory hallucinations result in Marcus obtaining < 3 hours sleep nightly.*
- *Decreased organizational skills result in Madison often forgetting to set cell phone alarm on school nights.*
- *Impaired judgment results in resident not calling for assistance when needing to use commode during the night.*
- *Impaired sensation and strength of B hands from multiple sclerosis result in Minah's need for mod A to manage bed linens in preparation for sleep.*
- *Impaired balance and decreased B UE strength limit mother's ability to pick up and position infant for nighttime breastfeeding.*
- *Decreased sequencing and memory limit client's ability to complete all steps of setting up overnight peritoneal dialysis.*

Education

- *Impaired sequencing and problem-solving skills result in Treyvon's need for step-by-step verbal cues to obtain lunch tray and pay attendant.*
- *Lack of familiarity with public transportation options limits Ava's ability to attend GED classes at local community center.*
- *Sensory-seeking behaviors and decreased attention result in Mateo's inability to complete classroom assignments in a timely manner.*
- *Slow handwriting speed related to juvenile idiopathic arthritis results in Yosef's inability to keep up with notetaking during college lectures.*
- *Bilateral incoordination results in Aaliyah's need for mod A to complete an art assignment requiring the use of a ruler.*
- *Tactile defensiveness results in Beckett's inability to tolerate unexpected touch from peers during circle time.*
- *Decreased balance and limited B UE strength limit Varun's ability to safely access playground equipment during school recess.*

Work

- *Preference for clothing with rips, tears, and offensive slogans limits Andrew's ability to find employment.*
- *Grip strength of 3# in R hand results in client's inability to perform carpentry work.*
- *Pain level of 7/10 with dominant L hand finger flexion results in decreased ability to grasp and hold tools required for job as landscaper.*
- *< 60° AROM in R shoulder abduction limits client's ability to perform work tasks.*
- *Daily methamphetamine use results in Josiah's inability to hold a job.*
- *Inattention to personal hygiene interferes with consumer's ability to find employment.*
- *Decreased vision limits Sofia's ability to complete online job applications without assistance.*
- *Impaired endurance from COPD results in client's inability to complete volunteer activities at hospital gift shop.*
- *Decreased sequencing and problem-solving skills limit client's ability to safely utilize farm equipment.*
- *Inability to accept constructive criticism limits Julian's success during job skills training.*

> Depending on the practice setting, funding sources may not consider problem statements and goals for play, leisure, and social participation medically necessary. However, examples are provided here to cover all areas of occupation identified in the *OTPF-4* (AOTA, 2020).

Play

- *Preoccupation with aligning objects limits Oliver's pretend play interactions with preschool classmates.*
- *Sensory processing deficits limit Jada's ability to engage in age-appropriate play activities with preschool peers.*
- *Limited attention span and decreased bilateral coordination limit teen's ability to participate in online gaming.*
- *Inattention to R side of body results in need for max verbal and tactile cues to transfer toys from one hand to the other.*
- *Impulsive behaviors result in teen's need for mod verbal cues for turn taking during group board games.*
- *Decreased fine motor skills limit Anika's ability to don dress-up clothes with peers during pretend play.*

Leisure

- *Impaired coordination of R hand results in resident's inability to complete needlework.*
- *Impaired problem-solving skills limit consumer's ability to utilize public transportation to attend weekly bowling league.*
- *Limited grasp patterns with dominant R hand limit Lorraine's ability to complete word puzzles.*
- *Decreased fine motor skills result in client's need for mod A to manage camera functions when taking pictures.*
- *Impaired figure ground and visual tracking skills limit Emma's ability to keep her place when reading novels.*
- *Decreased B UE strength and coordination limit Isabella's ability to participate in crafting activities with siblings.*

Social Participation

- *Belief in government conspiracy limits consumer's willingness to participate in social activities in the community.*
- *Anxiety in crowds limits Jose's willingness to leave home for participation in social events.*
- *Individual's aggressive behavior results in limited success in establishing and maintaining social relationships.*
- *Drug-seeking and drug-using behaviors limit client's social participation in non–drug-related activities.*
- *Progressive oral motor weakness resulting from muscular dystrophy limits Maddox's ability to communicate with peers orally.* (Please note that while communication skills are addressed by our speech-language colleagues, occupational therapy practitioners may also be involved in augmentative and alternative communication [AAC] evaluations to determine how the client will access the communication device.)

REFERENCES

American Occupational Therapy Association. (2015). *AOTA fact sheet: Occupational therapy's role in skilled nursing facilities.* https://www.aota.org/

American Occupational Therapy Association. (2016). *AOTA fact sheet: Occupational therapy's role in school settings.* https://www.aota.org/

American Occupational Therapy Association. (2020). Occupational therapy practice framework: Domain and process (4th ed.). *American Journal of Occupational Therapy, 74*(Suppl. 2), 7412410010. https://doi.org/10.5014/ajot.2020.74S2001

Amini, D. (2016). *AOTA documentation series—Module 2: Occupation-based goal writing for OT practice* [Online continuing educational module]. American Occupational Therapy Association. https://www.aota.org/

Cahill, S. (2021). *Research update on telehealth: Client outcomes and satisfaction, occupation-based coaching, and stroke rehabilitation.* American Occupational Therapy Association. https://www.aota.org/

Finni, B., & Karr, K. (2022). *"Audit-proof" your documentation: Capturing the "skill" of value-based occupational therapy in SNF and long-term care facilities* [Conference presentation]. AOTA Inspire 2022 Annual Conference & Expo, San Antonio, TX, April 2, 2022.

Gerber, H. (2019). *School occupational therapy goals to consider.* Sunbelt. https://www.sunbeltstaffing.com/

Millacci, T. S. (2021, June 26). *School-based occupational therapy and its goals explained.* PositivePsychology.com. https://positivepsychology.com/school-occupational-therapy/

Moll, C. M., Billick, M. N., & Valdes, K. (2018). Parent satisfaction of occupational therapy interventions for pediatrics. *Pediatrics & Therapeutics, 8*(1), 1-8.

Rose, C. (2021, June 29). *What to expect when you are—or aren't—expecting occupational therapy.* https://www.foxrehab.org/what-is-occupational-therapy/

Saito, Y., Tomori, K., Nagayama, H., Sawadai, T., & Kikuchi, E. (2019). Differences in the occupational therapy goals of clients and therapists affect the outcomes of patients in subacute rehabilitation wards: A case-control study. *Journal of Physical Therapy Science, 31*(7), 521-525. https://doi.org/10.1589/jpts.31.521

Stephenson, B. (2021). *Benefits of occupational therapy for worker's comp injuries.* https://rehabselect.net/

Suc, L., Svalgeer, A., & Bratun, U. (2020). Goal setting among experienced and novice occupational therapists in a rehabilitation center. *Canadian Journal of Occupational Therapy, 87*(4), 287-297. https://doi.org/10.1177/0008417420941979

WORKSHEET **6-1**

Identifying the Contributing Factors

Complete each of the following functional problem statements with at least three possible contributing factors. (Hint: It may be helpful to refer to Table 6-2 for potential contributing factors.)

1. **Area of Occupation = Work**

*   _____ *results in consumer's inability to sustain employment longer than 2 weeks.*

*   _____ *results in consumer's inability to sustain employment longer than 2 weeks.*

*   _____ *results in consumer's inability to sustain employment longer than 2 weeks.*

2. **Area of Occupation = ADLs**

*   _____ *results in veteran needing 90 minutes to complete grooming tasks.*

*   _____ *results in veteran needing 90 minutes to complete grooming tasks.*

*   _____ *results in veteran needing 90 minutes to complete grooming tasks.*

3. **Area of Occupation = Education**

*   _____ *limits Avery's ability to complete grade-appropriate written worksheets.*

*   _____ *limits Avery's ability to complete grade-appropriate written worksheets.*

*   _____ *limits Avery's ability to complete grade-appropriate written worksheets.*

WORKSHEET 6-2
Writing Occupation-Based Problem Statements

Use the following descriptions to write occupation-based problem statements for each client. Make them specific enough to:
- Show the area of occupation that is a concern
- Show the contributing factor/s that affect this area of occupation
- Serve as a baseline against which to measure progress

Use the formula provided in this chapter for writing the functional problem statements.

1. *The client has an acquired injury to his brain. As a result, he is not able to pay attention to task for very long at a time, and he is having trouble completing his morning routine. Typically, he can pay attention to what he is doing for about 2 minutes and needs to be redirected back to the task after that.*

2. *Jerrica is having trouble in school because she has difficulty staying within the lines when she is writing. She habitually grips her pencil in a gross grasp, although with help (someone's hand placed over hers) she can hold it with her thumb and two fingers.*

3. *The resident is not very cognitively aware. About 40% of the time, she has trouble figuring out what to do first if she has to complete a self-care task, and she doesn't remember what she has just been told.*

4. *Mr. J has recently sustained a R CVA. His L arm is flaccid, and he forgets that it is there. He needs physical and verbal help with ADL tasks about 60% of the time.*

5. *The consumer has had trouble finding a job. His appearance is unkempt, and he has a strong body odor, neither of which seem troubling to him.*

6. *The client is unable to transfer safely w/c to/from toilet without someone to remind him that he needs to follow his total hip precautions.*

WORKSHEET 6-3

Revising Problem Statements

Consider the following problem statements. Decide what is needed to make each one better, and then rewrite the sentences into a better format.

1. *Trunk instability results in inability to complete LE dressing independently.*

2. *Decreased activity tolerance results in child not tolerating much classroom activity.*

3. *Consumer acts out.*

Chapter 7

Writing Measurable Occupation-Based Goals and Objectives

Goals and objectives used in a treatment plan must be written in occupation-based, measurable, observable, action-oriented terms. They must also be realistic for the client and achievable in a reasonable amount of time within the client's current practice setting. Goals are formulated from the problem list compiled in collaboration with the client. For successful intervention, it is critical to work on goals that are important to the client. Occupational therapy practitioners have a responsibility to include clients in discussions regarding the goals and interventions that will direct their care (Cahill, 2021; Moll et al., 2018; Saito et al., 2019; Suc et al., 2020).

Occupational therapy goals must focus on **functional improvements in occupational performance**. The client factors that contribute to such progress, such as strength and range of motion, are much less important to a third-party payer than **what the client can actually do**, even though the gains in those contributing factors may be essential to achieving the functional outcomes.

Lamb (2014) emphasized the importance of "demonstrating the distinct value of occupational therapy through documentation" and encouraged practitioners to "approach documentation as an ethical and fiscal responsibility, as a marketing tool, and as a means of obtaining data for current and future research projects" (pp. 1, 5). Over the past few decades, the occupational therapy profession, along with all health care professions, has experienced a demand for **evidence-based practice**, which involves combining the best available research, clinical expertise, and client preferences to make informed decisions about evaluation and intervention to address clients' needs and goals (Dang et al., 2022; Juckett, 2022; Skaletski, 2021). More recently, health care leaders have focused on knowledge translation, "a broad term often used to describe the process of integrating research findings into routine practice" (Juckett, 2022, para. 1). Occupational therapists combine scientific research evidence with information gathered through interviews and observations of clients and use their clinical expertise to identify problem statements and goals that serve as a baseline of functional performance and a way to measure progress with skilled occupational therapy intervention. Documentation "provides justification for the services provided to the client and allows the third-party payer to know what and why they are paying for the essential therapy service" (American Occupational Therapy Association [AOTA], 2021, p. 1).

GOALS

Goals in an intervention plan are also called *long-term goals* (LTGs) or *outcomes*. These are usually discharge goals—what the client hopes to accomplish by the time of discharge from occupational therapy services in the current setting (Sames, 2015). For each problem you have identified, you will have at least one LTG, and often more than one.

Gateley, C. A. *Documentation Manual for Occupational Therapy, Fifth Edition* (pp. 77-99). © 2024 Taylor & Francis Group.

Figure 7-1. Steps to the ultimate LTG.

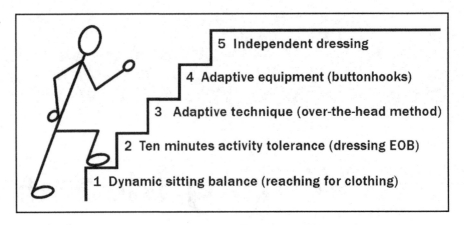

5 Independent dressing

4 Adaptive equipment (buttonhooks)

3 Adaptive technique (over-the-head method)

2 Ten minutes activity tolerance (dressing EOB)

1 Dynamic sitting balance (reaching for clothing)

OBJECTIVES

Objectives are also called *short-term goals* (STGs). These are goals that are met in smaller increments while progressing toward the discharge goals.

For example, if your LTG is:

Client will complete 3-step stove top meal preparation independently using walker within 1 week.

then one of your STGs might be:

Client will retrieve and transport items from refrigerator to stove using walker and wheeled cart with CGA within 3 days.

If your LTG is:

Client will move 35# objects needed for work from table to counter without increase in pain by discharge in 2 weeks.

then one of your STGs might be:

Client will be able to lift 10# objects needed for work without increase in pain within 1 week.

You may have several STGs (objectives) for each LTG. For example, suppose you are treating Mr. Hawkins, a 45-year-old executive who sustained a right CVA a few days ago and now demonstrates left hemiplegia. On evaluation, you find that he is oriented x 4, verbal, intelligent, able to learn, and has a supportive wife. After talking with him about what he would like to achieve in occupational therapy, you and he decide upon a goal of independence in upper body dressing with adaptive equipment and adaptive techniques. You believe that this is a realistic goal, if he receives skilled instruction in adaptive strategies and the necessary adaptive equipment. You set the following series of STGs:

1. Seated edge of bed, client will reach for and obtain clothing items at arm's length with CGA to maintain dynamic sitting balance by the end of the 3rd treatment session.

2. By the 6th treatment session, client will participate in dressing activities for > 10 minutes without rest break seated EOB with CGA.

3. After skilled instruction, client will don shirt seated EOB using one-handed techniques with min verbal cues by the 8th treatment session.

4. Client will be able to button shirt using a button hook with 2 or fewer verbal cues by 10th treatment session.

5. Client will complete all upper body dressing tasks independently using adaptive equipment and one-handed techniques seated EOB by discharge in 2 weeks.

As you can see, each of these STGs is measurable, observable, and action-oriented. The first four STGs are steps to the ultimate LTG (Figure 7-1).

An intervention plan is always a work in progress. Unexpected events and conditions affect the progress your client will be able to make toward their goals. If you determine that a goal you originally set is now unrealistic for your client, you need to modify it. It is not useful to continue with a plan that is not working. For example, suppose the client described above begins to have some motor function return in his involved L UE. You now know that he may be able to dress his upper body without adaptive techniques or equipment, and he wants very much to do that. You would need to write a new set of STGs for him.

Table 7-1

EXAMPLES OF GOAL FORMATS ACROSS HEALTH PROFESSIONS

A	Actor	S	Specific
B	Behavior	M	Measurable
C	Conditions	A	Achievable
D	Degree	R	Relevant (or Realistic)
E	Expected Time	T	Timebound
R	Relevant	T	Time Frame
U	Understandable	I	Individual
M	Measurable	C	Change Expected
B	Behavioral	K	Key Issues
A	Achievable	S	Supports

Data sources: Parkinson & Brooks, 2021; Quinn & Gordon, 2016.

GOAL WRITING IN THE HEALTH PROFESSIONS

There are several formats for goal writing, along with acronyms to remember each component (Table 7-1). You may encounter any of these formats in a client's health record, and you may be expected to use any of these formats in your fieldwork or practice setting. As you can see, each format involves a combination of some, or all, of the following components:

- Who
- What
- Where/How
- Amount of Assistance
- When

OCCUPATIONAL THERAPY GOAL WRITING: THE COAST METHOD

Although any of the above goal formats are acceptable, in this manual I advocate the use of a format I first introduced in the third edition this textbook (Gateley & Borcherding, 2012): the COAST method. The COAST method was designed around the premise that occupational therapy is both client-centered and occupation-based (AOTA, 2020). The COAST method is now widely accepted across the occupational therapy profession as an effective way to ensure that all essential elements are present in client goals and that goals are **focused on occupation** (Amini, 2016; Chamberlain, 2022; Fusion Web Clinic, 2022; The OT Minute, 2021; The OT Toolbox, 2021). Here are the components of a COAST goal:

- C—Client   Client will …
- O—Occupation   Perform which occupation?
- A—Assist Level   With how much assistance/independence?
- S—Specific Conditions Under what conditions?
- T—Timeline   By when?

There has been considerable debate about the concepts of *occupation, activity,* and *task,* with definitions varying between conceptual models and frames of reference (Cole & Tufano, 2020). It is not within the scope of this textbook to engage in that debate. For purposes of this textbook, you can assume that the "O" in the COAST goal acronym encompasses any activity or task that is related to the performance of an area of occupation as defined in the *Occupational Therapy Practice Framework: Domain and Process, Fourth Edition (OTPF-4;* AOTA, 2020). You can refer to Table 9-1 regarding how *occupation* and *activity* are differentiated in the *OTPF-4* in terms of intervention types.

To write goals and objectives in a way that can be measured, the elements to be included are very specific. Let's take a closer look at each category.

C—Client

In writing treatment goals, the **client** is the key player. Goals should be written in terms of what the client will do, not what the therapist will do (Sames, 2015). The therapist's actions are documented later, under intervention strategies. As discussed in Chapter 5, use the term that is considered most appropriate for your setting. Examples include *client, patient, student, child, infant, resident, individual,* or *veteran,* just to name a few. You may also use the client's name or initials. For example:

- *Client will ...*
- *Child will ...*
- *Mrs. G will ...*

O—Occupation

This component of a COAST goal involves the specific **occupation**, or component thereof, that you want the client to demonstrate. The "O" of your goal statement should relate to one of the problem statements that you already established. Improving an individual's ability to engage in occupation is the core of occupational therapy practice. It is the first thing you think of in writing goals. The "O" should be the essential focus of the goal statement. You may need to insert an action verb here to accompany the occupation, such as *perform* or *complete.* For example:

- *Client will <u>perform a 3-step cooking process</u> ...*
- *Mrs. G will <u>complete upper body dressing</u> ...*
  In other cases, the "O" already involves an action verb such as retrieve, cut, don, or participate. For example:
- *Patient will <u>retrieve clothing items from closet</u> ...*
- *Child will <u>cut out a 4" diameter circle</u> ...*
- *Veteran will <u>don L UE prosthesis</u> ...*
- *Aiden will <u>participate in circle time</u> ...*
  A word of caution—**whenever you find yourself writing "will demonstrate the ability to," ask yourself if there is a more concise way to phrase the "O."** For example, rather than say:
  Client will <u>demonstrate the ability to put on socks</u> ...
  simply say:
  Client will <u>don socks</u> ...
  In another example, rather than say:
  Sherry will <u>demonstrate the ability to place shirt on hanger</u> ...
  simply say:
  Sherry will <u>place shirt on hanger</u> ...
  Let's also discuss what should **not** be the "O" of your goal. To reiterate a statement from earlier in this chapter, third-party payers are more interested in **what a client can do** because of your occupational therapy intervention than they are in changes in client factors such as increased strength, improved range of motion, or decreased pain. Those changes certainly will be documented in the Objective portion of your SOAP note, but your **goals should**

focus on something the client will be able to do because of increased range of motion or decreased pain. I understand that you will encounter goals focused on biomechanical client factors in some practice settings, particularly hand therapy clinics. However, as students or new practitioners learning to write goals, I challenge you to remain focused on occupation.

A—Assist Level

This is where you specify the **level of assistance** expected, which ultimately translates into the level of independence that the client is expected to demonstrate. This should include the physical and/or verbal cues that will be required for the client to complete the activity. See Table 7-2 for a list of commonly accepted assistance levels in therapy and their respective abbreviations and description.

Table 7-2

LEVELS OF ASSISTANCE

ASSIST LEVEL	ABBREVIATION	DESCRIPTION
Independent	I	Client completes activity **without any assistance from caregiver**, whether or not equipment, adaptive strategies, or extra time were required.
Set-Up	No abbreviation	Client requires **only set-up and/or clean-up** assistance, but caregiver does not need to be present during completion of the activity.
Supervision	No abbreviation	Client requires caregiver to be **present in same room** and ready to provide verbal cues if necessary, but **physical assistance is not anticipated**.
Standby Assistance	SBA	Caregiver needs to be right next to the client for duration of activity due to potential need for physical assistance, consistent verbal cueing, or other safety concerns. **Physical assistance is not provided** at this level.
Contact Guard Assistance	CGA	Client is putting forth full physical effort, but caregiver needs to have **hands on** the client or gait belt for steadying assistance.
Minimal Assistance	min A	Client performs **75% or more of the effort** for the activity, but caregiver is providing **more than just steadying assistance**.
Moderate Assistance	mod A	Client performs **50% to 74% of the effort** for the activity.
Maximal Assistance	max A	Client performs **25% to 49% of the effort** for the activity.
Dependent	D	Client performs **less than 25% of the effort** for the activity, or **two or more caregivers** are needed to provide assistance.

Data sources: AOTA, 2022a; OTDude, 2020; Stromsdorfer & Ferri, 2022.

Please note that all physical assistance levels from contact guard assistance to dependent assistance imply that verbal cues were also provided. There is no need to state, "with moderate assistance and verbal cues." However, when physical assistance is not provided nor anticipated, in other words when verbal cues are the primary form of assistance, it is helpful to specify the amount of verbal cues needed. Some practitioners use a similar scale for verbal cues as they do for physical assistance levels. For example, *min verbal cues* indicates that verbal cues were provided for approximately 25% of the task, *mod verbal cues* indicates that verbal cues were provided for approximately 50% of the task, and so on. Other practitioners prefer to specify the exact number of verbal cues in a goal. For example:

Client will perform a 3-step cooking process <u>with 2 or fewer verbal cues for sequencing and safety</u> …

This distinction really comes down to practitioner preference. For students learning how to write goals, I recommend you ask your professor or fieldwork educator what their preference is when including verbal cues in a goal. You may get different responses from different people who will be grading or critiquing your documentation, and you will need to adapt your documentation to those expectations. For new practitioners, I recommend you ask your colleagues what their standard practice is in that particular work setting.

As previously explained in Chapter 5, **this textbook does not include the use of the term modified independence (mod I) in sample goals or notes**. That assistance level was part of the old Functional Independence Measure (FIM) previously used by the Centers for Medicare & Medicaid Services (CMS) as a means of rating a patient's functional performance in post-acute settings. The new Section GG, currently used by CMS in post-acute settings, does not include modified independence as an assistance level (AOTA, 2022a), although you may still see the term used in practice or embedded in electronic documentation systems. With the new Section GG codes, patients are considered independent regardless of adaptive equipment, adaptive strategies, or extra time required for an activity. However, these extra supports may become part of the "S"—Specific Condition of your goal.

Be careful not to mix levels of assistance. This is a common mistake made by students when they are first learning to write goals. For example:

Client will perform a 3-step cooking process <u>independently with 2 or fewer verbal cues</u> …

Inherent in the definition of independence is that no verbal cues are required. You cannot use both levels of assistance in the same goal. Here are a few more examples of assistance levels:

- *Patient will retrieve clothing items from closet <u>with CGA for trunk balance</u> …*
- *Child will cut out a 4" diameter circle <u>with hand-over-hand assistance for bilateral coordination</u> …*
- *Veteran will don L UE prosthesis <u>with set-up</u> …*
- *Aiden will participate in circle time <u>with 2 or fewer verbal cues for redirection to task</u> …*

Note that in most of the examples above, I provide additional information about what the assist level is for. When you are writing goals and get to the assist level, always **ask yourself why the assistance is needed**. Min A for what? Min A to maintain grasp on utensil. Verbal cues for what? Verbal cues for sequencing. In rare cases, like the example above regarding set-up of the prosthesis, no additional information is needed.

One final word of caution when setting assist levels for your client's goals: **You should set assistance levels based on the client's expected level of performance at the time of discharge from the specific setting in which you are seeing the client**. If you are seeing the client in an acute care setting, and you anticipate the client will go to a skilled nursing facility (SNF) setting at discharge because she lives alone and is not expected to be independent within the next few days, do not set goals for the client to be independent. Set goals for her to be just one or two levels better than her current performance. For example, if she currently needs max A for lower body dressing after an elective hip surgery, and you know from chart review of social work notes that she will be discharging to a SNF in 1 to 2 days, it does not make sense to set goals for her to be independent. Instead, set the lower body dressing goal for her to be either at mod A or min A at discharge based on your clinical expertise. This helps support her need for continued therapy in the next setting. If you set the goal for her to be independent, you are communicating to the insurance company that you think she can meet that goal and will not need SNF, which could negatively impact her discharge planning process.

S—Specific Conditions

This is where you **specify any other conditions** under which the client is expected to perform the desired action such as location, adaptive equipment, or modified technique. Think of the specific condition as the **how, where, with what, or with whom** component of the goal. In my nearly 15 years of teaching documentation, students consistently have struggled most with the "S" part of COAST goals. I explain that **the "S" part of the goal <u>helps the reader picture</u> exactly where, how, and with what or with whom the client will be performing the occupation in question**. A student who forgets to include the "S" portion of the goal may simply write:

Client will complete grooming tasks with min A for B hand coordination ...

My questions back to the student go something like this: "Will she complete grooming while riding a unicycle down the street? Will she complete grooming while standing on her head in the living room? Will she complete grooming while hanging upside down from a trapeze bar?" These silly scenarios help the student understand how better to describe the specific condition:

- *Client will complete grooming tasks with min A for B hand coordination <u>seated in w/c at sink</u> ...*
- *Client will complete grooming tasks with min A for B hand coordination <u>while seated EOB</u> ...*
- *Client will complete grooming tasks with min A for B hand coordination <u>standing at sink with wheeled walker</u> ...*

Each of the examples above suggests varying levels of trunk control and gives the reader a very different picture of what the client is expected to do. The client needs more trunk control to maintain balance on the edge of the bed than when seated in a supportive wheelchair. The client needs even more trunk control and lower extremity function to stand at the sink for grooming tasks.

Here are a few more examples of how the specific condition significantly changes the expectation of the client's performance:

- *Client will perform a 3-step cooking process with 2 or fewer verbal cues for sequencing and safety <u>from w/c level in rehab kitchen</u> ...*
- *Client will perform a 3-step cooking process with 2 or fewer verbal cues for sequencing and safety <u>while navigating kitchen with a hemi-walker</u> ...*
- *Infant will reach for and grasp toys with affected R hand with min A to cross midline <u>while prone on floor</u> ...*
- *Infant will reach for and grasp toys with affected R hand with min A to cross midline <u>in tall kneeling position at couch</u> ...*
- *Norma will don button-up shirt with min A for R hand grasp <u>using button hook</u> ...*
- *Norma will don button-up shirt with min A to thread over R UE <u>while adhering to post-surgical shoulder precautions</u> ...*
- *Norma will don button-up shirt with min A for positioning clothing <u>utilizing one-handed dressing techniques</u> ...*
- *Hai will cut out a circle with min A <u>using adaptive scissors with 2 or fewer deviations from line</u> ...*
- *Hai will cut out a circle with min A <u>using standard scissors with no line deviations from line</u> ...*

The "A" and "S" together make your goal statement **measurable** and allow you to show your client's progress. Other examples include the following:

- *... by using a dressing stick with 2 or fewer verbal cues*
- *... using wheeled walker with CGA*
- *... with mod A using sliding board*
- *... 3 out of 4 attempts without verbal cues*
- *... independently from standing position*
- *... with weekly supervision for set-up of medication organizer*
- *... independently 3 out of 5 attempts during evening meal*
- *... with SBA using tub bench and long-handled sponge*
- *... during group sessions without use of profanity*
- *... seated EOB with CGA for balance*

In rare cases, it is acceptable to omit either the "A" or the "S," **but never both**. You may write a goal for a task that either can or cannot be done, and assistance would not be applicable. For example, suppose you have a client who presents with pain in her R CMC joint. She can complete most IADL tasks independently, but she reports pain during tasks such as opening doorknobs. Your LTG may look like this:

Client will open doorknobs using R hand without report of wrist pain within 2 weeks.

In this example, no assist level is mentioned, but "without report of wrist pain" makes this goal measurable. Another example:

Client will complete all dressing tasks I by discharge.

In this example, the assistance level (or in this case the lack of assistance level) is stated, but there are no other specific conditions that are necessary for this goal.

T—Timeline

> Please note that in many of the examples throughout this book, when specific dates are used, the examples provide only a month and day. However, if you use this method in your practice setting, **you should also provide the year**, such as *by 3-25-24*.

This is the time frame within which the goal is expected to be accomplished. For a LTG, this may be the anticipated discharge date.

For example:

- *Client will perform a 3-step cooking process with 2 or fewer verbal cues for sequencing and safety from w/c level in rehab kitchen by March 20th.*
- *Client will perform a 3-step cooking process with 2 or fewer verbal cues for sequencing and safety from w/c level in rehab kitchen within 2 weeks.*

Depending on your setting, the timeline for your STGs may be daily, weekly, or by number of sessions.

For example:

- *Client will prepare a sandwich with 2 or fewer verbal cues for sequencing and safety from w/c level in rehab kitchen by March 16th.*
- *Client will prepare a sandwich with 2 or fewer verbal cues for sequencing and safety from w/c level in rehab kitchen within 1 week.*
- *Client will prepare a sandwich with 2 or fewer verbal cues for sequencing and safety from w/c level in rehab kitchen by 5th treatment session.*

It is important to remember that the time frame for the client's LTG must be realistic to the setting in which you are working. For example, if you work in an acute care hospital setting where the average length of stay is only a few days, it does not make sense to write a goal about what the client will do in 3 weeks. By that time, the client may be working with a home health or outpatient occupational therapist. **We only write goals for our own setting!** The next occupational therapist will set goals for what the client will accomplish in the next setting. You must estimate what you will be able to accomplish in the time frame that is typical for your setting. This sounds challenging, but it does get easier with experience. See Table 7-3 for a rough guideline of maximum time frames for common occupational therapy practice settings. **See Table 11-1 in Chapter 11 for an expanded discussion of requirements in each setting.**

Please note that the time frames listed are general guidelines for the maximum time frame for LTGs. This does not mean that every client's condition will justify that length of time. Your time frames should be driven by your best estimate of how long it will take your specific client to achieve maximum function in your particular setting. Consistently setting the same time frame on goals for every client you see can be a red flag to claim reviewers (Valdes, 2014).

EXAMPLES OF GOAL STATEMENTS

The COAST method is useful as you are learning to write, although the order may need to be changed slightly in order for your sentence to make sense or flow well. If all of the required elements are present, it does not matter with which element you begin your sentence. Let's take a look at a few examples:

C:	*Client will*
O:	*feed self 50% of meal*
A:	*with min A to scoop*
S:	*using built-up spoon*
T:	*within 3 tx sessions.*

The elements of this goal statement can be rearranged without changing the meaning of the goal:

- *Within 3 tx sessions, client will feed self 50% of meal using built-up spoon with min A to scoop.*
- *Using built-up spoon, client will feed self 50% of meal with min A to scoop within 3 tx sessions.*

Table 7-3

TIMELINE FOR LONG-TERM GOALS IN COMMON OCCUPATIONAL THERAPY PRACTICE SETTINGS

SETTING	TIMELINE FOR LONG-TERM GOALS BASED ON AVERAGE LENGTH OF STAY
Inpatient Acute Care	Typically **just a few days**. As soon as the patient is medically stable, they likely will be discharged to a different setting such as SNF, inpatient rehabilitation, home with home health therapy services, or home with outpatient therapy services.
Long-Term Acute Care Hospital (LTACH), also known as Long-Term Care Hospital (LTCH)	Typically **25 days or more** (CMS, 2019). Patients in this setting have complex medical needs requiring prolonged acute care, such as ventilator use, intensive respiratory care, multiple intravenous medications or transfusions, ongoing dialysis, complex wound or burn care, post-surgical acute care, infection management, and post–organ transplant care.
Inpatient Rehabilitation Facility (IRF)	A **few weeks** depending on the setting and severity of impairments (Medicare Payment Advisory Commission, 2021). Rehabilitation hospitals specializing in TBI and SCI rehabilitation may have longer average lengths of stay.
Skilled Nursing Facility (SNF)	A **few to several weeks** depending on the setting and severity of impairments. Average length of stay ranged from approximately 18 to 28 days in a recent study (Fitch et al., 2021). SNF length of stay often is influenced by payer source and the beneficiary's ability to pay a portion of the cost. For example, Original Medicare Part A covers SNF stays at 100% for the first 20 days, then at 80% for days 21 to 100. Medicare Advantage and other private insurance plans may only authorize short periods of time and require frequent documentation updates before authorizing additional days.
Home Health	A **few to several weeks** depending on the setting and severity of impairments. Three or 4 weeks is a good estimate for LTGs.
Inpatient Psychiatric Hospital	Short-term psychiatric hospitals focus on stabilization of a crisis situation and typically keep patients only **3 to 5 days** (University of Maryland Medical Center, 2022). Long-term psychiatric hospital stays may range from **several weeks to several months, and possibly even years**. State psychiatric hospitals typically "provide inpatient and residential services to individuals committed by the criminal or probate courts" (Missouri Department of Mental Health, 2022, para. 1).
Outpatient Clinic	A **few to several weeks.** Funding sources may require updates every 30 days, so 4 weeks is a good estimate of time for LTGs. Other funding sources may require updates after a particular number of visits.
School	**Yearly basis.** If a child requires special education services and occupational therapy is listed in the child's plan as a related service in the Individualized Education Program (IEP), LTGs are updated annually.
Early Intervention	Early intervention services span anywhere from birth through a child's third birthday (Center for Parent Information & Resources, 2021), but you likely will write LTGs for **a few to several months** in the child's Individualized Family Service Plan (IFSP). Each state sets its own rules regarding IFSP documentation requirements.
Community-Based Practice	**Varies greatly** depending on type of setting and client population.

Here is another example:

C:	*Client will perform*
O:	*bed-making activity*
A:	*with min verbal cues*
S:	*while adhering to post-surgical back precautions*
T:	*by discharge in 2 days.*

The elements of this goal statement can be rearranged without changing the meaning of the goal:

With min verbal cues, client will perform bed-making activity while adhering to post-surgical back precautions by discharge in 2 days.

Although acceptable to rearrange some elements of the COAST goal, the "C" and the "O" should always be kept together to help keep the focus on the occupation.

- Incorrect example: *Client will use adaptive equipment with SBA to complete lower body dressing within 2 days.*
- Correct example: *Client will complete lower body dressing using adaptive equipment with SBA within 2 days.*

In the first example, the focus is on the adaptive equipment rather than the occupation of lower body dressing. Make it easy for the insurance reviewer to discern the most important part of your goal. The client will do what? The client will complete lower body dressing.

Activities of Daily Living (ADLs)

- *Halinka will don coat using over-the-head method independently within 1 month.*
- *Client will fasten 3 buttons in 2 minutes using button hook with min verbal cues by May 2nd.*
- *Within 3 treatment sessions, Mr. S will complete toileting using raised toilet seat with min A for balance during clothing adjustment.*
- *Pt. will complete posterior hygiene using toilet tongs with min verbal cues to adhere to post-surgical back precautions by discharge in 2 days.*
- *Using adapted handles, Vivian will apply make-up independently within 1 week.*
- *Pt. will complete bathing tasks seated on tub bench using long-handled sponge with SBA within 3 days.*
- *Owen will feed self 50% of meal using adaptive spoon with mod A to prevent spillage within 3 weeks.*
- *Client will retrieve and transport clothing from closet using walker with CGA for balance by November 30th.*
- *Caregiver will apply client's post-surgical back brace independently during upper body dressing tasks by end of 2nd treatment session.*
- *Within 1 week, resident will complete grooming tasks from w/c level with min tactile cues to attend to left side.*
- *By discharge tomorrow, patient will demonstrate car transfer using wheeled walker with CGA from spouse while adhering to posterior hip precautions.*
  - Please see text box regarding functional mobility goals.
- *Client will verbalize understanding of safe positions for sexual intimacy that adhere to post-surgical hip precautions by time of discharge in 2 days.*
  - Education regarding sexual activity falls within the purview of occupational therapy (AOTA, 2020). I typically prefer to see students and practitioners write goals that involve the client demonstrating an occupation rather than verbalizing understanding of education provided. For obvious reasons, this is an area of occupation where writing goals for verbalizing understanding is sufficient.

Functional mobility is listed in the *OTPF-4* as an occupation under ADLs (AOTA, 2020). However, our physical therapy colleagues also address functional mobility, and we must collaborate with them to avoid **duplication of service** in our client sessions and documentation (Mastrangelo, 2016). In many settings, occupational therapists write goals for car transfers, toilet transfers, and tub or shower transfers. However, if in your practice setting physical therapy typically scores the mobility portion of Section GG, which includes toilet transfers and car transfers (AOTA, 2022a), then physical therapy may be the discipline writing goals for those activities. In that case, rather than write an occupational therapy goal for the toilet transfer, write an occupational therapy goal for toileting, which includes clothing management and hygiene:

- PT goal: *Client will complete toilet transfer with CGA using raised toilet seat and wheeled walker by next treatment session.*
- OT goal: *Client will complete clothing management and toileting hygiene with CGA using raised toilet seat and wheeled walker by next treatment session.*

Here is another ADL example:

- PT goal: *Client will complete sit to stand with SBA using quad care within 1 session.*
- OT goal: *Within 1 session, client will don pants with SBA for balance during clothing adjustment over hips in standing, using quad cane for support.*

The same holds true for IADLs and other areas of occupation. **Don't write goals that the "client will ambulate."** Write goals related to the performance of an occupation and **let the mobility portion become your specific condition**, in other words **how** the client will complete the occupation. For example:

- PT goal: *Client will ambulate 50′ using wheeled walker with CGA for balance within 1 week.*
- OT goal: *Client will transport items in kitchen using wheeled walker and walker tray with CGA for balance within 1 week.*

The overlap between occupational therapy's scope of practice and the scopes of practice of physical therapy, speech-language pathology, and other health professions remains a contentious issue (AOTA, 2022b). AOTA works continuously to articulate occupational therapy's domain and defend our scope of practice via advocacy to state regulators and payers. Within our various practice contexts, we must each find a balance between continuing to advocate for occupational therapy's purview, working collaboratively with our interprofessional colleagues to meet client needs, and making sure we all get paid for the important work of each discipline.

Instrumental Activities of Daily Living (IADLs)

- *By June 23rd, client will transfer 10 laundry items from washer to dryer with 3 or fewer verbal cues to adhere to post-surgical back precautions.*
- *Client will change infant's diaper using adaptive one-handed methods with 2 or fewer verbal cues within 2 weeks.*
- *Mackenzie will analyze bill statement and accurately complete online bill pay process with min verbal cues by August 19th.*
- *Resident will identify and navigate safe route independently from bedroom to exit of residential care facility using 4-wheeled walker by July 5th.*
- *Aniyah will locate phone number for apartment complex maintenance via online search with 2 or fewer verbal cues by next session.*
- *Using oven mitts, Rhea will remove hot pan from oven with SBA within 1 week.*
- *Lorenzo will navigate public bus system from home to doctor's office with supervision during next treatment session.*
- *Within 2 weeks, Mrs. S will make bed independently while incorporating energy conservation techniques.*
- *With SBA, Monique will carry full 1-gallon drink pitcher from refrigerator to kitchen table without spillage within 2 sessions.*
- *By next visit, Eli will identify safety concerns in 4 out of 5 written or visual scenarios without additional prompts.*
- *Within 2 weeks, Maria will kneel on padded surface and safely return to standing position with CGA from spouse for balance, in preparation for return to church services.*

- *Shoshanah will place online order for grocery delivery with 2 or fewer verbal cues by January 27th.*
- *During next visit, Kwan will use credit card successfully to obtain snack from vending machine with min A for bilateral coordination during wallet management.*
- *With moderate verbal cues, Felix will develop a weekly grocery shopping list that stays within a $200 budget, within 4 visits.*

Health Management

- *By April 30th, Shantelle will attend indoor walking group at community recreation center at least twice weekly for 3 out of 4 consecutive weeks with minimal encouragement from group home staff.*
- *Pt. will empty catheter leg bag with min verbal cues for technique within 1 week.*
- *Consumer will complete weekly medication set-up using pill organizer independently without errors before tomorrow's case manager check-in visit.*
- *Jamie will complete blood sugar checks independently with glucometer using one-handed technique by next home health visit.*
- *Within 4 sessions, Peyton will select appropriate after-school snack, adhering to daily carbohydrate restrictions for her type 1 diabetes, with min verbal cues from parent.*
- *Seated at sink in wheelchair, Scarlett will place both contact lenses into eye with nondominant L hand without dropping them within 1 week.*
- *Following written handout, client will complete self-ROM home exercise program for flaccid R UE with min tactile cues for correct positioning and movement, before discharge in 3 days.*
- *Seated EOB, veteran will replace hearing aid batteries with min A for bilateral coordination, within 1 week.*
- *Within 2 weeks, patient will complete ostomy care with min verbal cues while seated in w/c.*
- *Before discharge home in 2 days, Ahmed will pull portable oxygen tank 50' with supervision, without bumping into obstacles.*

Please note that although we typically write goals for the client, occasionally we need to write a goal for the caregiver to demonstrate an aspect of the client's care in preparation for return home. For example:

- *Caregiver will don/doff client's resting hand splint correctly at all recommended intervals without reminders during independent living trial in rehab unit apartment this weekend.*
- *Following written instructions, spouse will correctly set up, place, and remove client's overnight peritoneal dialysis by discharge in 5 days.*
- *By discharge in 2 days, patient's daughter will apply B thigh-high compression stockings using plastic bag technique over foot to reduce friction.*

Rest and Sleep

- *Using visual checklist as memory aid, Taylor will remember to lock doors before bedtime on 5 consecutive nights by September 21st.*
- *Consumer will go to bed before midnight at least 75% of weeknights within 2 weeks to obtain adequate sleep for effective participation at job.*
- *Within 1 month, teen will complete 3-step bedtime routine using visual schedule with 2 or fewer verbal cues.*

Education

> Note: Therapists working in school settings use slightly different terminology and methods writing for goals. In IEPs, goals for 1 year may be referred to as objectives or behavioral objectives. Educational goals often are not measured by time, such as by 5/7/25 or within 3 weeks. Since the IEP is written annually, time frame for the objectives is assumed to be 1 year from the date the IEP is established. Children often exhibit a new behavior or skill inconsistently before it is really established. Therefore, measurement for children is more likely to reflect whether the behavior or skills is established. For example:
>
> *From wheelchair, Li Mei will obtain and transport lunch tray to table with distant supervision 9 of 10 consecutive days.*

- *Na'Kyra will cut out circle independently during classroom activities using supinated grasp on scissors with < 2 deviations from line on 75% of attempts.*
- *Child will maintain seated position at desk for 5 minutes with 2 or fewer verbal cues 4 of 5 consecutive days.*
- *Abdul will print upper case alphabet independently on wide-ruled notebook paper, demonstrating proper letter formation and staying on line, with < 3 errors 75% of attempts.*
- *Student will don/doff coat without physical assistance 90% of the time to be independent with beginning and end-of-day school routine.*
- *Addison will take turns on playground equipment without adult intervention 3 of 4 consecutive days.*
- *Dyani will copy 10 math problems from whiteboard to paper with < 2 errors and no verbal cues 80% of attempts.*
- *Lamar will complete assigned classroom tasks within allotted time with fewer than 3 verbal cues 75% of the time.*
- *Using pencil with adaptive grip, Reyna will copy a square from a visual model with 80% accuracy, 3 of 4 trials.*
- *Isla will remain in line keeping hands to self without requiring adult intervention when class walks between school locations on 4 of 5 trials.*
- *Gentry will place coat and backpack on classroom wall hook with min verbal cues to follow visual schedule by end of school year.*
- *Mia will participate in group activities for up to 10 minutes without exhibiting aggressive behaviors toward class-mates 4 of 5 consecutive days.*
- *Cedric will comply with teacher's verbal instructions within 1 minute, with only 1 additional prompt, for 3 consecutive days.*
- *Kezia will open combination lock on her locker independently 100% of the time.*
- *Hendon will enter username and password to access school Wi-Fi on tablet with no more than 1 verbal prompt, 90% of attempts.*
- *Jalin will remain on worksheet task for 5 minutes, ignoring classroom distractions, with 2 or fewer prompts from paraprofessional, 75% of attempts.*
- *Hallie will maintain engagement in physical activities during PE class for at least 10 minutes before taking a rest break, 80% of trials.*
- *During cutting tasks, Joaquin independently will achieve and maintain a supinated grasp on scissors with elbow at side, 3 out of 4 observations.*
- *Ashna will type 15 words per minute on keyboard during school writing tasks, 75% of opportunities.*
- *With visual model on desk, Jaxson will copy 10 spelling words onto lined paper demonstrating correct letter formation and spacing with 80% accuracy, with no more than 1 cue from paraprofessional, on 4 of 5 consecutive attempts.*
- *Using reminders on cell phone, Anna will turn in at least 80% of homework assignments on time at beginning of class, before additional prompting by classroom teacher or para.*
- *Kyung Mi will exhibit appropriate pressure with pencil and eraser when completing worksheets, as evidence by no broken pencil lead and no tears in paper, 4 of 5 trials.*
- *From a visual model on vertical whiteboard, Francisco will replicate a 6+ word sentence on paper with proper letter formation, spacing, and spelling with 80% accuracy, 3 of 4 consecutive attempts.*

Work

- *Without staff support, Malik will request at least one job application from a restaurant within 1 week.*
- *Lane will transfer 10# boxes from floor to shelf during simulated work tasks, demonstrating proper body mechanics without verbal cues by October 17th.*
- *By May 4th, client will count correct change from a $20 bill without verbal cues to return to position as volunteer in hospital gift shop.*
- *Within 2 weeks, Emmett will utilize tools to remove/replace parts without assistance during simulated mechanics tasks.*
- *Alejandro will identify at least 2 opportunities for community volunteer service independently by next group session.*
- *Client will navigate power w/c in work environment without bumping into objects or people within 3 weeks.*
- *Jonah will arrive to work and clock in on time independently for 90% of shifts within 1 month.*
- *Natalia will type 20 words per minute during simulated work tasks using B wrist cock-up splints within 2 weeks.*
- *Using adaptive nail holder, Caleb will hammer 10 nails into board within 5 minutes, missing head of nail on hammer swings no more than 10% of attempts, within 3 weeks.*
- *Within 5 minutes of receiving instructions, Blake will follow 2-step verbal directions to complete work task accurately with 2 or fewer verbal prompts from job coach, by end of 30-day employment trial.*
- *Within 3 weeks, farmer will carry 10-lb bucket independently from barn to feed trough and pour into feed trough with no more than minor spillage.*
- *Following restaurant computer screen, Imani will make 10/10 drinks correctly without cues from job coach, within 1 week.*
- *Using ergonomic desk chair, Ryleigh will complete seated typing task for 20 minutes without complaint of back pain, exhibiting appropriate body mechanics throughout activity, within 2 weeks.*
- *Using hand control adaptations, Luke will navigate tractor around 5 obstacles successfully with min verbal cues from AgrAbility coach, within 4 sessions.*

> As noted in the previous chapter, some funding sources do not consider problem statements and goals for play, leisure, and social participation medically necessary. However, examples are provided here to cover all areas of occupation identified in the *OTPF-4* (AOTA, 2020).

Play

- *Infant will engage in play with parent or sibling by visually tracking a toy 45 degrees past midline in both directions by June 30th.*
- *Within 2 months, Jorge will stabilize pop-up toy with L UE while activating toy with R hand with min physical facilitation.*
- *Child will place 3 shapes into puzzle board with no verbal cues within 3 months.*
- *Katrina will engage in pretend play activity with peers for >3 minutes with minimal adult facilitation by February 28th.*
- *Infant will engage in B UE play activity while independently sitting unsupported >1 minute by December 10th.*
- *Child will catch tennis ball in B hands on 8 of 10 attempts when tossed from 10 feet within 3 weeks.*
- *Lauren will stack 6 or more 1" blocks independently using R hand to stabilize tower within 1 month.*
- *Asia will take turns during board game without emotional outbursts during 3 of 4 family game nights, by December 31st.*
- *Within 1 week, Ryker will play online video game independently for 15 minutes with teen peers using adapted controller, based on client and family report.*
- *In supported sitting on parent's lap with R hand restricted, Patrick will place and remove toys from container using L hand to reach to various heights, within 4 weeks.*
- *Theo will play with stuffed animals or action figures in a functional way during pretend play with preschool peers, for 3 consecutive sessions within 3 months.*

Social Participation

- *Consumer will choose and participate in at least one social activity per week independently, 3/3 weeks within 1 month.*
- *With mod verbal cues, consumer will ask roommate to smoke outside the building next time the situation arises.*
- *Matias will make at least 2 verbal contributions to group discussions with min verbal prompts 5/5 days within 1 week.*
- *Within 2 months, Liam will tolerate unexpected touch from peers during circle time without demonstrating aggressive behaviors 80% of the time per day care provider report.*
- *Using visual schedule and min verbal cues, Myah will transition between home and preschool environment without expressing anxiety or fear at least 50% of the time within 3 months.*
- *Within 1 week, Kenya will engage in conversations with family members without yelling, at least 60% of attempts.*
- *With 1 verbal prompt, Eleanor will initiate interaction with peers at least one time during day care outdoor recess during 75% of opportunities by May 31st.*
- *Kyra will share crafting supplies with other group home residents without staff intervention during 3 out of 4 craft groups, within 3 months.*

Leisure

- *Independently, Erick will identify at least 3 leisure activities that are not associated with drinking by September 8th.*
- *Client will complete gardening tasks independently, consistently implementing energy conservation techniques, within 2 weeks.*
- *Within 3 weeks, client will manipulate toothpaste caps, buttons, and knitting needles independently, demonstrating sufficient coordination for task success with extra time.*

Medical Necessity

As occupational therapists, we view a client holistically, considering the whole person with their needs, interests, problems, strengths, and priorities. We know that leisure is an important part of the total picture. When this is the client's priority, we might be inclined to write problem statements and goals focusing on leisure skills and interests, such as:

- **Problem:** *Client is unable to crochet due to decreased AROM and increased pain in R wrist.*
- **LTG:** *Client will crochet without wrist pain within 6 weeks.*

However, we know that both Medicare and private insurance are very frugal with our health care dollars and approve expenditures only for medical necessity. Since even adaptive equipment such as a raised toilet seat is not always considered medically necessary, treatment focused on a client's leisure goals is likely to be denied under our current reimbursement system. In consideration of the client's holistic needs and the reimbursement limitations, we may address some of the contributing factors that enable the client to perform a variety of functional tasks in the intervention plan. Documentation would focus on goals and interventions that provide the client with skills for self-care, IADLs, and work, as well as the leisure activities that are so important to the quality of life.

In the previous example about crocheting, we might suspect that the client is also having difficulty with household or work tasks requiring R UE use. It would be more appropriate to write an IADL goal, such as:

Client will lift pots and pans during dishwashing without wrist pain in 6 weeks.

Interventions would be targeted toward the client factors of active range of motion and pain, and improvements in these client factors would result in an increased ability for the client to pursue her leisure interests as well. In fact, the client's preferred leisure activity of crocheting would be a great occupation-based intervention to address the deficits in client factors that also impact IADLs.

Note: **DO NOT** use participation in treatment as a goal. For example:

Client will do 20 reps of shoulder ladder with 1-lb wt. to increase endurance for IADLs.

The shoulder ladder, although it may be a preparatory exercise before you move toward occupation-based interventions, is just that: **an intervention**, NOT a goal. The client's funding source does not care about shoulder ladder repetitions, and the reviewer may not even know what that means anyway. Instead, write a goal that specifies the amount of endurance the client needs to demonstrate for an occupation-based activity:

From standing position, client will place dishes from dishwasher into overhead cabinets for 3 minutes without requiring a seated rest break, within 1 week.

Another thing to remember about COAST goal writing is to **focus on the occupation rather than the treatment media**. Consider the following goal:

Client will place 8 half-inch screws and washers on a block of wood with holes with min A by next session.

This goal emphasizes the treatment media and is not occupation-based. Written in a different way, the targeted occupation of work becomes evident, and the treatment media becomes the **specific condition** rather than the focus of the goal:

By the end of the 2nd treatment session, client will complete work simulation task with min A for dexterity by placing 8 half-inch screws into a block of wood in < 5 minutes.

GOALS IN DIFFERENT SETTINGS

The COAST format works well in many occupational therapy settings. This method of goal writing allows you to demonstrate the specific need for occupational therapy services by focusing on areas of occupation affected by the client's condition. Once you learn the important components of COAST goals, you can adapt your goal format to fit other practice settings. In some settings, problem statements and goals are written differently due to the nature of services provided.

Mental Health and Substance Use Disorders

In mental health and substance use disorder practice settings, problem statements and goals are often interprofessional and are written to be addressed by the treatment team rather than by one specific discipline. For example:

- **Problem:** *Alcohol use*
- **Behavioral Manifestation:** *Kyle admits to drinking at least 8 oz. of liquor and 7 to 8 beers nightly, resulting in failing grades and involvement with the law due to physical violence toward peers.*
- **Goal:** *By next group session, Kyle will identify 2 leisure activities not associated with drinking.*
- **Goal:** *By end of next individual session, Kyle will create list of upcoming area Alcoholics Anonymous meetings he can attend to reinforce sobriety.*
- **Goal:** *By discharge within 1 week, Kyle will identify at least 3 relapse prevention strategies for use in future stressful situations with min verbal cues from addiction recovery staff.*

Another example:

- **Problem:** *Noncompliant behavior*
- **Behavioral Manifestation:** *Talia is noncompliant with family rules and social norms (attending school, abiding by the law), resulting in assignment to a parole officer and 3 failed foster home placements.*
- **Goal:** *Talia will demonstrate willingness to cooperate with family norms by entering into a behavioral contract with her foster parents within 1 week.*
- **Goal:** *Within 2 weeks, Talia will attend school 5 out of 5 consecutive days without truancy.*
- **Goal:** *During next 30 days, Talia will abide by set curfew by returning home at appropriate time from school functions or social events, with less than one incidence of breaking curfew.*

Early Intervention

In recent years, early intervention programs that provide services for children from birth to 3 years of age have moved toward a family-centered, transdisciplinary model of service delivery (McCarthy & Guerin, 2022; Raver & Childress, 2015). One aspect of a family-centered approach is that, rather than the professionals setting the goals for the child, **families identify the "child outcomes"** that they hope their child will achieve. IFSP child outcomes are written in the family's words and may not contain all the elements of COAST goals that you have learned. For example, the family may identify child outcomes such as the following:

- *Jaden will use words during playtime and meals to express his needs.*
- *Charlotte will express her emotion in positive ways when she is excited.*
- *Levi will show interest in potty training.*
- *Isabella will walk up and down the stairs at home unassisted.*
- *Jack will use a spoon to feed himself at least half of his meal.*
- *Zion will play with brother after school without hitting him with toys or other objects.*
- *Aurora will tolerate riding in shopping cart during grocery shopping outings with Mom.*
- *Kayden will brush teeth for at least 2 minutes each night before bed, with or without parent help.*
- *Rowan will try at least one bite of new foods without having a tantrum.*
- *Aria will allow parents to dress her in the morning without hitting or biting them.*
- *Finn will allow his fingernails to be clipped without crying.*
- *Thea will sit and play with toys by herself in the living room while parents fix dinner.*
- *Malachi will show interest in exploring books and turn pages on his own.*
- *Hudson will tolerate new babysitters by calming self within 10 minutes of parents' departure.*
- *Reese will scribble with a crayon in a coloring book.*
- *Skyler will feed herself small snacks such as dry cereal and crackers.*
- *Maverick will let Grandma and Grandpa hold him during weekend visits.*

The transdisciplinary aspect of early intervention means that families will interact directly with only one or two individuals of the team on a regular basis, with other disciplines providing services on a consultative basis. Occupational therapists providing early intervention services under a transdisciplinary model may encounter the need for role release, which involves setting aside disciplinary boundaries and working collaboratively to support the needs of the child and family, even when that means addressing established outcomes that typically fall under the purview of other disciplines (Therapies for Kids, 2022). If you work in an early intervention setting, your documentation and interventions should reflect the service delivery model required by the agency.

REFERENCES

American Occupational Therapy Association. (2020). Occupational therapy practice framework: Domain and process (4th ed.). *American Journal of Occupational Therapy, 74*(Suppl. 2), 7412410010. https://doi.org/10.5014.ajot.2020.74S2001

American Occupational Therapy Association. (2021). *AOTA's knowledge translation toolkit: Documentation strategies.* https://www.aota.org/

American Occupational Therapy Association. (2022a). *Section GG self-care (activities of daily living) and mobility items.* https://www.aota.org/

American Occupational Therapy Association. (2022b). *Advocacy issues: Scope of practice.* https://www.aota.org/

Amini, D. (2016). *AOTA documentation series—Module 2: Occupation-based goal writing for OT practice* [Online continuing educational module]. American Occupational Therapy Association. https://www.aota.org/

Cahill, S. (2021). *Research update on telehealth: Client outcomes and satisfaction, occupation-based coaching, and stroke rehabilitation.* American Occupational Therapy Association. https://www.aota.org/

Center for Parent Information & Resources. (2021). *Writing the IFSP for your child.* https://www.parentcenterhub.org

Centers for Medicare & Medicaid Services. (2019). *What are long-term care hospitals?* https://www.medicare.gov.

Chamberlain, M. (2022). *Occupational therapy goal writing and goal bank guide for adults.* Seniors Flourish.

Cole, M. B., & Tufano, R. (2020). *Applied theories in occupational therapy: A practical approach* (2nd ed.). SLACK Incorporated.

Dang, D., Dearholt, S. L., Bissett, K., Ascenzi, J., & Whalen, M. (2022). *Johns Hopkins evidence-based practice for nurses and healthcare professionals* (4th ed.). Sigma Theta Tau International Honor Society of Nursing.

Fitch, K., Broulette, J., & King, K. (2021). *Variability in average length of stay for skilled nursing facilities—Opportunities exist for more efficient management*. Milliman. https://www.milliman.com/en/insight/variability-in-average-length-of-stay-for-skilled-nursing-facilities

Fusion Web Clinic. (2022). *Getting SMART about formatting pediatric therapy goals*. OT Accelerator. https://seniorsflourish.com/contact/

Gateley, C., & Borcherding, S. (2012). *Documentation manual for occupational therapy: Writing SOAP notes* (3rd ed.). SLACK Incorporated.

Juckett, L. (2022). *An introduction to AOTA's knowledge translation toolkit*. American Occupational Therapy Association. https://www.aota.org/

Lamb, A. J. (2014). *Documenting the distinct value of occupational therapy through documentation*. Presentation at the 2014 AOTA Specialty Conference—Effective Documentation: The Key to Payment & Articulating Our Distinct Value, September 12-13, 2014, Alexandria, VA.

Mastrangelo, K. (2016, April 25). *Top 5 must-know to prevent duplication of therapy services*. Harmony Healthcare International. https://www.harmony-healthcare.com/blog/top-5-things-to-know-to-prevent-duplication-of-therapy-services

McCarthy, E., & Guerin, S. (2022). Family-centred care in early intervention: A systematic review of the processes and outcomes of family-centred care and impacting factors. *Child: Care, Health, and Development, 48*(1), 1-32. https://doi.org/10.1111/cch.12901

Medicare Payment Advisory Commission. (2021). *Report to the Congress—Medicare payment policy: Inpatient rehabilitation facility services*. https://www.medpac.gov/

Missouri Department of Mental Health. (2022). *State operated psychiatric hospitals and facilities*. https://dmh.mo.gov/

Moll, C. M., Billick, M. N., & Valdes, K. (2018). Parent satisfaction of occupational therapy interventions for pediatrics. *Pediatrics & Therapeutics, 8*(1), 1-8.

OT Dude. (2020, December 26). *Occupational & physical therapy levels of assistance*. https://www.otdude.com/

Parkinson, S., & Brooks, R. (2021). *A guide to the formulation of plans and goals in occupational therapy*. Routledge.

Quinn, L., & Gordon, J. (2016). *Documentation for rehabilitation: A guide to clinical decision making in physical therapy* (3rd ed.). Elsevier.

Raver, S. A., & Childress, D. C. (2015). *Family-centered early intervention: Supporting infants and toddlers in natural environments*. Paul H. Brooks Publishing Company.

Saito, Y., Tomori, K., Nagayama, H., Sawadai, T., & Kikuchi, E. (2019). Differences in the occupational therapy goals of clients and therapists affect the outcomes of patients in subacute rehabilitation wards: A case-control study. *Journal of Physical Therapy Science, 31*(7), 521-525. https://doi.org/10.1589/jpts.31.521

Sames, K. (2015). *AOTA documentation series—Module 1: The nuts and bolts of effective OT documentation* [Online continuing educational module]. American Occupational Therapy Association. https://www.aota.org/

Skaletski, E. (2021). *Start here: A straight forward guide to searching for evidence*. American Occupational Therapy Association. https://www.aota.org/

Stromsdorfer, S., & Ferri, B. (2022). *Must-know occupational therapy medical abbreviations*. My OT Spot. https://www.myotspot.com/

Suc, L., Svalgeer, A., & Bratun, U. (2020). Goal setting among experienced and novice occupational therapists in a rehabilitation center. *Canadian Journal of Occupational Therapy, 87*(4), 287-297.

The OT Minute. (2021). COAST goal writing method: How to write easy and clear OT goals [Video]. YouTube. https://www.youtube.com/watch?v=1uepV5iXmg4

The OT Toolbox. (2021). *Occupational therapy documentation tips*. https://www.theottoolbox.com/

Therapies for Kids. (2022). *How we work: Transdisciplinary teamwork*. https://therapiesforkids.com.au/

University of Maryland Medical Center. (2022). *Short-term inpatient psychiatric hospitalization*. https://www.umms.org/

Valdes, K. (2014). *How to comply with Medicare documentation requirements for Part B therapy services*. Summit Professional Education seminar, August 23, 2014, Columbia, MO.

WORKSHEET 7-1

Choosing Goals for Medical Necessity

Imagine you are on fieldwork in an outpatient clinic and you have a client who has stated a priority of getting back to leisure interests. Your problem statement and goals may look like this:

- **Problem:**   *Client unable to perform sewing due to 2+/5 strength in R hand musculature.*
    - ◦ **LTG:**   *Client will perform embroidery independently for 20 minutes within 8 weeks.*
    - ◦ **STG:**   *To improve performance of embroidery, client will use needle continuously for 5 minutes within 2 weeks.*

However, when your fieldwork educator reviews your draft problem statement and goals, her response is, "It's great that you are thinking holistically about the client's needs, but Medicare doesn't care whether the client can complete embroidery. You need to address problems and goals that are considered medically necessary." She sends you back to revise your problem and statement and goals.

Think about the contributing factors that are impacting the client's ability to complete her preferred leisure task, and answer the following questions:

1. What other occupational performance problems might this woman have due to decreased strength in her R hand?

2. What LTG might you use that would show medical necessity for increasing R UE strength?

3. What STG might be used as a step to achieve that LTG?

WORKSHEET 7-2

Evaluating Goal Statements

Refer to the COAST elements to determine which of the following goals has each of the necessary components to be useful in occupational therapy documentation. For each goal that you find to be incomplete or inaccurate in some way, indicate what is missing and rewrite a better COAST goal.

1. *By the time of discharge in 2 weeks, client will dress himself with min A for balance using a sock aid and reacher while sitting in w/c.*

   _____ This goal has all of the necessary COAST components.

   _____ This goal lacks:

2. *Client will tolerate 10 minutes of treatment daily.*

   _____ This goal has all of the necessary COAST components.

   _____ This goal lacks:

3. *Client will demonstrate increased coping skills in stressful situations within 2 weeks.*

   _____ This goal has all of the necessary COAST components.

   _____ This goal lacks:

4. *Client will demonstrate 15 minutes of activity tolerance without rest breaks using B UEs to complete ADL tasks before breakfast each morning.*

   _____ This goal has all of the necessary COAST components.

   _____ This goal lacks:

5. *OT will teach lower body dressing using a reacher, dressing stick, and sock aid within 2 treatment sessions.*

   _____ This goal has all of the necessary COAST components.

   _____ This goal lacks:

6. *Patient will demonstrate ability to budget for the month.*

   _____ This goal has all of the necessary COAST components.

   _____ This goal lacks:

WORKSHEET 7-3

Writing Client-Centered, Occupation-Based, Measurable Goals

Write goals for the following scenarios that are client-centered, occupation-based, and measurable. Please remember that we set goals <u>with</u> the client. Assume for this worksheet that you have already collaborated with the client regarding goals.

1. Ayana is not able to attend to task for more than a few minutes, which makes IADL activities difficult for her. Since she likes to cook and plans to return to cooking after discharge, you have been working with her in the kitchen. You would like to see her able to attend to a task for 10 minutes by the time she is discharged next week. Write a goal that addresses Ayana's attention span during cooking.

    C:

    O:

    A:

    S:

    T:

2. Now write a goal for Ayana to be able to follow directions so that she can read the back of a boxed meal, and eventually a recipe, when she is cooking.

    C:

    O:

    A:

    S:

    T:

3. Scott is having trouble dressing himself after his stroke. You have been teaching him an over-the-head method for putting on his shirt. Write a dressing goal for Scott.

    C:

    O:

    A:

    S:

    T:

WORKSHEET **7-3** (CONTINUED)

Writing Client-Centered, Occupation-Based, Measurable Goals

4. Nikki is very weak, and she wants to be able to go back to work as a receptionist. She also wants to be able to care for her 4-month-old child. Write a goal that addresses her activity tolerance during an occupation-based activity.

    C:

    O:

    A:

    S:

    T:

5. Demarco wants to live independently in the community, but he lacks basic money management skills. Write a goal for Demarco to improve his money management skills.

    C:

    O:

    A:

    S:

    T:

6. Taylor has become increasingly more depressed over the past several weeks and was admitted after a suicide attempt. You estimate that you will have her in group for 1 week. You would like to see her mood change in that week. Write an occupation-based goal that will indicate an improved mood.

    C:

    O:

    A:

    S:

    T:

WORKSHEET 7-4

De-Emphasizing the Treatment Media

Remember to de-emphasize the treatment media in your goal statements. Rewrite the following goals statements to emphasize the change in occupational performance that you want the client to demonstrate rather than emphasizing the intervention.

1. *Client will assemble a clock craft project independently using appropriate materials by anticipated discharge in 1 week.*

2. *Consumer will spend at least 30 minutes lacing a leather billfold during next 45-minute craft group session.*

3. *Within 1 month, child will place 10 cotton balls into a jar independently to demonstrate improved dexterity for school activities.*

Chapter 8

Writing the "S"—Subjective

As discussed in Chapter 2, the SOAP approach is only one method for writing notes. It is the method you will learn over the next several chapters. Even if your practice setting uses a different format or an electronic documentation software system, you should be able to take the key elements of a SOAP note (e.g., what the client said, what you observed and did for the client, your interpretation of the client's situation and performance, your plan moving forward) and adapt them to a different format.

The first section of the SOAP note contains **subjective** information obtained from the client, giving their perspective on their condition or treatment. Subjective data are information that usually cannot be verified or measured during the treatment session. In this section, the therapist records the client's report of limitations, concerns, and problems, as well as what the client said that was relevant to treatment, such as significant complaints of pain; fatigue; or other expressions of feelings, attitudes, concerns, goals, and plans. When direct quotes are used in the Subjective section of the SOAP note, it is understood that the statement came from the individual receiving therapy unless otherwise stated.

The information obtained from the client will be of greater significance and relevance to your note if it is specific in nature. For instance, if your client tells you, "My shoulder hurts," you may question him further, asking, "How much does it hurt?" or "When does it hurt?" so your note can communicate more detailed information on his condition. You may either use a direct quote or summarize what the client has said, so his description might be written as:

"My right shoulder hurts when I try to put my shirt on."

or

Client reports R shoulder pain 7 out of 10 when he tries to put his shirt on.

EXAMPLES OF "S" STATEMENTS

- *"I don't need therapy."*
- *Resident reports pain in R shoulder when reaching up to comb hair.*
- *Patient asked for help when it was needed during the session.*
- *Client reports, "I keep blowing up at home and yelling at everyone, and I don't know what to do about it."*
- *"I can't wash the dishes or zip my coat."*

Gateley, C. A. *Documentation Manual for Occupational Therapy, Fifth Edition* (pp. 101-107). © 2024 Taylor & Francis Group.

- *Veteran reports that his fingers "feel kind of dead."*
- *Pt. reported that he needed to go meet someone and get to work when the session began. When asked questions such as "Can you hear me?" he often responded, "I need to go."*
- *Resident reports he feels "pretty good" now and his goal is to "get back as independent as I can."*
- *Consumer reports being fearful of leaving her home.*
- *Client reports that his doctor has ordered "some home health for a few days to help me learn how to take care of myself."*
- *Client reported that her shoulder feels better after application of kinesiotape to reduce subluxation. "My short-term goal is to be able to write, and my long-term goal is to return to work."*
- *Cindy called the emergency room last night to report a burning sensation in her "gut," which made her afraid she was going to die. Today she reports that she has been worrying about dying and has not showered for 2 days.*
- *Resident reports being able to bathe and dress self independently but does not open dresser drawers and closet doors due to a recent fall from opening a dresser drawer that resulted in a R hip fx. She was able to state the correct day and month when asked.*
- *Pt. commented that she used to use her L hand to hold a cup but now is unable to do so. Pt. also complained of soreness in L shoulder and inquired about agencies that can help with housekeeping tasks when she returns home.*
- *Client stated that she has experienced several episodes of bladder incontinence when trying to make it to the bathroom in the middle of the night.*
- *Consumer reports that the hardest feelings for her to deal with are worry and fear about her physical problems, which might go undetected. She reports being unable to function at home (cannot cook, keep house, or do laundry) when she is "sick with depression," but wants to do these things again. Consumer reports that exercise, prayer, and volunteer work are her primary coping strategies, and that she would like to learn more about relaxation techniques.*
- *Student reports frustration with handwriting tasks, stating, "I'm just no good at it. I hate writing!"*

As part of the initial evaluation process, an occupational therapist works toward establishing a collaborative relationship with the client by interviewing the client about their concerns and priorities and developing an occupational profile. The occupational profile is "a summary of the client's occupational history and experiences, patterns of daily living, interests, values, needs, and relevant contexts" (American Occupational Therapy Association, 2020, p. 80). Additional information for the occupational profile may be gathered from discussions with family or caregivers and through the review of existing health records. In an evaluation note, the "S" may contain all or part of the client's occupational profile.

For example:

Client reports that she was admitted after a fall that resulted in confusion and left-sided weakness. Prior to admission, she was living alone in a one-story home and was independent in all ADLs. She reports that she is a retired librarian, widowed 10 years ago. She says she values her independence and fully intends to return to her own home. She reports that her activities are primarily sedentary, including sewing, reading, and playing cards with friends. She says her daughter lives two blocks away and provides transportation when needed.

Another example:

The client talked about his current symptoms and the events leading up to his hospitalization. He reports losing his job with a construction company after not reporting to work for 2 weeks due to depression, having an argument with his wife, and taking an overdose. He says that he has always "worked construction" and does not know how to do anything else. He reports concerns that his former employer will not give him "a decent reference." He says he really has no leisure interests except "going out drinking with the guys after work" and sometimes going hunting in the fall.

Sometimes the client is nonverbal, does not make any relevant comments, or communicates in other ways. In such cases, include that information in the "S" section.

For example:

- *Client unable to communicate verbally due to expressive aphasia.*
- *Client did not speak without cueing.*
- *Using her augmentative communication device, pt. reported that she wanted to be able to take care of herself.*

- *Resident does not clearly verbalize during treatment, but smiles and nods appropriately when asked questions.*
- *Client nonverbal throughout most of session but did express frustration and displeasure with therapy tasks through facial expressions, gestures, and occasional vocalizations of "No, no, no."*
- *Child did not articulate full sentences but did use several two-word phrases including "more swing," "want Mama," and "big ball" during session.*

Sometimes you will include information that the family or caregiver provided about the client if this is pertinent to the session or the client's progress. This is common when treating infants and very young children.

For example:

- *Mother reports difficulty with diapering and dressing the infant, stating, "He just gets all stiff and arches his back."*
- *Foster parents report that child exhibits excessive energy, constantly running around the house and jumping on furniture. They also report that child is aggressive toward foster siblings and the family pet, and he will not remain seated at mealtimes.*
- *Parents report child has difficulty remaining in upright seated position for feeding in standard highchair. "She just keeps falling to the right side."*

Although the "S" is primarily reserved for the client's view, occasionally it is acceptable to report comments from caregivers and other professionals if the comments are directly related to the client's occupational therapy services (Kettenbach & Schlomer, 2016). This allows you to demonstrate the collaborative efforts of the treatment team. Incorporating caregiver comments may also be relevant when there is a discrepancy between client and caregiver reports. Here are some examples of including caregiver report:

- *Pt. tearful throughout session, with very little verbalization. Social worker reports pt.'s family just informed pt. they cannot care for her at home and that she will have to go to a skilled nursing facility.*
- *Classroom teacher reports significant improvement in child's ability to remain seated at desk since implementing use of sensory-cushion in chair to provide additional proprioceptive input. Child states, "I love the bumpy feel of it!"*
- *Physical therapist reports patient should use sliding board for all transfers because she is unable to maintain weight-bearing precautions for stand pivot transfers with wheeled walker. Patient states, "I can use that board getting from the wheelchair to the bed, but I'm afraid I'll fall off if I use it to get to the toilet."*
- *Client reports no difficulty with financial management, but spouse reports multiple errors in bill paying and banking account management in recent months.*
- *Pt. reports he is adamantly opposed to SNF placement, but spouse reports, "I just can't care for him at home. I can't lift him when he falls, and we don't have any family nearby to help me out."*
- *Paraprofessional reports child's behavior in classroom and other school environments has improved over the past month with implementation of visual schedule.*

COMMON ERRORS

Not Using Communication Time With Client Effectively

The most common error that students and new therapists make in gathering subjective information is failing to make good use of time when communicating with the client during treatment sessions. Instead of using the time in therapy to talk socially, a good therapist will use the time to listen effectively and to ask questions that will provide pertinent information about the client's attitudes and concerns. This information can be used to ensure effective treatment as well as appropriate documentation. Instead of talking to your client about the weather or *Monday Night Football*, why not ask them how they think they are doing in therapy or what their feelings are related to their upcoming discharge placement? As therapists gain experience, they begin to use the treatment session to gather relevant data regarding occupational history, functional status, prior level of functioning, motivation, priorities, and family support.

Effective communication and interviewing during treatment sessions can seem just like a conversation on the surface. However, as a skilled therapist, you are directing the conversation to topics that are meaningful to client care rather than allowing it to remain superficial. Use this opportunity to expand your occupational profile of the client and to gather data that are vital to providing the very best occupational therapy possible. In having a conversation with your client, guide the discussion to your client's history, problems, needs, strengths, support systems, living situation, and goals for treatment. Without knowing this information from your client's point of view, you will have difficulty planning effective treatment. When a therapist does not listen effectively during treatment, the "S" may read:

- *Client talked about grandchildren visiting.*
- *Patient reports he is reading a good book.*

While these statements are within the scope of the "S," they are not particularly helpful pieces of information to spend the time and space reporting, and they offer nothing to help provide additional information or context for the scrutinous eyes of insurance reviewers.

Not Writing Concise, Coherent Statements

The second most common error made by new therapists writing the Subjective section of the note is simply listing all remarks that the client makes about their condition. For example, during one treatment session, the following subjective information was gathered:

- *Client said, "I can't feel anything with my hands."*
- *Client stated, "I'm as wobbly as all get out today."*
- *Client expressed dizziness after bending down to touch the floor while in a seated position.*
- *Client acknowledged improvement in his sitting balance in comparison to the previous week.*

Many of the statements above have to do with stability, balance, and safety. Although the quotations are a very objective way of reporting data, and all the statements are relevant to the intervention session, it is more effective to summarize the client's remarks in a concise and coherent manner instead of listing each of these statements separately in the "S" section of the note.

For example:

Client expressed lack of sensation in both hands and dizziness in sitting position with dynamic movement (a "wobbly" sensation). He also acknowledged improvement in sitting balance since last week.

or

Client acknowledged improved sitting balance compared to previous week. However, he experienced dizziness after bending down while sitting and reported feeling "wobbly." Client also reported inability to feel anything with his hands.

Repeating the Client's History Rather Than Something the Client Communicated

Unless you are including the client's occupational profile in the "S" of an evaluation note, **there is no reason to repeat the client's history in the "S" when it is readily available in other sections of the client's health record.** In my own documentation course, we use several videos to practice documentation, and I often give the students a brief client history. Students frequently repeat something from the history in the "S" in their first attempts at SOAP notes. I tell them I want to see them **report something specific that the client said or otherwise communicated** during the session.

REFERENCES

American Occupational Therapy Association. (2020). Occupational therapy practice framework: Domain and process (4th ed.). *American Journal of Occupational Therapy, 74*(Suppl. 2), 7412410010. https://doi.org/10.5014.ajot.2020.74S2001

Kettenbach, G., & Schlomer, S. L. (2016). *Writing patient/client notes: Ensuring accuracy in documentation* (5th ed.). F. A. Davis.

WORKSHEET 8-1

Choosing a Subjective Statement

An occupational therapist wrote the following observation after treating Mrs. W, a 62-year-old woman who had a stroke 3 weeks ago:

O: *Client participated in 45-minute OT session in hospital room and rehab gym for UE activities to increase AROM in R shoulder, activity tolerance, UE strength, and dynamic standing balance, to increase independence in ADL tasks.*

__ADLs:__ In room, client was instructed in safety techniques and adaptive equipment use in toileting. Client needs B grab bars in bathroom for safe sit to stand transition during toileting. Client attempted to stand by pulling on walker and one grab bar. Client was educated on safety issues and the use of B grab bars; she verbalized understanding of recommendations.

__Performance Skills:__ Client required CGA for balance during sit to/from stand. To address activity tolerance, dynamic standing balance, and increase AROM in R shoulder, client moved canned goods from counter to cupboard for 5 minutes before needing a 2-minute seated rest break. After resting, she participated in activities to increase dynamic standing balance by pouring liquid from a pitcher while standing with CGA for balance. After a 1-minute seated rest, client continued activities to increase dynamic standing balance and safety by retrieving objects from floor using reacher while ambulating with wheeled walker and CGA.

__Client Factors:__ R shoulder abduction AROM < 90°. R shoulder abduction PROM WFL.

The treatment session included all of the following. Which would be best to use as the Subjective portion of the SOAP note?

1. *Client was very cooperative and engaged in social conversation throughout the tx session.*

2. *Client remarked that her grandson will be coming to visit later in the week, and that she will be very glad to see him.*

3. *Client reports that she feels "pretty good" today.*

4. *Client says she has difficulty moving R UE, although she does not know why it will not move. She reports, "It really doesn't hurt. It's just tight."*

5. *Nursing staff report client is incontinent at night.*

WORKSHEET 8-2

Writing Concise, Coherent "S" Statements

1. Mrs. P is recovering from a total hip replacement. During a treatment session, she makes the following statements:
   - *"I used that dressing stick and sock aid like you showed me to get dressed without bending down this morning."*
   - *"My hip doesn't hurt when I stand up or sit down, especially with that new toilet seat you got for me."*
   - *"It's getting easier for me to get dressed now."*
   - *"My daughter said they delivered all that bathroom equipment to her house yesterday."*

   Using these statements, write your own concise and organized version for the "S" portion of the SOAP note.

2. Tanner is a 14-year-old recently admitted to an inpatient adolescent psychiatric unit following an unsuccessful suicide attempt by overdose with his mother's sleeping pills. During a group session, he makes the following comments:
   - *"I have nothing to live for."*
   - *"I don't have any friends."*
   - *"My family would be better off without me anyway."*
   - *"The teachers at my school all hate me."*
   - *"Maybe next time I should do it right and just use a gun!"*

   Using these statements, write your own concise and organized version for the "S" portion of the SOAP note.

WORKSHEET 8-2 (CONTINUED)

Writing Concise, Coherent "S" Statements

3. Wesley is at a SNF recovering from a recent R BKA. He makes the following comments during an ADL session:
    - *Client told OT he has really bad arthritis in his R shoulder and L knee.*
    - *Client rates pain at the site of his R BKA as 8 out of 10.*
    - *Client said, "It hurts to stand on my left leg."*
    - *Client stated, "It [sliding board] needs to be moved further up on the seat."*
    - *When asked if he was okay after the transfer, he said, "I'm just tired."*
    - *Client stated, "I'm through," and requested help to get closer to the bed.*
    - *When client transferred to the bed for dressing tasks, he said, "This is the hardest part."*
    - *Client stated he prefers to transfer toward the R side so he can push off with his L LE and avoid bumping his R BKA on the tire-rim of the w/c.*

    Using these statements, write your own concise and organized version for the "S" portion of the SOAP note.

4. Kira is a 3-year-old girl who recently transitioned from early intervention services at home into an Early Childhood Special Education (ECSE) classroom through her local public school. During your initial evaluation, you make the following notes for the "S" of your evaluation report:
    - *Child cries for first 15 minutes after parent drop-off to classroom.*
    - *Child does not use intelligible words.*
    - *Child yells "Eee eee!" when she is happy about something.*
    - *Kira does not use her augmentative communication device unless prompted by classroom teacher.*
    - *Child attempts to get attention of peers by yanking on their clothing during play activities.*
    - *Kira points to desired object when given a choice between two toys.*
    - *Parent states, "I just don't know how I will be able to leave her. She's never been away from me for this long."*
    - *Teacher asks for recommendations about calming activities to help Kira prepare for seated work and circle time.*

    Using these statements, write your own concise and organized version for the "S" portion of the SOAP note.

Chapter 9

Writing the "O"—Objective

The next part of the note is the **Objective** section, where you will record all measurable, quantifiable, and observable data obtained during the session. In this section, you will present a picture of the skilled session you have provided. Once you start looking at things with your professional eyes, they can look quite different. Instead of seeing a child playing with a toy, now you begin to note the child's asymmetrical posture, lack of bilateral hand use, difficulty crossing midline, and immature grasp and pinch patterns. The trick in writing the "O" is knowing what kind of material to include and what to omit. At first your "O" may tend to be longer than that of an experienced therapist, but with time you will learn to write notes that are both complete and concise.

STEPS TO WRITING GOOD OBSERVATIONS

There are four important steps to remember when writing the "O" section of your SOAP note:
1. Begin with a statement about the length, setting, and purpose of the session.
2. Next, provide a brief overview of the key deficits that are affecting the client's performance.
3. Follow the opening statements with a summary of what you observed.
4. Be professional, concise, and specific.
   We will look at each of these steps more in depth in the following sections.

Step 1: Begin With a Statement About the Length, Setting, and Purpose of the Session

This opening statement gives the reader an introduction to the remainder of the "O" section. It explains the "where," "what," "how long," and "why" about the client's occupational therapy services. Your documentation is the basis for answering any questions about the services that a client received. In Chapter 3, you learned about Current Procedural Terminology (CPT) codes. Most CPT codes are based on the number of minutes of each specific service the client received. Although not all settings charge for occupational therapy by the number of minutes provided, it is still best practice to state the total length of the therapy session in the opening statement of the "O" section.

Gateley, C. A. *Documentation Manual for Occupational Therapy, Fifth Edition* (pp. 109-126). © 2024 Taylor & Francis Group.

Table 9-1

TYPES OF OCCUPATIONAL THERAPY INTERVENTIONS

TYPES OF OCCUPATIONAL THERAPY INTERVENTIONS	DESCRIPTION
Occupations and Activities	**Occupations** occur in context and are "broad and specific daily life events that are personalized and meaningful to the client" (AOTA, 2020, p. 59). **Activities** are "components of occupations that are objective and separate from the client's engagement or contexts. Activities as interventions are selected and designed to support the development of performance skills and performance patterns to enhance occupational engagement" (AOTA, 2020, p. 59).
Interventions to Support Occupations	This category includes physical agent modalities (PAMs), mechanical modalities (such as manual lymphatic drainage), orthotics and prosthetics, assistive technology and environmental modifications, wheeled mobility, and self-regulation. These interventions may be used "in preparation for or concurrently with occupations or activities" (AOTA, 2020, p. 59).
Education and Training	**Education** focuses on sharing knowledge and information, and the goal is enhanced understanding. **Training** focuses on helping the client or caregiver acquire concrete skills, and the goal is enhanced performance. Education and training are often used in conjunction with each other.
Advocacy	This category involves the practitioner and/or the client (self-advocacy) seeking and obtaining "resources to support health, well-being, and occupational participation" (AOTA, 2020, p. 61).
Group Interventions	This type of intervention involves two or more people working together to improve skills for occupational participation.
Virtual Interventions	This type of intervention includes telecommunication and information technology for service delivery. This category also includes the use of simulations.

Data source: American Occupational Therapy Association, 2020.

Sames (2015) suggested that practitioners move away from the passive terminology of the client was "seen" in occupational therapy, and instead state that the client "participated in" the occupational therapy session (p. 15). This distinction is important because funding sources want evidence that the client is actively participating in the habilitation or rehabilitation process. Additionally, funding sources want to know why your session was important. As occupational therapy practitioners, of course our focus is helping our clients improve occupational performance. One of the most effective ways to do that is by using occupations as interventions (American Occupational Therapy Association [AOTA], 2020). However, occupations are only one type of intervention identified in the *Occupational Therapy Practice Framework: Domain and Process, Fourth Edition* (OTPF-4). See Table 9-1 for a brief description of each category of intervention that you may need to describe in the "O" section of your SOAP note. Each of these will be explained in more depth in Chapter 12.

If you are utilizing occupations or activities (AOTA, 2020), use the following format for your opening statement:

Client participated in ____- minute OT session _____ for _____.
            #   **in what setting**   **occupation or activity**

For example:

- *Client participated in 45-minute OT session in rehab kitchen for meal preparation activity.*
- *Pt. participated in 30-minute OT session in rehab gym bathroom to practice tub bench transfer and simulated use of hand-held shower and long-handled sponge for increased safety and independence during bathing.*
- *Grayson participated in 30-minute OT session on school playground to facilitate social interaction skills with peers during outdoor recess.*
- *Consumer participated in 2-hour supervised outing involving use of public transportation system for community mobility.*
- *Zion participated in 60-minute OT session at brain injury day program to address financial management skills.*
- *Pt. participated in 30-minute OT session in hospital room for completion of morning bathing, dressing, and grooming routine using adaptive equipment.*
- *Anya participated in 45-minute OT session at home to facilitate development of play skills.*
- *Curt participated in 60-minute OT session at work hardening clinic to complete work simulation tasks while incorporating ergonomic principles.*

If your session focuses on interventions to support occupations (see Table 9-1), education and training, advocacy, group interventions, or virtual interventions as described in the *OTPF-4* (AOTA, 2020), then explain the relevance of your intervention to occupation in your opening statement:

Client participated in ____- minute OT session _____ for _____ for _____.
          #   **in what setting**   **intervention**   **what occupational gain**

For example:

- *Child participated in 30-minute OT session in outpatient clinic focusing on improving postural control and B UE coordination for increased success in play activities.*
- *Ashlyn participated in 30-minute OT session in classroom with focus on improving sensory processing and selective attention needed for engagement in classroom activities.*
- *Client participated in 30-minute OT session in hospital room for skilled instruction in energy conservation during IADLs.*
- *Carter participated in role-playing during 30-minute assertion group in outpatient mental health setting to explore alternative ways to meet his social needs.*
- *Client participated in 30-minute OT session in outpatient hand clinic to address R hand strengthening and scar desensitization in preparation for return to construction work.*
- *Shoneia participated in 30-minute OT session in therapy room to increase strength and dexterity needed to improve handwriting at school.*
- *Client participated in 30-minute OT session in hospital room with emphasis on caregiver training to assist client with ADLs and IADLs in preparation for return home.*
- *Marquez participated in 60-minute OT session in his home for training in use of switches to increase independence in activating electronic toys during play activities with family members.*
- *Navya participated in 45-minute OT group session to address self-advocacy skills needed for successful transition from high school to community college.*

- *Client participated in 45-minute OT session in hand therapy clinic for electrical stimulation and splint fabrication to facilitate return to administrative assistant work duties following carpal tunnel surgery.*
- *Pt. participated in 30-minute IADL session in rehab kitchen to increase dynamic standing balance and attention to L side for safety when ambulating around kitchen to prepare meals.*
- *Patient and caregivers participated in 15-minute bedside OT session for education on positioning client to prevent skin breakdown and further contractures.*
- *Client participated in 45-minute session in home to select positioning strategies to improve seated posture for mealtimes.*

It is essential that you show **the need for your skill as an occupational therapy practitioner** in this opening statement. So rather than simply saying, "*Client participated in 45-minute OT session at bedside for ADL training,*" you might instead say:

- *Client participated in 45-minute OT session at bedside for skilled instruction in compensatory dressing techniques.*
- *Resident participated in 45-minute OT session at bedside for skilled instruction in use of adaptive equipment to increase safety during ADL tasks.*
- *Veteran participated in 45-minute OT session at bedside to facilitate attention to L side during self-care activities.*

Step 2: Provide a Brief Overview of the Client's Key Deficits

In an ideal world, other team members and insurance reviewers would read every note that you have written to gain a full understanding of your client's deficits. Realistically, a therapist taking over your client might read only your most recent note to get an idea of what to do next, or an insurance reviewer might be reviewing certain dates of claims to determine whether payment for your services will be issued. The best documentation paints a picture of the client (Mayer & Poppert, 2019; Syzek, 2022). In other words, if there are multiple clients seated in a rehabilitation gym or working with therapists in an outpatient clinic, someone reading your documentation should be able to pick out your client based on what you have described about their appearance, function, or behavior. Provide a one- to two-sentence description of your client's key deficits. For example:

- *Client seated in w/c and presents with dense hemiparesis of L UE and L LE, edema of L hand, and severe L neglect.*
- *Client presents with R BKA with protective brace in place; B shoulder AROM limited to 90° due to severe osteoarthritis.*
- *Client supine in bed upon therapist's arrival; wound VAC in place on nonhealing incision from lumbar discectomy and fusion.*
- *Infant presents with R torticollis and positional plagiocephaly with molding helmet in place.*
- *Child exhibited significant sensory seeking behaviors throughout session; also demonstrated escape behaviors when therapist attempted to engage him in functional activities seated at desk.*
- *Client presents with severe B hip flexor, elbow flexor, and finger flexor contractures related to spastic quadriplegia CP.*
- *Client presents with decreased strength, sensation, and proprioception of L LE and L UE.*

Please note that experienced therapists often eliminate Step 2 because the client's deficits are well explained in Step 3. However, it has been my experience in years of teaching documentation that students and new practitioners often get so caught up in describing the details of **what** the client did that they fail to convey the details of **how** the client performed a functional activity. I may read a note and have no idea that a client had a CVA and has flaccid paralysis of one side.

Some of the examples in this chapter and throughout the book will have a distinct statement of the client's key deficits, while other examples will have that information embedded into the summary of what was observed. Either method is acceptable, as long as the reader has a clear picture of the client's functional performance. For clients who do not have distinct physical characteristics, your statement of deficits might summarize behaviors such as eye contact, sensory seeking or avoiding behaviors, response to frustration, engagement with peers, etc.

Step 3: Follow the Opening Statements With a Summary of the Client's Performance and Skilled Interventions

After you have established the setting and purpose and provided a very brief overview of the client's deficits, you will discuss the interventions that were completed and the client's response to those interventions. There are different ways that are acceptable in organizing the information of the "O":

- **Chronologically:** Discuss each treatment event in the order it occurred during the treatment session.
- **Categorically:** Organize the information according to categories. The categories you select will vary depending on the client and the purpose of the treatment session. You can refer to the *OTPF-4* (AOTA, 2020) for potential categories. For example, it may be helpful to organize the objective information by areas of occupation, client factors, or performance skills:
  - Areas of occupation (e.g., ADLs, IADLs, work, social participation)
    - Note how each of the performance skills and client factors observed affect performance in the relevant areas of occupation. Include assist levels and set-up required, adaptive equipment or techniques used, types of cueing provided, caregiver education, related positioning and mobility issues, and client's response to the treatment provided. Describe client's awareness of others in group, initiation of conversation, and interaction with peers in a group setting.
  - Client factors (e.g., ROM, strength, edema, sensation, attention, reflexes)
    - Provide specific measurements such as girth or volumetric measurements for edema, grip and pinch strength, PROM and AROM, type of sensation that is intact or impaired, length of attention to task, involuntary motor reflexes observed or elicited.
  - Performance skills (e.g., balance, coordination, cognition, behavior)
    - Note whether balance was static or dynamic. Consider whether the client leans in one direction, has rotated posture, or has uneven weight distribution. Describe hand dominance, types of prehension used, purposeful grasp and release, and gross motor versus fine motor ability. Report on orientation, task initiation, ability to stay on task, sequencing, judgment, and ability to follow directions. Document client's frustrations, lethargy, affect, compulsivity, anxiety, or demanding behaviors.

Let's take a look at a few examples of the different ways to organize the "O."

Chronologically

One way to organize the "O" section of your SOAP note is to document events in the order in which they happened during the treatment session. Think of this method as giving the reader a "play-by-play" of the session.

For example:

- *Client participated in anger management group for 45 minutes today to improve social interaction skills and ability to maintain employment. Initially required verbal prompting from nursing staff and security aides to attend group. Presented with disheveled appearance, kept arms crossed throughout group, and made limited eye contact with other group participants. He displayed displeasure at being asked to attend the group by using profanity. During the group, client related 2 instances in which individuals on the unit consistently bother him and discussed the way he usually handles the situation. Client receptive to peer feedback about alternative strategies.*

- *Client participated in 30-minute evaluation in OT clinic for assessment of low back pain and instruction in proper body mechanics during IADLs. Winced in pain when transitioning sit to stand and sits with weight shifted to L hip. Client demonstrated the way she usually removes items from the refrigerator, washes dishes, cleans the floors, and lifts. Client received instruction in proper body mechanics for completing IADL tasks including using a golfer's lift, squats, stepping toward the item she wished to retrieve, facing the load, and keeping it close to her body. Client demonstrated techniques with min verbal cues and was provided with educational handouts to remind her of correct positioning.*

Categorically

Many students and new practitioners initially prefer to arrange the "O" chronologically. However, the resulting "O" can be too lengthy. Alternatively, you may choose to organize your information into categories. There is no "right" list of categories to use. Use what makes sense for the individual client and situation. Ask yourself, "What was important about this session?" For example, suppose that today you saw a client in the kitchen for a cooking session in preparation for discharge. She plans to cook when she returns home, but you are not certain of her safety or her ability to perform all the steps of the activity from her wheelchair. You wonder if her strength, activity tolerance, and ability to use her involved hand and arm are sufficient for cooking, and you also want to assess her judgment and ability to problem solve. You therefore choose the following categories, using a combination of client factors and performance skills:

- Functional Mobility
- UE Range of Motion and Strength
- Hand Function and Strength
- Functional Endurance
- Cognition

Your note might look like this:

O: *Client participated in 1-hr. OT session in clinic kitchen for skilled instruction in compensatory techniques for safe and independent cooking. Pt. uses w/c for functional mobility due to decreased balance and decreased endurance following MS exacerbation.*

Functional Mobility: Min verbal cues required for maneuvering w/c in kitchen and appropriate placement of w/c to reach items. Min A needed to stabilize items while transporting them in lap and maneuvering w/c simultaneously.

UE ROM and Strength: WFL for reaching items in drawers, opening oven door, and putting dishes in the sink independently. UE strength adequate for opening refrigerator door and stirring batter independently. Min A required to open plastic storage container.

Hand Function and Strength: Adequate for unscrewing lids, cracking egg, opening muffin box, using baking tools, setting oven dial, and placing muffins in oven independently.

Functional Endurance: Client independently took a break after approximately 20 minutes of activity.

Cognition: Client correct on 3/3 questions about recipe instructions. Problem-solved repositioning her w/c independently 75% of tx time. Demonstrated good safety awareness in asking for assist to remove muffins from hot oven.

Let's look at another example of a note organized by category. Suppose you work in a school setting, and you have a child on your caseload who has been receiving occupational therapy services on a consultative basis one time monthly. During your monthly visit, you consult with the classroom teacher and the child's paraprofessional and observe the child in the classroom. Although the child's handwriting performance and ability to meet classroom expectations without disruptive behaviors appear much improved following previous occupational therapist recommendations, staff report a new concern that the child is displaying aggression toward classmates when going through the lunch line. You then observe the child during lunch and make recommendations to the teacher and paraprofessional. Your note might look like this:

O: *30-minute monthly consultation completed this date including observation of student in classroom and cafeteria, and recommendations to teacher and paraprofessional to help improve child's ability to participate effectively during lunch. Lucas calms to deep pressure sensory input but reacts aggressively to unexpected touch.*

Classroom Observations: Remained seated at desk to complete worksheet for 8 minutes while wearing weighted vest for increased proprioception. Now writes all letters of the alphabet legibly using adaptive paper with alternating highlighted lines and a rubber pencil grip.

Cafeteria Observations: Exhibited verbal and physical aggression (pushing) twice toward classmate when inadvertently bumped in line. Follow-up questioning with Lucas indicates that he perceives unexpected touch as "painful."

Staff Education: Classroom teacher and paraprofessional educated regarding sensory processing deficits related to unexpected touch. Recommendation made to either allow Lucas to leave classroom a few minutes early to go to cafeteria or to have him stand at the beginning or end of the line to reduce the chances of classmates bumping into him. Staff verbalized understanding and plan to implement suggestions tomorrow.

Students and new practitioners often have difficulty discerning what goes in "S" versus what goes in "O" when occupational therapy sessions are primarily verbal in nature. In behavioral health settings and cognitive rehabilitation, much of the evaluation and intervention involves talking with the client rather than performing physical tasks. However, it is still important to distinguish what is the **subjective** report of the client and what are the **objective** findings of the session that can be used for future comparison. Categorical organization of the "O" can be very helpful in this process. For example:

S: *Client states that she would like to live on her own. However, family expresses concern about teen's residual cognitive deficits from TBI 1 year ago. During challenging tasks presented during evaluation, client stated, "This is stupid. I don't know why my family is making me do this."*

O: *Client participated in 45-minute evaluation in outpatient setting to assess cognitive abilities in ADL and IADL performance. Throughout session, client had difficulty maintaining attention to task more than 2 minutes and frequently pushed activities away when she was unsuccessful.*

* **Memory:** Correctly named all members of immediate family. Repeated 3 of 3 words immediately; recalled only 1 of 3 words after 5-minutes of engaging in other tasks.*

* **Problem Solving:** During grocery list activity, client listed only 3 of 8 items required for recipe, despite reading it aloud correctly.*

* **Money Management:** Able to correctly count out specified amounts of money involving only one type of coin or bill (e.g., 10 cents, 50 cents, $5.00, $20.00). Max verbal cues to count out given amounts of money involving multiple coins and/or bills (e.g., 72 cents, $1.42, $17.87).*

* **Safety Awareness:** Identified 4 of 10 home safety hazards from pictures. Required mod verbal cues to identify potential solutions to those safety hazards.*

* **Medication Management:** Unable to state name, purpose, or correct dosage of her 3 daily medications. Required max verbal cues to fill weekly pill organizer based on directions on medication labels.*

* **Daily Routines:** Mod verbal cues needed to list the steps of her typical morning routine in preparation for going to school.*

Step 4: Be Professional, Concise, and Specific

The "O" section does not need to be written in complete sentences. Give complete information in the most concise form possible. Some details must be included. For example, ROM must be specified as active, passive, or assistive and must indicate the joint at which the movement occurred. You always must indicate R, L, or B when discussing UEs or LEs. You must specify the level of assistance that was provided. The following are some examples of wording change that make your documentation more professional, concise, and specific.

Rather than saying: *Resident flopped down onto the bed short of breath, closed her eyes, and moaned. Resident lay in bed with min A to position herself.*
You might say: *Resident fatigued and SOB following tx session; required min A for positioning in bed.*

Rather than saying: *Veteran had to use a trapeze to sit up.*
You might say: *Supine to sit using trapeze.*

Rather than saying: *Client put the board in place to make a sliding board transfer.*
You might say: *Client positioned sliding board for transfer.*

When documenting test results, it is helpful to put them into a chart like the following one, rather than burying them in narrative:

L Hand Sensation	
Hot/Cold	Intact
Sharp/Dull	Impaired over volar surface; intact over dorsal surface
Stereognosis	Absent

When you are first learning to write client observations, it is hard to decide what to include and what to leave out. At first, it is better to include too much data rather than taking a chance of omitting something important. As your observational skills become more refined, it will become second nature to include all important data, and the "O" section of your notes will begin to be more concise. Here is a client observation written by an inexperienced therapist. To include all of the necessary data, she wrote a note that was too wordy.

O: *Client participated in 30 minutes of R UE strengthening in outpatient therapy gym to prevent future shoulder dislocation. Client is no longer required to wear the brace she wore previously after surgery, but she still held R UE in a protective position close to her body against her abdomen when she was seated. Client maintained same R UE position when ambulating in gym. Client was asked to clasp hands together and raise arms above head x 30. Client was then instructed to cross her midline and touch her opposite shoulder with R UE x 30. Client required 6 rest periods for completion. Client completed tasks independently. Client was then introduced to weight and pulley system. Client was asked to specify how much weight she thought she could do. She responded with 5#. Client did 30 repetitions of the pulley system with 5# in shoulder flexion to strengthen her rotator cuff to decrease the probability of dislocating her shoulder again. After strengthening exercise, client had 3 heat packs applied to shoulder to decrease pain.*

A more experienced therapist might have written:

O: *Client participated in 30 minutes of R UE strengthening in outpatient therapy gym to prevent future shoulder dislocation. Client no longer required to wear post-surgical immobilizer but noted to hold R UE in guarded position across her body when seated and during functional mobility. Client completed the following:*

- *B clasped-hand shoulder flexion and extension x 30 repetitions*
- *Horizontal adduction R hand to L shoulder x 30 repetitions*
- *R shoulder flexion pulleys with 5# wt. x 30 repetitions*

3 hot packs applied to R shoulder to decrease pain after tx.

You will notice, however, that there is another problem with this note besides the fact that the original note is wordy. Despite the opening line of the "O," it sounds like a physical therapy note rather than an occupational therapy note. This note needs to have a functional component added in the opening statement of the "O" section. For example:

Client participated in 30 minutes of R UE strengthening in outpatient therapy gym to prevent future shoulder dislocation during ADLs, IADLs, work, and sports activities.

Adding in a statement from the client in the "S" about what she is unable to do with an injured rotator cuff and a statement in the "A" and/or "P" indicating functional problems/goals would suffice to make it a good occupational therapy note.

Notice that being more concise means knowing what information can be omitted without compromising the quality of the observation. It is possible to be too concise, omitting necessary information. For example, consider the following "O" from a community mental health center evaluation:

O: *Client evaluated in office using COPM. Client required 45 minutes to complete COPM. Client responded to directive questions regarding self-care, productivity, and leisure.*

This "O" does not provide much information. When additional information is added, we learn much more about the evaluation session with this client:

O: *Client participated in evaluation in office using the Canadian Occupational Performance Measure (COPM), which she completed in 45 minutes. She arrived 45 minutes late to the appointment, well-groomed and neatly dressed. Questions regarding productivity and leisure were answered with clear enunciation and animated tone, but questions about self-care (particularly those about scar management) were declined or given short answers with sad tone and no eye contact. Client frequently touched scars on trunk during the evaluation.*

TIPS FOR MAKING YOUR DOCUMENTATION SOUND MORE PROFESSIONAL

There are several ways to make your documentation sound professional. The following are some tips to remember when writing your note:

- Focus on occupation.
- Focus on the client's response to the treatment provided rather than on what the therapist did.
- Write from the client's point of view, leaving yourself out.
- Be specific about assist levels.
- Avoid making a list of actions and assist levels.
- De-emphasize the treatment media.
- Make it clear that you were not just a passive observer in the session.
- Avoid judging the client.
- Use only standard abbreviations.

Let's look at some examples of each of these recommendations.

Focus on Occupation

Be sure that occupation is integral to the note. In a treatment session devoted to self-care activities, function is obvious. However, in a session devoted to addressing client factors such as strength or endurance, in a session where modalities are used, or in a co-treatment session, function must be addressed separately to justify **skilled** occupational therapy. For example, although the following note is an observation of a session that was devoted to performance components, it contains a statement about the functional intent of the exercises.

O: *Veteran participated in 30-minute OT session in room for AROM and strengthening of L UE to regain ability to dress self. L UE AROM 90° with min verbal cues to avoid trunk substitution. Completed self-ROM exercises from standing and seated position with SBA for balance and verbal instructions to correct errors. Theraputty exercises x 5 minutes using L hand with minimal resistance putty to improve strength for ability to manipulate clothing fasteners.*

Focus on the Client's Response to the Treatment Provided

Rather than saying: *Client was reminded about hip precautions.*
You might say: *Client required 4 verbal cues for correct hip alignment when donning shoes.*

Rather than saying: *Client was asked orientation questions pertaining to the time of day.*
You might say: *Client unable to correctly identify time when cued to look at watch.*

Rather than saying: *Client reminded to relax.*
You might say: *UE tone moderately increased but decreases with tactile cue for repositioning.*

Rather than saying: *Child was given a puzzle to play with.*
You might say: *Child placed simple shapes into inset puzzle with min A to reposition pieces.*

Write From the Client's Point of View

The focus of good professional writing is always on the client. Turn your sentences around so that the client is the subject of your sentence.

Rather than saying: *The OT put the client's shoes on for him.*
You might say: *Client required dep A to don shoes.*

Rather than saying: *OT instructed the client and family in energy conservation techniques.*
You might say: *Following skilled instruction, client and family incorporated energy conservation techniques into ADL activities with min verbal cues.*

Be Specific About Assist Levels

When documenting assist levels, be sure to note **what part of the activity** the client needed physical assistance or verbal cues to perform. For example:

- *Veteran doffed night garment with min A **to untie strings in back**.*
- *Child needed HOH assist **for accuracy in staying on line** when cutting with scissors.*
- *Client required verbal cues **to sit down** for safety when doffing socks.*
- *Consumer able to follow bus schedule with min verbal cues **to identify correct time**.*
- *Resident completed supine to sit in bed with min verbal cues **to roll to R side**.*
- *When transitioning stand to sit using a standard walker, pt. required min tactile and verbal cues **to bring walker completely back to w/c and reach back for armrest before sitting**.*
- *Infant able to roll supine to prone with min tactile cues **to initiate movement**.*
- *Pt. required 5 verbal cues **for sequencing of tasks** during morning ADL routine.*
- *Client required mod A **to follow total hip precautions** while washing lower legs and feet with long-handled sponge.*
- *Client completed sit to stand during dressing with mod A **for balance and to maintain TTWB precautions**.*

Avoid Making a List of Actions and Assist Levels

In trying to be concise, sometimes inexperienced therapists make the mistake of writing an "O" that contains only a list of actions with assist levels. Simply writing a list of activities or assist levels does not show the skilled occupational therapy being provided and is an incorrect method for the "O." Consider this occupational therapist's observation:

O: *Client participated in 1-hr. OT session in shower room to increase activity tolerance and improve balance during showering. Client presents with SOB upon exertion and ataxic movements of trunk and all extremities. Client was shown a smaller shower that simulated her home shower, to prepare for discharge in 1 week.*

Client alert and oriented x 4.

Client required verbal cues for safety to sit in w/c rather than standing to doff socks and to dry off B LEs; min physical assist also needed to complete both tasks.

Client spontaneously rinsed soap off hands before gripping grab bar while showering.

Client used walker going to and coming from shower room.

Client tolerated standing with SBA during entire shower.

Client instructed in home showering.

Now let's take a look at the same observation, rewritten in a more useful format:

O: *Client participated in 1-hr. OT session in shower room to improve activity tolerance and balance during showering. Client presents with ataxic movements of trunk and all extremities following cerebellar CVA. Client completed shower in smaller shower stall that simulates her home shower to prepare her for safe and independent showering after discharge in 1 week.*

Functional Balance and Mobility: *Pt. ambulated to/from shower room and completed standing portion of dressing/undressing with supervision using standard walker for stability. Stood for 5-minute shower with SBA to prevent slipping on wet surface with no SOB.*

Cognition: *Client oriented x 4.*

ADLs: *Min A required to doff socks and dry B LEs, as well as verbal cues to sit rather than stand during these tasks to reduce fall risk. Independently rinsed soap off hands prior to gripping grab bar during shower. SBA for all shower tasks in standing. Client received skilled instruction in safe technique to use in her single shower stall, and recommendations provided re: grab bar placement. Client voiced understanding of all recommendations.*

De-Emphasize the Treatment Media

To improve a client's performance skills, you may use various treatment media, such as equipment or activities that will help the client reach functional goals. However, when documenting your observations of these treatment sessions, you should de-emphasize the media used and focus instead on the performance skills needed for function. For example, an inexperienced therapist might write the following:

Client worked on placing pegs into a pegboard.

This statement may accurately describe what a casual observer would see, but as a trained professional, you need to look beyond the treatment media used and explain what the client was really accomplishing. The media used here are pegs and a pegboard, but what is the performance skill? Placing pegs into a pegboard is not a skill this client needs to be able to care for herself. However, the performance skills she practices during this activity may well be crucial to achieving independence. Suppose the therapist had written:

Client worked on tripod pinch using pegs and a pegboard.

Notice that in this example the therapist did not simply add the performance skill to the statement "*Client worked on placing pegs into pegboard to increase tripod pinch,*" but actually turned the sentence around so that the tripod pinch received the emphasis, and the media was mentioned only for clarification. Suppose the therapist had written:

Client demonstrated multiple repetitions of tripod pinch to be able to grasp objects needed for ADL tasks.

In this case mention of the media becomes optional. They could also have written:

Client demonstrated multiple repetitions of tripod pinch using pegs and a pegboard to be able to grasp objects needed for ADL tasks.

Which of the three preceding examples do you think best describes the skilled instruction that is occurring in this treatment session? This may seem like a minor distinction, but it is important in demonstrating the need for skilled occupational therapy and the emphasis on functional outcomes in therapy. **One of the most common errors among inexperienced occupational therapy practitioners is focusing on the media used rather than on the performance skill and area of occupation that are being improved by use of the media.** Consider this occupational therapist's observation:

O: *Client participated in 30-minute OT session at outpatient rehab clinic for standing balance activities. Client relies on wheeled walker for functional mobility and demonstrates decreased static and dynamic standing balance without walker for support. Client used R UE to hit balloon and was able to reach to R and L sides approximately 7 out of 10 tries. Activity was continued for 3 minutes. Client requested rest break and sat for 30 seconds. Client then stood with walker with mod A and hit balloon with L UE for 3 minutes. Client was able to hit balloon approximately 6 out of 10 times and spontaneously switched to R hand x 2 when balloon was to her far right. Client sat for another break and to switch activities. Client stood with CGA to toss beanbags with R hand for 4 minutes. Client scored 240 points with R hand by throwing beanbags at target. Once all beanbags were thrown, client sat for a 30-second break. Client stood with CGA for balance to toss beanbags with L hand for 3 minutes, 30 seconds. Client scored 150 points with L hand by throwing beanbags at scoring target. Once all beanbags were thrown, client sat and session was ended.*

When this note is rewritten to focus on the performance skills, notice the difference in professionalism and the way the note reads:

O: *Client participated in 30-minute OT session at outpatient rehab clinic to address standing balance needed for ADL and IADL tasks. Client uses wheeled walker for functional mobility and decreased static and dynamic standing balance. Client stood with walker with mod A for dynamic standing balance needed for independent showering, using a balloon toss activity. Client held walker with L hand and used R UE to reach to both R and L sides approximately 7/10 attempts. Client sustained activity for 3 minutes continuously before requiring a 30-second seated rest break. Client completed additional 3 minutes of continuous standing with walker with mod A for weight shifting and balance while engaged in UE activity. Client able to reach to R and L sides for moving object approximately 6/10 times. Client spontaneously weight-shifted 2 times to reach object. Additional 30-second seated rest required before next activity. Client completed 2 additional trials of continuous dynamic standing balance during beanbag toss activity with CGA using wheeled walker, for 4 minutes and 3.5 minutes with 30-second seated rest in between.*

Make It Clear That You Were Not Just a Passive Observer in the Session

This will be a critical factor in reimbursement. Although you should write from the client's point of view as described previously, **we do not get paid to watch a client do something**. To show that the skill of an occupational therapy practitioner is needed, you must be actively involved in intervention, such as evaluating or modifying the activity, or it will be considered unskilled.

| Rather than saying: | *Client compensated for shoulder flexion by leaning forward with entire body during prehension activities.* |
| You might say: | *Client required skilled facilitation to avoid compensation at the shoulder during prehension activities.* |

| Rather than saying: | *Client performed home exercise program.* |
| You might say: | *Client's performance of home exercise program was assessed for accurate movement patterns and modified to accommodate for progress.* |

Avoid Judging the Client

| Rather than saying: | *Client was cooperative.* |
| You might say: | *Client followed 3-step directions and sequence without redirection.* |

When you are working with a client who is difficult or whose opinions or behavior you do not agree with, it is easy to judge the client and to reflect your judgments in your observation. The following is a note written by a student who was in a difficult situation. The client "went off" on the student, refusing a sponge bath, lying about having already bathed, throwing her washcloth across the room so the student would have to pick it up, refusing to put on her slacks, and announcing that therapy was "stupid." In spite of all this, the student wrote an observation that was nonjudgmental of the client:

Client required max encouragement to participate in 30-minute therapy session this am. Client independent with transfers and ambulation during ADLs. Client completed simulated bathing activity using long-handled sponge standing at sink with supervision. Client retrieved washcloth from floor independently using a reacher. Client donned socks with sock aid and shoes with shoehorn with supervision. Client declined to don slacks.

Use Only Standard Abbreviations

You may only use the abbreviations **approved by your facility**. Please note that the list of abbreviations provided in Chapter 5 is for purposes of learning to document using the exercises in this workbook. Do not use any other abbreviations, even if they seem common to you. This is particularly important as many students have grown up in an age where abbreviations are commonly used in texting and social media communications. If you try to read a note containing abbreviations with which you are unfamiliar, you will understand instantly how important this is.

Remember that your documentation must be read by those unfamiliar with the "shorthand" that health professionals use so freely. Suppose your chart is being read by someone who is from a different background, such as an insurance reviewer, attorney, or committee from a local community organization that is considering funding a piece of equipment for your client. To make your note understandable to all readers, be judicious in applying abbreviations and keep them very standard. A good rule to follow: **When in doubt, write it out!**

REFERENCES

American Occupational Therapy Association. (2020). Occupational therapy practice framework: Domain and process (4th ed.). *American Journal of Occupational Therapy, 74*(Suppl. 2), 7412410010. https://doi.org/10.5014.ajot.2020.74S2001

Mayer, S., & Poppert, N. (2019, March 7). *Paint a picture with your documentation.* The Note Ninjas. https://thenoteninjas.com/

Sames, K. (2015). *Documenting occupational therapy practice* (3rd ed.). Prentice Hall.

Syzek, T. (2022). *Paint a picture: EMR documentation of appearance and activity.* The Sullivan Group. https://thesullivangroup.com/

WORKSHEET 9-1

Using Categories

Consider the following chronological observation:

O: *Child participated in 60-minute OT session at day care to address feeding skills and reach/grasp/release during play. Child demonstrated strong R hand preference, flexed position of L UE, and did not spontaneously initiate use of L UE as a functional assist during self-care or play. With min A for facilitation of extension at elbow, child demonstrated ability to use L UE to reach, grasp, and release 5 objects with 1-2 verbal cues per object and restriction of R UE movement. Child was able to feed self independently with ~50% spillage, but demonstrated significant limitations in chewing action after ~3 rotary chews and swallowing ~90% of food without chewing. Child required verbal cues throughout session to maintain attention to task. Child wore soft spica thumb splint for entire session.*

How would you divide this information into categories to make it easier to read? Choose three to four categories and redistribute the information above into the categories you have chosen.

WORKSHEET 9-2

Being More Concise

Revise the following note to be complete but more concise.

O: *Pt. participated in 60-minute OT session bedside to complete morning ADL routine. Pt. presented with decreased standing balance and safety awareness. Pt. ambulated ~36 inches to shower with SBA for safety. Pt. instructed to complete shower while sitting. Pt. performed shower with SBA to manage IV line. Pt. able to wash upper and lower body with SBA and dry entire body with SBA after completing shower. Pt. required ~20 minutes to complete shower. Pt. then ambulated ~36 inches to chair and sat. Pt. needed verbal cues to remain seated while donning underwear and pants. Pt. able to dress upper and lower body with set-up after verbal cues to sit for safety. Pt. demonstrated good sitting balance but needed SBA for standing balance. Following shower, client was assisted back to bed for a nap.*

WORKSHEET 9-3

Writing Good Opening Lines

Rewrite the following opening statements to show how your skill as an occupational therapist is important in each situation and to indicate the primary deficits addressed in the session.

1. *Client seen in room for 45 minutes for self-care activities.*
   Additional information: Client is on total hip precautions, which raises safety concerns during mobility, especially during toilet transfer. Adaptive equipment is available if needed. Client has underlying memory deficits.

2. *Client seen at sheltered workshop for 1 hr. to work on job skills.*
   Additional information: Client has deficits in sequencing tasks, which decreases his ability to work independently. Bilateral coordination problems interfere with client completing essential job function of opening/closing boxes. Sensory registration deficits contribute to client's high distractibility during task completion.

3. *Client seen bedside for 30 minutes for morning dressing.*
   Additional information: Deficits include decreased balance and decreased bilateral motor control of UEs that limit ability to safely complete ADL activities and use a manual w/c for mobility during ADLs.

4. *Client seen in kitchen for 1 hr. to work on independence in cooking.*
   Additional information: Client's problems include decreased dynamic standing balance and inattention of affected L UE, which raise safety concerns.

WORKSHEET 9-4

Being Specific About Assist Levels

When noting assist levels in your observation, it is not enough to state just the level of assistance required. You also need to describe the part of the task that required assistance. For example:

- *Resident donned pants with min A **to pull up over hips**.*
- *Client propelled w/c from room to OT clinic but required verbal cues **to avoid running into other clients**.*

Do each of the following statements include the specific part of the task requiring assistance?

_____ *Child required HOH A to stay in the lines when following path with crayon.*

_____ *Client needed mod verbal cues to participate in discussion during life skills group.*

_____ *Resident needed min A to don socks due to pain.*

_____ *Client required max A x 2 bed to bedside commode and bed to w/c transfers; dependent for toileting.*

Rewrite the statements below to provide a part of the task that required assistance. Since you have not seen the client, you cannot know what part really required assistance. In professional practice, making things up is fraud, so please keep in mind that the client you are about to imagine is just an exercise in creativity. For this exercise, you will create a client in your mind and imagine that client doing the task described. As you watch your client in your mind, notice what parts of the task required assistance, and modify the sentences below accordingly.

1. *Client completed supine to sit with min A; bed to w/c with mod A.*

2. *Client required SBA in transferring w/c to/from toilet.*

3. *Client retrieved garments from low drawers with min A.*

4. *Client required max A to brush hair.*

5. *Client completed dressing, toileting, and hygiene with min A.*

WORKSHEET 9-5

De-Emphasizing the Treatment Media

Rewrite the following statements to emphasize the skilled occupational therapy that is actually occurring in the treatment session.

1. *Client played catch using B UEs to facilitate grasp and release patterns.*

2. *Resident put dirt into pot to halfway point, added seedling, and filled remainder of pot with dirt transferred by cup. Resident completed 3 more pots while standing 8 minutes before requiring a 5-minute rest. Resident resumed standing position to water completed pots for approximately 5 minutes.*

3. *Client painted some sun catchers in crafts group to be able to see that she could do something successfully.*

4. *Pt. cut out magazine pictures that indicated her emotions and glued them onto construction paper.*

5. *Child picked up beans with tweezers and placed them in pill bottle to work on tripod grasp in preparation for handwriting.*

WORKSHEET 9-6

Revising the "O"

Rather than rewriting this note to improve it, just write down at least five suggestions for what it needs to make it better.

O: **Toilet Transfers:**   *max A*

  Toileting: *max A due to inability to support self with L arm and to dress*

  UE Dressing: *min A, verbal cues, set-up, independent in pulling shirt over head*

  LE Dressing: *min A pants to hips; max A pants to waist*

  Dons L shoe independently with elastic laces; dons R shoe independently with elastic laces

  R Hand Status: *R fingers: small spasticity (index finger greatest amount)*

  Thumb: CMC joint painful in abd and flex

  R wrist: flaccid

Suggestions for improvement:

-

-

-

-

-

Chapter 10

Writing the "A"—Assessment

The third section of the note is the **Assessment**, which contains the therapist's appraisal of the client's occupational performance limitations, progress, and expected benefit from occupational therapy services. In the Assessment section of the note, you will use your professional reasoning to **interpret the meaning** of the data you have presented in the "S" and "O" sections. You will describe what it means in your professional judgment and its potential impact on the client's ability to engage in meaningful occupations. In the Assessment section of your note, you will note the three Ps:

- Problems
- Progress
- Potential

You might also point out inconsistencies, discuss psychosocial components, or present some reason that something was not done as planned. Finally, the Assessment section is where you justify continuation of occupational therapy services.

The Assessment is the "heart" of your note. If you could write only six lines, the Assessment section of your note would contain the six lines you would choose. This is the section that demonstrates your professional reasoning as an occupational therapy practitioner. Anything you see a client do is an observation and goes in the "O" section of your SOAP note. **The meaning of that observation, in terms of your client's occupational performance, is your assessment** and becomes the "A" section of your SOAP note.

ASSESSING THE DATA

To assess the data, go through the information presented in the "S" and the "O" sentence by sentence, and ask what the information means for the client's ability to engage in meaningful occupation. Note the problems, progress, and potential for rehabilitation you see.

Gateley, C. A. *Documentation Manual for Occupational Therapy, Fifth Edition* (pp. 127-146). © 2024 Taylor & Francis Group.

Problems

Some notes will show progress and/or potential for improvement and some will not, but almost all notes will show problem areas. The problem areas are what justify continued occupational therapy services. Problems may include the following:

- **Safety risks:**
  - *Attempt to stand without locking w/c brakes raises safety concerns for falls during ADL transfers.*
  - *Poor problem solving when using the stove raises safety concerns for staying home alone.*
  - *Limited coping strategies for dealing with stress raise concerns for continuing to demonstrate self-destructive behaviors.*
- **Inconsistencies between client report and objective findings:**
  - *Client's lack of insight regarding left-side neglect presents safety risks to return home alone.*
  - *Motor planning deficits create a barrier to ADL performance despite client's willingness to complete ADLs.*
  - *Decreased behavioral control when reward incentives are unavailable limit client's ability to progress toward stated goal of next level of responsibility at halfway house.*
- **Contributing factors that can be influenced by occupational therapist intervention:**
  - *Left-side weakness interferes with standing balance while showering.*
  - *Left-side neglect necessitates verbal cues to attend to left side during ADL tasks.*
  - *Deficits in cognitive processing create a need for constant verbal cues to perform kitchen tasks safely.*

The most common problem area that you will be assessing is the impact of a contributing factor on the ability to engage in occupation. When therapists are first learning to write SOAP notes, they may find it difficult to distinguish observations from assessments. In Chapter 6, you learned a formula for writing functional problem statements that makes the limiting factor the subject of the sentence, followed by how that factor affects the client's ability to engage in an area of occupation. This formula is the basis for your problem statements in the "A" of a SOAP note:

_____ results in (or limits) _____.
          Contributing factor/s   **area of occupation affected**

This is not the only way to write an assessment of problem areas, but the formula is a good one when you are first learning to help you refrain from simply repeating an objective statement. As you identify each contributing factor (e.g., limited AROM, sequencing deficits, unstable balance), ask yourself, **"So what?"** Is the area of difficulty you observed today an indicator of problems the client may have in other areas of occupation? For example, is the decreased AROM you observed today in grooming also a problem in other ADL activities? Will the client's inability to count change correctly impact other money management tasks? Do the deficits you observed today put the client's safety at risk? The answer to your "So what?" question is your **assessment** of the situation.

You may want to refer back to Chapters 1 and 6 to review the aspects of occupational therapy's **domain** as described in the *Occupational Therapy Practice Framework: Domain and Process, Fourth Edition* (*OTPF-4*; American Occupational Therapy Association [AOTA], 2020b) and to identify contributing factors related to client factors, performance skills, performance patterns, and contexts. In addition to the potential contributing factors from these *OTPF-4* categories, you should also consider **activity and occupation demands** that affect a client's participation in occupation. According to the *OTPF-4*, "*Activity demands* are what is typically required to carry out the activity regardless of client and context. *Occupation demands* are what is required by the specific client … to carry out an occupation" (AOTA, 2020b, p. 57). Activity and occupation demands can act as barriers to occupational participation. See Table 10-1 for examples of problem statements based on components from the *OTPF-4*.

Table 10-1

EXAMPLES OF PROBLEM STATEMENTS

OTPF-4 COMPONENT	PROBLEM STATEMENT EXAMPLES
Client Factors: Values, beliefs, and spirituality; body functions; body structures	• *Deficits in UE strength and activity tolerance* limit client's ability to complete basic self-care tasks. • *Lack of forearm supination and active elbow flexion against gravity* interfere with child's ability to perform age-appropriate developmental play activities. • *Pain in L shoulder* limits client's ability to carry out child care and household management tasks.
Performance Skills: Motor skills, process skills, social interaction skills	• *Deficits in attention span* make IADLs difficult and potentially unsafe. • *Inability to manage anger* results in difficulty finding work and establishing successful intimate relationships. • *Decreased fine motor coordination* affects child's ability to write name.
Performance Patterns: Habits, routines, roles, rituals	• *Perseveration with lining up toys* limits child's social interaction with peers at school. • *Client's gambling habits* result in lack of financial resources to pay monthly rent. • *Client's routine of watching television for 12+ hours daily* limits performance of household management tasks.
Contexts: Environmental factors, personal factors	• *Extraneous noises in classroom* limit child's ability to attend to written work. • *Narrow doorways in home* inhibit client's ability to access the bathroom from w/c level for toileting and bathing. • *Lack of financial resources* affects client's ability to purchase clothing necessary to obtain employment.
Activity and Occupation Demands: Objects used and their properties, space demands, social demands, sequencing and timing demands, required actions and performance skills, required body functions, required body structures	• *Need for assistance during multi-step sequences* limits independence with self-catheterization. • *One-handedness following traumatic amputation of R hand* limits ability to tie shoes. • *Inability to tolerate close proximity of classmates during circle time* interferes with child's ability to participate in group classroom activities.

Data source: American Occupational Therapy Association, 2020b.

The Assessment section is NOT the place to introduce new contributing factors. **Do not mention a new contributing factor in the "A" that has not been discussed in the "S" or "O."** If you find yourself wanting to make a statement in the "A" that is not supported by the data in your "S" or "O," ask yourself if you need to go back and add an important client/caregiver statement in the "S" or observation in the "O."

Although you should not introduce new contributing factors in the Assessment, **the "A" is the perfect place to discuss other areas of occupation that may be affected by the contributing factors you have identified**. This is an excellent way to show your professional reasoning. For example, if in your session you saw that a client's poor trunk balance and left side weakness impacted his ability to complete grooming tasks at the edge of the bed, you can use your professional reasoning to infer that those same contributing factors will also impact dressing, toileting, and other ADLs.

Progress

Think about whether the occupational therapy treatment being provided is effective. What improvements have you observed? **This may be progress that you observe within a single session or progress as compared to a previous session.** For example:

- *Weighted utensils decrease intention tremors by ~50% when eating.*
- *Brady's ability to prepare for outing, respect rules by following directions, interact socially with staff, and control his behavior indicate progress toward community re-entry.*
- *10-degree increase in AROM in L elbow this week allows client to don shirt with min A.*
- *Infant's ability to maintain seated position indicates improved postural control needed for engagement in play activities.*
- *Patient's ability to attend to ADL tasks for 3 minutes today demonstrates improvement from baseline attention span of 60 seconds.*
- *Client's spontaneous participation in group discussion shows good progress in developing social interaction skills.*
- *Improved prehension skills now enable child to zip coat.*

Sometimes progress is indicated by stating that previous goals have been met or modified:
- *STG #2 (buttoning ½-inch buttons x 3 on shirt) met this week.*
- *STG #3 upgraded to "complete grooming tasks, standing for at least 3 minutes at sink."*
- *STG #4 changed to "attend at least 2 group sessions daily."*

Sometimes you may need to explain why there has been a lack of progress:
- *Acute infection has resulted in patient being more dependent in ADL tasks this week.*
- *Client's need to care for terminally ill spouse has resulted in sporadic attendance of therapy sessions this month.*
- *Child's progress toward handwriting goals has been limited due to recent R radius fracture and casting of dominant R UE.*
- *Anesthesia from medical procedure earlier today impaired client's ability to remain alert during OT session.*

Potential

In addition to problems and progress, the "A" section is also where you should comment on the client's **potential** for future improvements in functional performance.
- *Ability to understand instructions and desire to return to living independently indicate good potential to return home alone at senior apartment complex.*
- *Patient's ability to recall and demonstrate 3/3 hip precautions shows good potential to adhere to hip precautions in ADLs and IADLs after discharge.*
- *Patient's intact cognitive skills indicate good potential for learning compensatory strategies for ADLs and IADLs.*
- *Willingness to consider alternative stress management strategies indicates good potential for improved success in work and part-time college enrollment.*

- *Participation in groups, including not interrupting, asking questions appropriately, and sharing experiences, indicates good potential to form successful social relationships.*
- *Student's progress in ability to use scissors indicates good potential to meet annual IEP goals.*
- *Consistent participation in therapy this week indicates good potential to tolerate and benefit from 3 hours of therapy daily for inpatient rehabilitation stay to improve functional independence prior to return home with family.*
- *Reduced verbal cueing to scan L environment during meals indicates good potential for greater independence in self-feeding.*

Note that in the examples of progress and potential statements, you do not see "Client demonstrated," "Client performed," or any Client + Verb combination to start the sentence. As a general rule, **Client + Verb is an observation statement that goes in the "O" section of your note**. If you find yourself using a Client + Verb combination in the "A" section, instead take the observation that came immediately after Client + Verb, and make that the subject of the sentence for your progress statement or potential statement, like the formula you used for problem statements:

_____ indicates _____
      Observation of improved performance   **potential and/or progress**

Rather than say: *Client demonstrated improved ability to grasp ADL items with affected L hand.*
Rearrange to say: *Improved ability to grasp ADL items with affected L hand indicates progress toward independent dressing.*

Rather than say: *Child held scissors in supinated position with fewer tactile cues this session.*
Rearrange to say: *Ability to use supinated grasp on scissors with fewer cues indicates good potential for greater independence and success with classroom craft activities.*

JUSTIFYING CONTINUATION OF OCCUPATIONAL THERAPY SERVICES

After you have documented the client's problems, progress, and potential, you should **end the "A" section of your note with a justification for continued occupational therapy services**. One very useful way of justifying continued occupational therapy treatment for your client is to end the "A" with the statement "*Client would benefit from …*" and complete the sentence with a justification of continued treatment that requires the skill of an occupational therapy practitioner. Not every therapist ends the "A" with this method, but for purposes of learning, we will use this method. This helps to make certain that justification for continued treatment is present in the note and is a good method for setting up the plan. Here are some examples:

- *Resident would benefit from environmental cues to orient him to the environment and skilled training to navigate w/c in room during set-up of dressing tasks.*
- *Consumer would benefit from instruction in problem-solving and anger management techniques needed for successful personal and social relationships.*
- *Client would benefit from further instruction in IADL tasks along with visual perceptual and problem-solving activities to increase safety.*
- *Veteran would benefit from activities that encourage trunk rotation to facilitate ADL transfers and dressing skills.*
- *Consumer would benefit from continued mental health education including recognition of his delusions, need for medication, how it can help him, and why it is essential to his recovery.*
- *Client would benefit from instruction in use of reacher, sock aid, and long-handled shoehorn to aid in LE dressing.*
- *Resident would benefit from skilled instruction in sequencing of tasks to increase safety while performing ADL tasks.*
- *Client would benefit from instruction in energy conservation techniques to perform meal preparation and clean-up.*
- *Child would benefit from continued use of modalities that decrease tactile defensiveness as well as establishment of home program for parents to carry out with child.*
- *Infant would benefit from therapeutic exercises on therapy ball to encourage trunk extension needed for postural control during play activities.*

A common mistake by students and new practitioners when learning to write the "A" is making the vague statement that the client would benefit from more of the same techniques that have already been provided without specifying the targeted outcome. **Don't just say the client needs more of the <u>same</u> intervention.** This is particularly important with the increased level of scrutiny by third-party payers as they review claims to determine if occupational therapy services will be reimbursed. **Ask yourself <u>what else</u> the client needs to work on.**

For example, imagine you evaluated a patient in intensive care unit for her very first occupational therapy session after surgery to remove a brain tumor, and the only thing she did during that session was transfer from supine to sit, sit edge of bed, and wash her face before returning to supine. It would not make sense to simply say, *"Pt. would benefit from continued grooming tasks seated EOB."* That suggests to whomever is reading your note that the only thing you plan to do with her in all future sessions is grooming tasks seated edge of bed.

Think about the rest of her hospital stay. What else might you address to make a discharge recommendation from acute care? A better justification statement would read, *"Pt. would benefit from continued OT for neuro re-education and skilled training in dressing, toileting, and other basic self-care activities."*

Make sure that you are **specific** with your description of what the client would benefit from and why it is important:

Too vague: *Client would benefit from continued ADL training.*
Better: *Client would benefit from instruction in use of tub bench and hand-held shower to increase safety during bathing.*

Too vague: *Student would benefit from continued visual perceptual activities.*
Better: *Student would benefit from visual memory activities to improve ability to copy math problems from board to paper.*

Too vague: *Consumer would benefit from continued OT services at behavioral health day program.*
Better: *Consumer would benefit from participation in OT groups focused on anger management and coping strategies to improve social participation and work behaviors.*

When you justify the need for continued occupational therapy services, you need to document the reason the service must be provided by an occupational therapist or occupational therapy assistant rather than by another professional or by nonprofessional personnel. The *Scope of Practice* (AOTA, 2021b), *Guidelines for Supervision, Roles, and Responsibilities During the Delivery of Occupational Therapy Services* (AOTA, 2020a), and *Definition of Occupational Therapy Practice for the AOTA Model Practice Act* (2021a) all outline the services that require an occupational therapy practitioner.

> Occupational therapists are responsible for all aspects of occupational therapy service delivery and are accountable for the safety and effectiveness of the occupational therapy services and service delivery process … Occupational therapy assistants deliver occupational therapy services within a supervisory relationship and in partnership with occupational therapists. (AOTA, 2020a, pp. 1-2)

Occupational therapists provide the following services (AOTA, 2020a):
- Directing the evaluation process, interpreting data, defining problems, determining goals, and developing intervention plans.
- Reviewing the effectiveness of the intervention and determining if the intervention plan should be continued, modified, or discontinued.

Within the provisions of each state practice act, occupational therapists *and* occupational therapy assistants are qualified to implement the following types of **skilled interventions to promote or enhance safety and occupational performance** (AOTA, 2021a, 2021b):
- Therapeutic use of occupations and activities
- Training in ADLs, IADLs, health management, and skills needed for work, school, and community engagement
- Remediation and compensation of physical, cognitive, sensory-perceptual, emotional regulation, pain management, developmental, motor planning, and behavioral skills
- Education and training of individuals, groups, and populations

- Services related to care coordination, case management, and transition
- Consultative services
- Virtual interventions including simulations and telehealth
- Modification of contexts and adaptation of processes
- Fabricating, fitting, and/or training in use of orthotics, prosthetics, and other assistive technology and adaptive devices
- Fitting and training in seating, positioning, and functional mobility related to occupational performance
- Exercises to improve client factors related to occupational participation, such as strength, ROM, and endurance
- Low vision remediation and compensation
- Interventions to improve driving and community mobility
- Management of feeding, eating, and swallowing performance
- Enhancement of performance skills via physical agent modalities (PAMs), mechanical modalities, manual therapy techniques, and wound care management
- Promoting occupational justice by empowering persons, groups, and populations to seek and obtain resources
- Group interventions to facilitate skill acquisition and learning

Skilled occupational therapy is **not** evident when the occupational therapist or occupational therapy assistant provides the following services:
- Continuing treatment after goals are reached or no further significant progress is expected
- Providing routine strengthening or exercise programs if there is no potential for functional improvement
- Carrying out daily programs after the adapted procedures are in place and no further progress is expected
- Presenting information in the form of handouts or videos without having the client or caregiver perform the activity (e.g., energy conservation techniques or donning procedures for post-surgical brace)
- Providing services to a client who has poor rehabilitation or habilitation potential
- Duplicating services with another discipline
- Carrying out a maintenance program, unless the occupational therapy practitioner clearly documents that "the specialized judgment, knowledge, and skills of a qualified therapist ('skilled care') are necessary for the performance of a safe and effective maintenance program" (Centers for Medicare & Medicaid Services, 2021, para. 3)

"Care is regarded as 'skilled' only if it is at a level of complexity and sophistication that requires the services of a therapist or an assistant supervised by a therapist. Services that do not require the performance or supervision of a therapist are not considered 'skilled' even if they are performed by a therapist" (PT Management Support Systems, 2018, para. 2).

Wording is critical to documenting the necessity for continued skilled occupational therapy. The occupational therapy practitioner **provides skilled instruction** to clients rather than **assisting** them. For example, an occupational therapist may provide instruction in methods of energy conservation and work simplification instead of helping the client perform a strenuous task. Occupational therapists **design** home programs and occupational therapists or occupational therapy assistants may **provide instruction** in home programs, which will then be carried out by clients, aides, or family members.

Why should a client's funding source reimburse you to watch a client carry out the home exercise program that they perform daily on their own? If you are **evaluating** their ability to do all the components of it correctly, or **modifying** it to compensate for recent progress, then your professional skill is clearly required. Analyze your professional reasoning and then document the principles and strategies used during a treatment session in justifying the continuation of skilled occupational therapy services. See Table 10-2 for a list of action words that help show that the skill of an occupational therapy practitioner is required.

Remember that the justification for continued treatment must support the frequency and duration of the plan that you will establish in the "P" section of your note. If the last sentence of your "A" reads, *"Client would benefit from information on energy conservation techniques,"* do not expect the payer to approve more than one more treatment session. If this is your last session, complete the sentence with what the client would benefit from after discharge. For example:

- *Following discharge from rehab unit, client would benefit from home health OT to assess need for home adaptations to accommodate use of w/c for ADLs and IADLs.*

- *Client would benefit from continued PROM provided by restorative aide to prevent R UE contracture and skin breakdown.*

- *Child would benefit from OT re-evaluation in 6 months to determine if fine motor skills are developing at an age-appropriate level.*

Table 10-2

ACTION WORDS THAT DEMONSTRATE THE NEED FOR SKILLED OCCUPATIONAL THERAPY

Accommodate	Create	Grade	Provide
Adapt	Cue	Guide	Reduce
Add	Customize	Identify	Re-evaluate
Adjust	Design	Implement	Regulate
Administer	Develop	Improve	Reinforce
Advance	Direct	Incorporate	Remediate
Advise	Downgrade	Increase	Restore
Advocate	Educate	Inhibit	Review
Analyze	Elicit	Initiate	Revise
Apply	Enable	Instruct	Select
Assess	Engage	Integrate	Sequence
Benefit	Enhance	Introduce	Simulate
Challenge	Establish	Manage	Stabilize
Change	Evaluate	Model	Stimulate
Coach	Expand	Modify	Strengthen
Collaborate	Explore	Organize	Support
Compensate	Fabricate	Orient	Tailor
Conduct	Facilitate	Position	Teach
Construct	Fit	Prepare	Train
Consult	Formulate	Prevent	Transition
Coordinate	Foster	Progress	Update
Correct	Generate	Promote	Upgrade

Data sources: AOTA, 2020b; Daulong, 2016; PT Management Support Systems, 2018; The Note Ninjas, 2022.

WRITING THE ASSESSMENT

As you read carefully through the material in your "S" and "O," it is sometimes helpful to make a quick list of things you want to discuss in the "A" section of your note. For example, consider this "S" and "O":

S: *Client stated that he gets bored during the day when he has nothing to do, and said, "I wish I had a car so I could get out easier."*

O: *Client participated in 90-minute OT session in his home, on city bus, and at grocery store for community reintegration following discharge from inpatient facility. Client deficits include limited problem-solving and money management skills. Client demonstrated home management skills and ability to care for pets by simulation with min verbal cues. Client was able to identify which bus to catch to go to grocery store but needed reassurance that his choice was correct. At the grocery store, client independently chose lunch meat and fruit for lunches this week but needed SBA for payment.*

The therapist identified the following problems, progress, potential, and need for continued services:

- **Problems:**
  - Client is anxious about whether his bus choice is really correct.
  - Client is still unable to manage money independently.
- **Progress:**
  - Client is able to simulate care of home and pets.
  - Client is able to choose the correct bus to get to the grocery store.
  - Client is willing to choose healthier foods at the store this visit.
- **Potential:**
  - In this therapist's professional judgment, the progress shown to date is also a good indicator of rehab potential for this client.
- **Need for Continued Services:**
  - Client still needs to improve community mobility and money management skills to increase functional independence.

Putting all this together, the "A" might read like this:

A: *Anxiety level in selecting the correct bus and need for assistance in managing money continue to limit client's ability to live alone. Ability to demonstrate home and pet care activities as taught earlier shows good progress toward being able to live independently in the community. Ability to identify correct bus and willingness to choose healthier food items also indicate progress and potential to transition to less caregiver support. Client would benefit from money management training and supported outings to advance skills in community transportation access and navigation.*

Here are a few more examples of what a completed Assessment of a note might look like:

A: *Inability to don L LE prosthesis without assist limits independence with transfers and mobility needed for functional toileting. Ability to don prosthesis today with min A indicates progress from mod A needed yesterday. Recent progress and motivation are good indications of potential to be independent with prosthesis management and toileting. Client would benefit from skilled instruction in use of pulley-like fasteners installed this date on prosthesis to allow one-handed closure.*

A: *Fear, isolation, and decreased activity tolerance limit Dominique's independent living skills. Emerging willingness to initiate conversation with others and to initiate daily bathing and grooming indicate good progress toward goals. Decreased hallucinations and improved hygiene indicate good potential to return to previous supported living situation. Dominique would benefit from skilled instruction in self-care skills as well as facilitation of socialization and physical activity to be successful with community re-entry.*

A: *Child's L neglect continues to limit her independence in self-care and play tasks. Spontaneous use of L hand as a functional assist 60% of the time demonstrates progress from less than 50% spontaneous use during prior visits. She would benefit from facilitation of more bilateral activities to increase use of L hand during play, as well as establishment of a home program for foster parents to carry out in between bi-weekly visits.*

A: *Client's spontaneous actions in groups, willingness to share verbally, and improved dress and hygiene indicate an improved mood this week. Progress also noted in unprompted attendance, which is up this week from 2/8 to 6/8 groups attended. Goals #1 (assertion) and #2 (communication) are met as of this date. Recent progress indicates excellent potential for successful community re-entry. Inability to identify preferred leisure tasks continues to limit client's ability to plan daily activities, both individually and involving interaction with others. Goal #3 (leisure skills) will be continued through discharge. Client would benefit from facilitation of social interactions with peers and coaching to formulate a plan for use of leisure time.*

Notice in the last example that the **problems, progress, and potential do not have to be in a particular order**. Sometimes it makes more sense to identify the progress first and then comment on the remaining problems that justify continued services. Let's walk through one more example in a step-by-step manner.

"A" EXAMPLE: MRS. W'S STROKE

Mrs. W is a 62-year-old woman who had a stroke 3 weeks ago. She lives with her husband of 40 years in a one-story home. Her husband works full time as an account manager at a local bank. She has good return in her involved LE and is getting some return in her UE as well. She intends to return home to live with her husband and will be alone during the day while he is at work.

S: *Client says she has difficulty moving R UE, although she does not know why it will not move. She reports, "It really doesn't hurt. It's just tight."*

O: *Client participated in 30-minute OT session in rehab gym for neuro re-education and R UE strengthening activities to increase independence in ADL tasks. Pt. presents with decreased AROM in R shoulder, decreased activity tolerance, limited R UE strength, and dynamic standing balance deficits.*

ADLs: In room, client was instructed in safety techniques and adaptive equipment use in toileting. Client needs B grab bars in bathroom for safe sit to/from stand transition during toileting. Client attempted to stand by pulling on walker and one grab bar. Client was educated on safety issues and the use of B grab bars; she verbalized understanding of recommendations.

Performance Skills: Client required CGA for balance during sit to/from stand. To address activity tolerance, dynamic standing balance, and increase AROM in R shoulder, client moved canned goods from counter to cupboard for 5 minutes before needing a 2-minute seated rest break. Client then completed activities to improve dynamic standing balance by pouring liquid from a pitcher while standing with CGA for balance. After a 1-minute seated rest, client continued activities to increase dynamic standing balance and safety by retrieving objects from floor using reacher while ambulating with wheeled walker and CGA.

Client Factors: R shoulder abduction AROM < 90°. R shoulder abduction PROM WFL.

How would you assess this information? What **problems** can you identify? Safety risks? Are there performance skills that are not WFL that occupational therapy might affect? Do you see evidence of **progress**? Is there any indication of the client's rehab **potential**? What would this client **benefit from**?

The therapist identified the following problems, progress, potential, and need for continued services:

- **Problems:**
  - Client is unsafe during toilet transfer.
  - Client has decreased AROM in R shoulder, decreased activity tolerance, and decreased dynamic standing balance.
- **Progress:**
  - Client verbalized understanding of safety instructions.
- **Potential:**
  - R UE PROM is WNL.
  - In this therapist's professional judgment, the client has good potential to return home with intermittent assist from her spouse.
- **Need for Continued Services:**
  - Client needs to improve AROM, strength, and activity tolerance and needs skilled instruction in safety and energy conservation techniques.

In preparing an Assessment of the data in this note, this therapist identified two main problem areas: the safety of transferring to/from the toilet, and the client factors that were not WFL. This therapist was particularly concerned about the safety issues and addressed those first. She also noted the rehabilitation potential that would be helpful to a reviewer in deciding whether the client's progress is sufficient to justify the expense of treatment.

A: *Impulsivity and decreased dynamic standing balance pose safety concern during toilet transfers and lower body clothing management. Ability to verbalize safety instructions demonstrates progress and indicates that the client has the potential to be home alone for short periods of time.*

Next, she addressed the professional reasoning behind devoting time to addressing client factors, in light of the client's rehabilitation potential:

A: *Impulsivity and decreased dynamic standing balance pose safety concern during toilet transfers and lower body clothing management. Ability to verbalize safety instructions demonstrates progress and indicates that the client has the potential to be home alone for short periods of time.* **Decreased R shoulder AROM, limited activity tolerance, and impaired dynamic standing balance all interfere with ability to complete ADL tasks safely and independently.**

She completes the Assessment by justifying continued treatment:

A: *Impulsivity and decreased dynamic standing balance pose safety concern during toilet transfers and lower body clothing management. Ability to verbalize safety instructions demonstrates progress and indicates that the client has the potential to be home alone for short periods of time. Decreased R shoulder AROM, limited activity tolerance, and impaired dynamic standing balance all interfere with ability to complete ADL tasks safely and independently.* **Client would benefit from R UE AROM and strengthening exercises along with skilled instruction in energy conservation techniques during ADLs and IADLs.**

In this case, the therapist decided that the client factors could be addressed in two different ways, both by working on improving AROM, strength, and activity tolerance and by teaching some energy conservation techniques. We know that payment for ongoing treatment of range and strength is often denied. In Chapter 11, you will see how this therapist plans to provide the services this client would benefit from in a cost-effective manner.

COMMON ERRORS IN WRITING THE ASSESSMENT
Repeating Observations

The difference between an observation statement and an assessment statement is often one of emphasis. Let's consider some examples of how an observation statement would be worded differently than an assessment statement. For example, suppose you are working with a client who tells you she plans to return home to live alone in her farmhouse. You have worked on teaching her some energy conservation techniques, but she forgets to incorporate those strategies into her morning dressing routine. What is the core problem for this client? Why does it matter? The following statement is an **observation** of the client's performance:

Pt. did not use energy conservation techniques during morning dressing due to memory deficit.

However, phrased differently, it becomes an **assessment** of what was observed:

Memory deficit interferes with client's ability to retain instructions in compensatory techniques such as energy conservation, which limits her ability to safely perform self-care tasks needed to return to prior independent living situation.

Note that in this assessment statement, the occupational therapist has identified the core problem as the client's inability to retain instructions she has been given. This might be followed by a recommendation to use memory cues of some kind. Otherwise, why should a funding source continue to pay for instruction that will not be remembered? You might also want to consider her safety in living alone if her short-term memory is impaired.

The assessment does not simply repeat what was observed. Instead, it begins with the contributing factor that is the problem, **broadens the scope of performance to include other relevant occupations**, and answers the question, "So what? Why does this matter in the client's life?"

Let's look at another example. The following is an **observation** of what the occupational therapist saw today:

Client needed verbal prompts for functional problem solving.

An **assessment** of the situation would sound like this:

Need for multiple verbal prompts to solve social problems limits client's ability to respond appropriately in unstructured social situations and to establish successful relationships with others. Ability to problem solve with decreased verbal prompting throughout session indicates progress toward and potential to reach stated goals.

Note that in the observation statement above, there was no area of occupation mentioned. In the assessment statement, the occupational therapist addressed the areas of occupation that are affected by the client's decreased problem-solving skills. Let's look at one more example. Here is an observation that tells what the client did:

Client tolerated vestibular and proprioceptive input well today as evidence by choosing the activity.

Yes, the client choosing the activity is an indication of his tolerance, and that is good professional reasoning, but there are more important things to assess. One is his progress in tolerating input, and the other is the effect that this progress has on his ability to engage in occupation.

Client's choice of activities with proprioceptive and vestibular components indicates progress in sensory tolerance necessary for participation and attention in the classroom.

Sweeping Assessment Statements

In the face of a busy schedule, time constraints, and productivity expectations, it is tempting to make concise and sweeping assessment statements, such as the following:

A: *Poor postural stability interferes with ADL performance. Improvement since last note shows good rehab potential. Client would benefit from continued activities to increase postural stability and ability to do personal ADL tasks.*

A: *Decreased strength and coordination prevent client from completing ADLs independently. Client's ability to follow instructions shows good rehab potential. Client would benefit from continued activities to increase strength, coordination, and fine motor skills.*

A: *Deficits in upper body strength, fine motor skills, and feeding limit Jordan's ability to be independent in home and classroom activities.*

While these assessments are accurate, they are limited and would benefit from some elaboration. An elaboration on Jordan's note might read:

A: *Deficits in upper body strength limit Jordan's ability to be independent in eating and dressing. Decreased fine motor skills impede typical classroom activities such as holding a pencil or crayon and manipulating small items. Recent emergence of supinated digital grasp on crayon indicates improvement from previous pronated mass grasp. Jordan's motivation to engage in classroom activities with peers indicates good potential for future progress in deficit areas. Jordan would benefit from continued upper body strengthening, reach-grasp-release activities, and feeding activities to reach developmental milestones more expediently.*

Here are two more examples of thorough assessments:

A: *Decreased cheek and lip range diminishes pressure in mouth needed for swallow, which results in inadequate swallow reflex. Poor suck and swallow pattern due to decreased oral musculature may lead to inadequate nutritional intake. Decreased head control with upright posture indicates poor head-righting skills, which will hinder Hannah during feeding. Demonstration of unfacilitated lip closure on bottle this session indicates improvement in feeding skills and potential to reduce supplemental tube feedings. Hannah would benefit from continued skilled OT for provision of oral motor stretches, facilitation of oral motor skills, and a home program for prone position activities to improve head and trunk control.*

A: *Ability to complete simple to complex bilateral eye coordination and visual scanning tasks in static position without verbal cues demonstrates improvements since last session. Eye coordination and visual scanning deficits during dynamic movement pose safety concerns during functional mobility for IADLs. Ability to perform L shoulder AROM with decreased pain indicates improvement since last session. Improved visual scanning indicates potential to complete ADL tasks with distant supervision from family. Client would benefit from further skilled OT in complex bilateral eye coordination and visual scanning activities during dynamic movement and progression of functional reaching tasks with L UE to increase functional ADL and IADL performance without pain.*

REFERENCES

American Occupational Therapy Association. (2020a). Guidelines for supervision, roles, and responsibilities during the delivery of occupational therapy services. *American Journal of Occupational Therapy, 74*(Suppl. 3), 7413410020. https://doi.org/10.5014/ajot.2020.74S3004

American Occupational Therapy Association. (2020b). Occupational therapy practice framework: Domain and process (4th ed.). *American Journal of Occupational Therapy, 74*(Suppl. 2), 7412410010. https://doi.org/10.5014.ajot.2020.74S2001

American Occupational Therapy Association. (2021a). *Definition of occupational therapy practice for the AOTA Model Practice Act.* https://www.aota.org/

American Occupational Therapy Association. (2021b). Occupational therapy scope of practice. *American Journal of Occupational Therapy, 75*(Suppl. 3), 751340030. https://doi.og/10.5014/ajot.2021.75S3005

Centers for Medicare & Medicaid Services. (2021). *Jimmo settlement.* https://www.cms.gov/

Daulong, M. (2016). *Key words to support skilled intervention.* PhysicalTherapy.com. https://www.physicaltherapy.com/

PT Management Support Systems. (2018, March 21). *PT/OT skilled therapeutic exercise documentation examples.* https://pt-management.com/

The Note Ninjas. (2022). *Documentation cheat sheet.* https://thenoteninjas.mykajabi.com/skilled-care-tips

WORKSHEET 10-1

Differentiating Between Observations and Assessments

Identify which of these statements are **observations** and which are **assessments**. Remember that an observation tells you what the client did. An assessment will tell you how the contributing factor affects an area of occupation.

_____ Client is unable to don AFO and shoe independently for ambulation.

_____ Inability to don AFO and shoe independently prevent client from completing IADLs required to live alone.

_____ Decreased sensory tolerance limits the client's attention to task in the classroom.

_____ Client required verbal cues to stay on task due to decreased sensory tolerance.

_____ Client was unable to incorporate breathing and energy conservation techniques, requiring several prompts to complete task.

_____ Inability to incorporate breathing techniques and energy conservation techniques into basic ADL tasks without verbal prompts limits her ability to live alone independently after discharge.

Next, you will be rewriting some observation statements to make them more effective assessment statements using the following formula:

_____ results in (or limits) _____.
Contributing factor/s   **area of occupation affected**

The following statements are **observations** of something the occupational therapist saw the client do. Rewrite them so that they become **assessment** statements using the formula above.

1. Client demonstrated difficulty with laundry and cooking tasks due to memory and sequencing deficits.

2. Client unable to complete homemaking tasks or basic self-care activities independently due to decreased endurance.

3. Decreased level of alertness observed during morning dressing activities, requiring redirection to task.

4. Client unable to follow hip precautions during morning dressing due to memory deficits.

5. Client problem solved poorly while performing lower body dressing, as evidenced by multiple attempts required to button pants and don socks successfully.

WORKSHEET 10-2

Justifying Continued Treatment

Which of the following require the skills of an occupational therapy practitioner?

_____ Evaluation of a client

_____ The practice of coordination and self-care skills on a daily basis

_____ Establishing measurable, behavioral, objective, and individualized goals

_____ Developing intervention plans designed to meet established goals

_____ Analyzing and modifying functional activities through the provision of adaptive equipment or techniques

_____ Determining that the modified tasks are safe and effective

_____ Routine exercise and strengthening programs

_____ Teaching the client to use the breathing techniques he has learned while performing ADLs

_____ Providing individualized instruction to the client, family, or caregiver

_____ Modifying the intervention plan based on a re-evaluation

_____ Donning/doffing of a client's resting hand splint on a regular schedule throughout the day

_____ Providing specialized instruction to eliminate limitations in a functional activity

_____ Developing a home program and instructing caregivers

_____ Making changes in the environment

_____ Teaching compensatory skills

_____ Gait training

_____ Adding instruction in lower body dressing techniques to a current ADL program

_____ Presenting informational handouts without having the client perform the activity

_____ Teaching adaptive techniques such as one-handed shoe tying

WORSHEET 10-3

Writing the Assessment—Ellie's Development

Ellie was born prematurely at 24 weeks' gestation. She is currently almost 7 months old, with an adjusted age of 3 months. She was referred to occupational therapy while in the NICU for facilitation of typical developmental sequence and continues to receive occupational therapy services because she is considered a high-risk infant.

S: *Parent reports that infant is gaining ~1 oz. per day and will probably be able to discontinue O_2 "in a couple days."*

O: *Infant participated in 30-minute OT session in home to assess visual skills and to increase mobility skills related to play (head righting, rolling supine to side lying, and push up in prone). Infant presents with low proximal and distal tone and poor head control. Infant oriented to black and white illuminated design by turning head. In supine, infant demonstrated visual tracking in horizontal plane 20° past midline. Infant unable to roll, right head, or push up in prone independently to engage with caregiver or toys. With facilitation of weight shift and proximal stability, infant could perform activities after about 20 seconds and hold position. Infant became fatigued and "fussy" after 20 minutes of treatment, with four 1-minute rest breaks.*

How would you assess this information? What **problems** can you identify? Are there any contributing factors that occupational therapy might affect? What influence do the limiting factors above have on Ellie's ability to engage in occupation that is appropriate for her age? Do you see evidence of **progress**? Is there any indication of Ellie's **potential for improvement**? What would she **benefit from**?

The therapist who is working with Ellie was concerned about the following:
- Inability to perform age-appropriate mobility skills independently during play
- Became fatigued after 20 minutes
- Lack of head righting responses
- Needs O_2

She was encouraged by the following:
- Need for O_2 is decreasing and she is gaining weight
- Ability to hold position if facilitated
- Ability to orient to a black-and-white image and to visually track horizontally

Write an **Assessment** to add to the "S" and "O" given above.

A:

WORKSHEET 10-4

Writing the Assessment—Ms. D's Social Participation Skills

Ms. D is a 35-year-old woman who has a diagnosis of bipolar disorder, although in a prior admission, she was diagnosed with schizophrenia. One of her goals is to talk to the mental health center staff about her problems rather than acting out her feelings. Today she was seen in social skills group with five other clients who also need help with relationship issues.

S: *Client reports that she understands the purpose of social skills group. She expressed a desire to attend all of the groups, saying that they are "fun."*

O: *Client participated in 60-minute social skills group focusing on friendship. Client appeared unkempt, with hair not combed and shirt rumpled. Client engaged in conversation with the other clients and the facilitator. Client interrupted others on 5 occasions. Client spontaneously verbalized her experiences with past friendships and her ideas of useful ways to make new friendships but had to be redirected to the topic twice during discussion.*

1. What problems do you see in the above "S" and "O"?

2. What areas of occupation do these problems affect?

3. What evidence of progress and/or potential do you see?

4. What would this client benefit from?

5. Write a complete Assessment statement for this note.

WORKSHEET 10-5

Writing the Assessment—Mr. Y's Functional Performance

Mr. Y is a 68-year-old man who had a L CVA 1 week ago. His R UE is getting some return, and occupational therapy was ordered yesterday. Your colleague who assessed Mr. Y yesterday is out sick today, and you are beginning treatment with him. Her initial note stated that his activity tolerance was less than 1 minute and she was not sure how much aphasia was present.

S: *Client stated, "I think my right arm is getting stronger. This morning I was able to wash my face using my right hand."*

O: *Client participated in 30-minute session in OT clinic to work on functional use of R UE in prep for ADL activities. Client deficits include R UE hemiparesis, decreased sitting balance, and decreased cognition. Client needed mod A in shifting weight to get to edge of w/c and max verbal cues to use correct posture and shift feet during stand pivot transfer w/c to mat. Client required max verbal cues to initiate grasp of small beanbag. Client needed mod A in reaching with R UE. Client able to complete R UE shoulder flexion required to toss beanbag ~2 ft. with max verbal cues. Client demonstrated cognitive understanding of activity with mod verbal cues by stating desired goal to be achieved by accurate aim. Client tolerated up to 3 minutes of activity before requiring rest break.*

Now assess the meaning of this information. Note the problems, progress, and potential that you see for this client.

- **Problems:**

- **Progress/Potential:**

Now write an "A" that assesses how engagement in occupation is affected. Include what the client would benefit from.

A:

WORKSHEET 10-6

Writing the Assessment—Marco's Visual Motor Skills

Now write an assessment for a school-aged child. Remember that treatment in public school always relates to the child's educational performance. Marco is a second grader who is receiving occupational therapy in the public schools. He has several problems, including low muscle tone, that contribute to his upper body weakness and decreased proximal stability. At the time of the last note, he was able to achieve 70% accuracy in letter formation with verbal cues.

S: *Child stated, "This is hard!" during a bilateral coordination exercise requiring UE strength and stability.*

O: *Child participated in 30-minute session in school therapy room to address skills related to handwriting and other visual motor classroom tasks. Child presents with deficits in oculomotor movements, fine motor skills, and upper body strength and stability necessary for dynamic UE function in the classroom.*

   Visual Tracking: *Child visually tracked a moving object 4x R to L @ 40% accuracy and L to R @ 20% accuracy. Child demonstrated 20% accuracy of eye convergence 4x staring 12" from nose and breaking at ~6" from nose.*

   UE Coordination: *Child performed B UE coordination activity (Zoom ball) at 80% accuracy with hyperextended knees and trunk movement to compensate for upper body weakness.*

   Handwriting: *Child able to write letters P, E, F, D, M, N, R from memory with 90% accuracy and 75% accuracy for staying in line boundaries with min verbal cues.*

What problems, progress, and/or potential do you see for Marco?

• **Problems:**

• **Progress/Potential:**

Now write an Assessment:

A:

WORKSHEET 10-7

Writing the Assessment—Mr. S's Social Participation Skills

Mr. S is a 35-year-old man who is in a maximum-security unit in a state psychiatric facility. He has criminal charges against him for a violent crime but was sent to the state mental institution rather than to prison. His current diagnosis is schizophrenia, R/O personality disorder. Today he participated in assertion group.

S: *Mr. S stated he knows what assertion is, but reports, "Manipulation and aggression have always worked better for me." When asked to explain assertion, Mr. S stated, "The problem with that is the sugar and fruit in the cake."*

O: *Mr. S attended 1-hr. assertion group this date for skilled instruction and role-play activities to improve assertion and effective self-expression skills. Mr. S was on time to the group, neatly dressed with hair combed. He was unable to correctly define assertion and did not respond to any of the 3 role-play activities, either by taking a role or by offering suggestions to others. During the role-play, Mr. S placed his head down and closed his eyes. Following the session, Mr. S quickly left the room.*

What problems, progress, and/or potential do you see for Mr. S?
- **Problems:**

- **Progress/Potential:**

Now write an Assessment:
A:

Chapter 11

Writing the "P"—Plan

The last section of a SOAP note is the **Plan**. In this section, you document the anticipated frequency and duration of your services and the specific interventions that will be used to achieve the client's goals. The plan should relate to the information presented in the "O" and the "A" and should address your assessment of what the client would benefit from. The "P" will inform your reader of your priorities regarding intervention strategies.

In an initial evaluation report, the "P" section will also contain the long-term and short-term goals. This will be covered in Chapter 12 when you learn more about intervention planning.

In some settings, you will see the "P" simply written as *"Continue plan of care."* For purposes of learning in this manual, *"Continue plan of care"* **is NOT a sufficient plan.** Your "P" should include the following:

- **Frequency** (how often; may also include length of session in some settings)
  - *Infant will be seen **2x/wk** …*
  - *Continue OT **daily** …*
  - *Client will be seen **30 minutes bid** …*
- **Duration** (how long occupational therapy will continue)
  - *Infant will be seen 2x/wk for **2 months** …*
  - *Continue OT daily for **2 days** …*
  - *Client will be seen 30 minutes bid for **1 week** …*
- **Purpose of continued therapy and/or specific interventions** (also include referral to other professionals or agencies if appropriate)
  - *Infant will be seen 2x/wk for 2 months **to address feeding skills. Treatment to include oral desensitization and caregiver training in use of adaptive bottles.***

Gateley, C. A. *Documentation Manual for Occupational Therapy, Fifth Edition* (pp. 147-160). © 2024 Taylor & Francis Group.

- *Continue OT daily for 2 days **for skilled instruction in ADLs and IADLs. Sessions will focus on education in post-surgical hip precautions and adaptive equipment to maximize safety and independence in preparation for return to independent living situation. OT will also contact social worker to explore options for home assistance with laundry and housekeeping. Referral also made to local Independent Living Center for assistance in obtaining necessary adaptive equipment due to client's limited insurance and financial resources.***

- *Client will be seen 30 minutes bid for 1 week **to address visual perceptual and cognitive skills necessary for safe performance of ADLs and IADLs. Environmental modifications will be made to improve visual scanning to L side during basic ADLs. Telephone book activity planned for afternoon session tomorrow.***

In each of the previous examples, another therapist could read your "P" and know exactly how to proceed with this client's treatment. Consider the following situations in which this would be crucial to providing quality care for your client:

- In acute care and rehabilitation settings, treatment may be provided 7 days per week, and the client will encounter multiple occupational therapy practitioners during their hospital stay. Writing a thorough "P" ensures that the next therapist to see the client will use the client's therapy time efficiently to work toward meeting goals rather than starting from scratch and trying to figure out what to do.

- In any setting where an occupational therapy assistant will be providing services, a thorough "P" is critical for communication and collaboration between the supervising occupational therapist and the occupational therapy assistant.

- Unexpected therapist absences happen in any setting. The "P" section of your note should allow another therapist to continue the client's treatment without interruption.

Note: There are three common errors in the "P" that students often make when they are first learning to document:

1. The first error is **failing to provide the anticipated duration of occupational therapy services**. In other words, when will the client be done with occupational therapy services? Students often think they have addressed the duration when they list the anticipated length of each session, such as *5x/wk for 60 minutes*, but that does not tell the reader when occupational therapy services will end. I tell my students when I am grading their notes that if they do not provide a duration, then I assume they plan to continue seeing the client forever. **Insurance reviewers want to see a clear plan for discontinuing occupational therapy services.** Or, for longer term clients, when will the client need to be re-evaluated to determine whether continued services are justified?

2. The second error is to keep using the words **plan to assess** in the "P" of the SOAP note. From an insurance reviewer's standpoint, most of your assessment should have taken place during the initial evaluation, and the expectation is that **future sessions will focus on intervention.** Unless you have specific assessments that you plan to complete in future sessions, such as standardized visual perceptual or cognitive tests, your "P" should focus on your planned interventions. It is implied that ongoing assessment is part of every session.

3. The third error is to list interventions in the "P" that are **not relevant for the client's current setting.** For example, if you are an occupational therapist in an acute care setting, your plan should not include interventions that will occur in the home health or outpatient setting. You should **only document what you can address in the current setting** in which you are treating the client.

Here are some more examples of a "P":

- *Resident to be seen for 2 more weeks for 30-minute bid sessions for skilled instruction in meal preparation and clean-up. Focus will be on independent use of microwave using wheeled walker for mobility.*

- *Child will continue to be seen 1x/wk for 30-minute sessions until IEP review in April to increase fine motor skills for better classroom performance. OT sessions to address handwriting and cutting skills.*

- *Client will continue to be seen in groups 5x/wk for 1 week to facilitate social participation. Group sessions to address assertion skills and anger management techniques.*

- *Consumer will continue sheltered workshop program 5 days/wk for 1 month to improve work skills. Target behaviors are improved attention to task and ability to follow 2-step directions.*

- *Continue 1-hr. daily sessions for 1 week for skilled ADL training. One-handed dressing techniques for donning shirt will be taught and button hook will be introduced.*

You must use your professional judgment when determining frequency and duration of services. In many cases, there are expected norms of frequency and duration based on setting, funding source, or physician's order. See Table 11-1 for examples. **Please note that these are general guidelines. Frequency and duration will vary greatly among settings and situations.** You must be familiar with the requirements, expectations, and general practices of your specific setting.

Funding sources may dictate the number of occupational therapy visits that will be paid, such as 60 minutes weekly for 8 weeks. Insurance companies may also limit the total number of therapy visits they will pay for in a calendar year. For example, it is common to see a limit of 60 outpatient visits per year for combined occupational therapy, physical therapy, and speech therapy visits. In such cases, it is important to communicate with other team members and the client to determine the optimal frequency and duration of therapy visits for your discipline.

COMPLETING THE PLAN FOR MRS. W

Now let us write a plan for the note on Mrs. W that we assessed in the last chapter. As you recall from Chapter 10, Mrs. W is a 62-year-old woman who had a stroke 3 weeks ago. She has good return in her involved LE and is getting some return in her UE as well. She intends to return home to live with her husband and will be alone during the day while he is at work.

S: *Client says she has difficulty moving R UE, although she does not know why it will not move. She reports, "It really doesn't hurt. It's just tight."*

O: *Client participated in 30-minute OT session in rehab gym for neuro re-education and R UE strengthening activities to increase independence in ADL tasks. Pt. presents with decreased AROM in R shoulder, decreased activity tolerance, limited R UE strength, and dynamic standing balance deficits.*

ADLs: In room, client was instructed in safety techniques and adaptive equipment use in toileting. Client needs B grab bars in bathroom for safe sit to/from stand transition during toileting. Client attempted to stand by pulling on walker and one grab bar. Client was educated on safety issues and the use of B grab bars; she verbalized understanding of recommendations.

Performance Skills: Client required CGA for balance during sit to/from stand. To address activity tolerance, dynamic standing balance, and increased AROM in R shoulder, client moved canned goods from counter to cupboard for 5 minutes before needing a 2-minute seated rest break. Client then completed activities to improve dynamic standing balance by pouring liquid from a pitcher while standing with CGA for balance. After a 1-minute seated rest, client continued activities to increase dynamic standing balance and safety by retrieving objects from floor using reacher while ambulating with wheeled walker and CGA.

Client Factors: R shoulder abduction AROM < 90°. R shoulder abduction PROM WFL.

A: *Impulsivity and decreased dynamic standing balance pose safety concern during toilet transfers and lower body clothing management. Ability to verbalize safety instructions demonstrates progress and indicates that the client has the potential to be home alone for short periods of time. Decreased R shoulder AROM, limited activity tolerance, and impaired dynamic standing balance all interfere with ability to complete ADL tasks safely and independently. Client would benefit from R UE AROM and strengthening exercises along with skilled instruction in energy conservation techniques during ADLs and IADLs.*

In the "A" section, the therapist has already justified the main things she intends to do and indicated the client's rehabilitation potential. Now she needs to be specific about how often the client will be treated and for what length of time. She first specifies the frequency and duration of treatment:

P: *Continue to treat client 5x/wk for 1 week …*

She could have specified the length of the treatment sessions (e.g., "*for 1-hr. sessions*"), but this therapist chose not to do that in this particular note. Next, she specifies how she plans to use the treatment time:

P: *Continue to treat client 5x/wk for 1 week **for skilled instruction in safe ADL transfers and toileting** …*

Since she anticipates discharge in 1 week, she has to prioritize her time. She chooses to work on balance and energy conservation as a part of functional mobility during ADL activities. Since she has already written in the "A" that the client would benefit from additional AROM and strengthening exercises, she now needs to specify how she plans to address this need as well:

P: *Continue to treat client 5x/wk for 1 week for skilled instruction in safe ADL transfers and toileting. **Plan to address dynamic standing balance during ADLs and to provide skilled instruction in energy conservation techniques. Home program for AROM and strengthening exercises for R shoulder will be taught.***

This note is now complete. This therapist has demonstrated professional reasoning in planning for discharge in advance of the discharge date. In later notes, she will indicate the client's progress in learning the home program since simply handing the client a set of printed exercises is not considered a skilled or billable service. The client's progress in learning the home program will also confirm that the therapist's assessment of the client's rehabilitation potential was on target.

Table 11-1	
TYPICAL FREQUENCY AND DURATION OF OCCUPATIONAL THERAPY SERVICES BY SETTING	
TYPE OF SETTING	**TYPICAL FREQUENCY AND DURATION**
Acute Care— General Medical	Patients who are admitted to an acute care hospital for general medical reasons such as pneumonia, cardiac issues, surgical procedures, or generalized weakness typically are **only in the hospital for a few days before discharging to another setting**. OT plays an important role in making recommendations about the safest discharge setting for the patient based on functional performance and available support. **It is common for recommended frequency to be provided as a range** rather than a set number to accommodate fluctuating hospital census and OT staffing. For example, recommended frequency may be 1-2x/wk or 3-5x/wk. This range allows OT practitioners to see the patient more frequently when staffing patterns allow and to triage patients when staffing patterns are stretched thin. Duration is implied to be for length of hospital stay until discharge unless the patient meets all goals or would no longer benefit from skilled OT services.
Acute Care— Orthopedics	Patients who have had an orthopedic surgery, whether planned/elective (e.g., spinal surgery or hip, shoulder, or knee replacement) or unplanned (e.g., to repair a fracture resulting from a fall) likely will have OT services **once or twice daily for the duration of their stay**, but this may vary depending on each surgeon's protocol for therapy services. **Total length of stay is often just a few days.** As with the general acute care population, OT plays a huge role in making discharge recommendations. As soon as patients are medically stable and appropriate discharge can be arranged by the care team, they will be discharged to a different setting, such as a skilled nursing facility, inpatient rehabilitation facility, or home with home health services.
Long-Term Acute Care Hospital (LTAC or LTACH)	Patients in an LTACH typically are in the hospital for **25 days or longer** due to their complex medical needs (CMS, 2019). Like general medical acute care, **frequency is often set as a range**, such as 2-5x/wk. Patients with lower activity tolerance or patients who already needed considerable assist before hospitalization may only be seen a few times per week, while patients with higher level of function who are closer to discharge home are seen more frequently.

(continued)

Table 11-1 (continued)

TYPICAL FREQUENCY AND DURATION OF OCCUPATIONAL THERAPY SERVICES BY SETTING

TYPE OF SETTING	TYPICAL FREQUENCY AND DURATION
Inpatient Rehabilitation Facility (IRF)	Patients in an IRF must receive **3 hours of therapy per day for 5 days each week**. The 3 hours is divided among OT, PT, and SLP (if needed), so OT typically is provided for 60, 75, or 90 minutes daily, 5x/wk. Each patient's "week" begins on the day of admission. For example, if a patient admits to an IRF on Friday, that patient's week will always run Friday–Thursday. If a different patient admits to the IRF on Wednesday, that patient's week will always run Wednesday–Tuesday. In rare circumstances, when the patient cannot tolerate 3 hours per day or there are other scheduling complications, **therapy may be spread out as 15 hours over 7 consecutive days** (CMS, 2018). An example of the 15 hours over 7 days exception might be a patient who is admitted to IRF following a below-knee amputation but has dialysis scheduled 3 mornings per week, thus limiting availability and endurance for therapy on dialysis days. **Documenting the exact number of therapy minutes provided is very important in an IRF**. Medicare and other insurance companies very closely scrutinize an IRF's adherence to this requirement. IRF lengths of stay are **typically a few weeks**, although IRFs specializing in TBI or SCI rehabilitation may have longer average lengths of stay (Medicare Payment Advisory Commission, 2021).
Skilled Nursing Facility (SNF)	Most patients in a SNF receive OT services five times per week. Some SNFs that specialize in short-term rehabilitation with a high return-to-home rate, such as those serving patients following elective orthopedic surgeries, may see patients 6x/wk for OT to maximize patient outcomes in a shorter length of time. The **average length of stay is 3 to 4 weeks** (Fitch et al., 2021), but it may be shorter or longer depending on the patient's funding source and needs. Many therapists have reported pressure to provide more group and concurrent therapy since Medicare SNF reimbursement is no longer tied directly to therapy minutes under the Patient Driven Payment Model (PDPM) that took effect in 2019 (Yamshon, 2020), although no more than 25% of the patient's total combined minutes can be provided in group or concurrent therapy sessions (Net Health, 2020). Original Medicare Part A covers SNF stays at 100% for the first 20 days, then at 80% for days 21 to 100. Medicare Advantage and other private insurance plans may only authorize short periods of time and require frequent documentation updates before authorizing additional days. All these factors may play a part in determining frequency and duration of OT services in the SNF setting.
Long-Term Care	"After 100 days in a nursing home, a resident will no longer be covered by Medicare Part A for certain services. It is at that point that Medicare Part B is utilized for physical therapy, occupational therapy, and speech-language pathology" (Zargar, 2021, para. 1). Long-term residents may require OT services **a few times per week for a few weeks** to address an issue related to positioning, splinting, recent falls, or decreased functional performance. Since they are long-term residents, the goal in this situation typically is not to improve the person's function in order to discharge to another location, but rather to maximize safety and independence in a supported living environment. Many facilities have a periodic screening method in place by nursing and/or therapy staff to determine which long-term residents would benefit from occupational therapy evaluation and treatment (Sullivan, 2021).

(continued)

Table 11-1 (continued)

TYPICAL FREQUENCY AND DURATION OF OCCUPATIONAL THERAPY SERVICES BY SETTING

TYPE OF SETTING	TYPICAL FREQUENCY AND DURATION
Home Health	As with all settings, frequency and duration for home health OT services varies, but home health OT visits are typically provided **a few times per week for a few to several weeks**. So, frequency and duration in your "P" might be *2x/wk for 4 weeks*, or if the plan is to taper services, the plan might be *2x/wk for 2 weeks* followed by *1x/wk for 2 weeks*. Some home health patients receive only an evaluation focused on home safety assessment and equipment recommendations. For patients needing home health OT services for a longer period of time, a functional reassessment is required at 30 days, and recertification is required at 60 days (Minnesota Home Care Association, 2022; National Government Services, 2021).
Inpatient Psychiatric Hospital	You may recall from Chapter 7 that **short-term psychiatric hospitals typically keep patients only 3 to 5 days for crisis stabilization**, whereas **long-term psychiatric hospital stays may range from several weeks to several months to several years** (Missouri Department of Mental Health, 2022; University of Maryland Medical Center, 2022). In either setting, the OT services may include a combination of group and individual therapy sessions. For example, your plan in a short-term psychiatric hospital might be *OT services 5x/wk through discharge to include 3 individual sessions and daily participation in relevant OT groups*. In a long-term psychiatric hospital, your frequency and duration will depend on the client's needs and the potential discharge situation. For example, a client who is approaching discharge to a halfway house may have a plan that reads *OT services 3x/wk for 4 weeks with emphasis on development of skills needed to transition to supported community living*.
Outpatient Clinic	Frequency is typically **a few times per week for a few to several weeks** (e.g., *2x/wk for 4 weeks*). Funding sources may dictate when reassessment or recertification is required. Funding sources may also limit the number of therapy visits covered per year, and this limit may be for the combination of OT, PT, and SLP services, so you will need to coordinate with your interprofessional colleagues.
Schools	The frequency of services will be determined at the child's annual IEP meeting date and will remain the same until the IEP is modified, unless there is a significant change mid-year requiring an increase, decrease, or discontinuation of OT services. Frequency of services are typically expressed in terms of the **number of minutes of OT services the child will receive on a weekly or monthly basis** (e.g., *60 minutes per week* or *120 minutes per month*). **Duration is implied to be for the year-long time frame of the IEP.**
Early Intervention	Frequency is set in the child's Individualized Family Service Plan (IFSP). Early intervention services vary greatly depending on the child's needs and the family's priorities. OT may provide consultative services on a monthly basis with a focus on caregiver training or see the child for direct intervention **up to a few times per week**. IFSP requirements vary among states, but IFSPs typically are **reviewed every 6 months** and **updated annually** (Center for Parent Information and Resources, 2021). Your plan for OT services might read *1x/month consultation with family for 6 months for home programming* or *direct OT services 1x/wk for 6 months to facilitation play and self-care skills*.
Community-Based Programs	**Varies greatly** depending on type of setting, client population and needs, and funding source.

REFERENCES

Center for Parent Information and Resources. (2021). *Writing the IFSP for your child.* https://www.parentcenterhub.org/

Centers for Medicare & Medicaid Services. (2018). *Inpatient Rehabilitation Facility (IRF) medical review changes.* https://www.cms.gov/

Centers for Medicare & Medicaid Services. (2019). *What are long-term care hospitals?* https://www.medicare.gov.

Fitch, K., Broulette, J., & King, K. (2021). *Variability in average length of stay for skilled nursing facilities—Opportunities exist for more efficient management.* Milliman. https://www.us.milliman.com

Medicare Payment Advisory Commission. (2021). *Report to the Congress—Medicare payment policy: Inpatient rehabilitation facility services.* https://www.medpac.gov/

Minnesota Home Care Association. (2022). *CMS provides guidance on 30-day reassessment requirements.* https://www.mnhomecare.org/

Missouri Department of Mental Health. (2022). *State operated psychiatric hospitals and facilities.* https://dmh.mo.gov/

National Government Services. (2021). *Home health billing basics.* https://www.ngsmedicare.com/documents/20124/121705/2110_0621_0722_hh_billing_basics_508.pdf

Net Health. (2020, October 6). *Group therapy: The answer to PDPM?* https://www.nethealth.com/

Sullivan, N. (2021, May 25). *Therapy screening.* PhysicalTherapy.com. https://www.physicaltherapy.com/

University of Maryland Medical Center. (2022). *Short-term inpatient psychiatric hospitalization.* https://www.umms.org/

Yamshon, L. (2020, February 10). *"Pendulum swung too far": Therapists raise concerns over layoffs, clinical changes under PDPM.* Skilled Nursing News. https://skillednursingnews.com/

Zargar, C. (2021, August 2). *Medicare Part B reimbursement in long term care.* Experience.care. https://experience.care/

WORKSHEET 11-1

Completing the Plan

You met each of the following clients in Chapter 10 when you wrote the "A" for their SOAP notes. Now you will develop a plan for each client that includes:
- Frequency
- Duration
- Purpose of continued therapy and/or specific interventions

Ellie's Development:

S: *Parent reports that infant is gaining ~1 oz. per day and will probably be able to discontinue O$_2$ "in a couple days."*

O: *Infant participated in 30-minute OT session in home to assess visual skills and to increase mobility skills related to play (head righting, rolling supine to side lying, and push up in prone). Infant presents with low proximal and distal tone and poor head control. Infant oriented to black-and-white illuminated design by turning head. In supine, infant demonstrated visual tracking in horizontal plane 20° past midline. Infant unable to roll, right head, or push up in prone independently to engage with caregiver or toys. With facilitation of weight shift and proximal stability, infant could perform activities after about 20 seconds and hold position. Infant became fatigued and "fussy" after 20 minutes of treatment, with four 1-minute rest breaks.*

A: *Decreased postural control and need for facilitation of weight shift limits infant's ability to perform early mobility skills needed for play. Limited mobility combined with her tolerance for less than 20 minutes of activity and the need for frequent rest breaks limit her ability to explore her environment and reach developmental milestones at a typical age. Ability to perform transitional movements with facilitation, orientation to black and white design, and ability to track in horizontal plane show good progress and potential for future developmental gains. Infant would benefit from continued OT services to stimulate developmental skills and from parent education in a home program.*

P:

Ms. D's Social Participation Skills:

S: *Client reports that she understands the purpose of social skills group. She expressed a desire to attend all of the groups, saying that they are "fun."*

O: *Client participated in 60-minute social skills group focusing on friendship. Client appeared unkempt, with hair not combed and shirt rumpled. Client engaged in conversation with the other clients and the facilitator. Client interrupted others on 5 occasions. Client spontaneously verbalized her experiences with past friendships and her ideas of useful ways to make new friendships but had to be redirected to the topic twice during discussion.*

A: *Client's unkempt appearance, interrupting behaviors, and need for redirection to topic of conversation interfere with her ability to engage in social participation with peers. Her expressed interest in groups and her willingness to engage in conversation and share her ideas show good potential to develop relationships and to express herself verbally in place of acting out. Client would benefit from participating in groups where conversational skills are stressed, from further facilitation of attention to social cues, and from instruction in ADLs stressing hygiene and appearance.*

P:

WORKSHEET 11-1 (CONTINUED)
Completing the Plan

Mr. Y's Functional Performance:

S: *Client stated, "I think my right arm is getting stronger. This morning I was able to wash my face using my right hand."*

O: *Client participated in 30-minute session in OT clinic to work on functional use of R UE in prep for ADL activities. Client deficits include R UE hemiparesis, decreased sitting balance, and decreased cognition. Client needed mod A in shifting weight to get to edge of w/c and max verbal cues to use correct posture and shift feet during stand pivot transfer w/c to mat. Client required max verbal cues to initiate grasp of small beanbag. Client needed mod A in reaching with R UE. Client able to complete R UE shoulder flexion required to toss beanbag ~2 ft. with max verbal cues. Client demonstrated cognitive understanding of activity with mod verbal cues by stating desired goal to be achieved by accurate aim. Client tolerated up to 3 minutes of activity before requiring rest break.*

A: *Deficits in motor planning, movement initiation, cognition, and muscle weakness in R UE result in decreased safety and independence in ADL tasks and functional mobility during ADLs. Ability to tolerate 3 minutes of activity at a time indicates progress over baseline of 1 minute activity tolerance. Client would benefit from skilled OT to increase balance, functional mobility, and grasp/release activities with involved UE to increase independence in self-care activities.*

P:

Marco's Visual Motor Skills:

S: *Child stated, "This is hard!" during a bilateral coordination exercise requiring UE strength and stability.*

O: *Child participated in 30-minute session in school therapy room to address skills related to handwriting and other visual motor classroom tasks. Child presents with deficits in oculomotor movements, fine motor skills, and upper body strength and stability necessary for dynamic UE function in the classroom.*

Visual Tracking: Child visually tracked a moving object 4 times R to L @ 40% accuracy and L to R @ 20% accuracy. Child demonstrated 20% accuracy of eye convergence 4x staring 12" from nose and breaking at ~6" from nose.

UE Coordination: Child performed B UE coordination activity (Zoom ball) at 80% accuracy with hyperextended knees and trunk movement to compensate for upper body weakness.

Handwriting: Child able to write letters P, E, F, D, M, N, R from memory with 90% accuracy and 75% accuracy for staying in line boundaries with min verbal cues.

A: *Decreased upper body strength and proximal stability limit the child's ability to use his upper extremities in an accurate and coordinated manner in class. Lack of fine motor and bilateral coordination limit the child's accuracy in schoolwork (including handwriting, art, and play activities). Inaccuracy in visual tracking and eye convergence interfere with ability to form letters and numbers or to complete written work from a book or whiteboard at grade level. Lack of visual tracking and convergence skills also limit ability to perform age-appropriate games safely. Improvement in accuracy of letter formation since last note and ability to remember 6 letter shapes indicate good progress and good potential to meet IEP goals. Child would benefit from continued work on postural stability to support functional UE use, as well as from continued work on visual and motor skills needed for classroom activities.*

P:

WORKSHEET **11-1** (CONTINUED)

Completing the Plan

Mr. S's Social Participation Skills:

S: *Mr. S stated he knows what assertion is, but reports, "Manipulation and aggression have always worked better for me." When asked to explain assertion, Mr. S stated, "The problem with that is the sugar and fruit in the cake."*

O: *Mr. S attended 1-hr. assertion group this date for skilled instruction and role-play activities to improve assertion and effective self-expression skills. Mr. S was on time to the group, neatly dressed with hair combed. He was unable to correctly define assertion and did not respond to any of the 3 role-play activities, either by taking a role or by offering suggestions to others. During the role-play, Mr. S placed his head down and closed his eyes. Following the session, Mr. S quickly left the room.*

A: *Poor ability to define assertive behavior and the statement that he prefers manipulation and aggression as relational skills limit Mr. S's ability to resolve conflicts and relate to others effectively, thus limiting his ability to function independently in a community setting. Lack of participation in group activity limits ability to explore alternate ways of communicating with others. Ability to manage time, willingness to remain in group until the end, and good dressing/grooming skills indicate good potential to meet stated goal of moving to next level of least restrictive environment. Client would benefit from group and individual OT sessions to address social communication skills with emphasis on alternative conflict resolution skills.*

P:

WORKSHEET 11-2

SOAPing Your Note

Now that you understand all the components of a SOAP note, indicate in which section of the SOAP note you would place each of these statements.

_____ *Supine to sit in bed independently.*

_____ *Client moved kitchen items from counter to cabinet independently using L hand.*

_____ *Decreased coordination, strength, sensation, and proprioception in L hand create safety risks in home management tasks.*

_____ *Client reports that his fingers are stiff this morning and that he is having trouble handling small items like buttons.*

_____ *Increase of 15 minutes in activity tolerance for UE activities permits client to prepare a light meal with supervision.*

_____ *Child participated in 60-minute eval. of hand function in OT clinic.*

_____ *Decreased proprioception and motor planning limit independence in upper body dressing.*

_____ *Continue retrograde massage to R hand for edema control.*

_____ *Correct identification of inappropriate positioning 100% of time indicates memory WFL.*

_____ *Client reports that she cannot remember hip precautions.*

_____ *Veteran would benefit from further instruction to incorporate total hip precautions into lower body dressing, bathing, and toileting.*

_____ *Client's improvement with repetition indicates good potential for successful access of augmentative communication device using eye gaze.*

_____ *Client did not make eye contact during group session.*

_____ *Client wrote check for correct amount to pay electric bill with 2 verbal cues.*

_____ *Client's request to take breaks demonstrates awareness of her limitations in endurance.*

_____ *Client completed weight shifts of trunk x 10 in each of anterior, posterior, left, and right lateral directions in preparation for standing to perform IADLs.*

_____ *3+ muscle grade of R wrist extension this week shows good progress toward goals.*

_____ *Continue OT 3x/wk for 2 weeks to address cognitive impairments that affect safe performance of IADLs.*

_____ *Unkempt appearance in mock interview situation indicates poor judgment and self-concept.*

WORKSHEET 11-3

Identifying Areas for Improvement in a Note

This worksheet will help you apply the principles of SOAP note writing described in Chapters 8 through 11. This note is **almost** good enough. In fact, it is quite good on the surface, but has major flaws in organization and professional reasoning. Mrs. B is a 78-year-old woman who has had a L CVA and has R hemiparesis. You do not have to rewrite this note, but as you read through it, keep track of suggestions that you have for improving it.

S: *Client reports stiffness in her R hip, but improvement from previous pain. She states a preference for transferring to her L side. Client states she is willing to do "whatever it takes to get out of the hospital."*

O: *Client participated in 45-minute session in room to work on dressing and functional mobility during ADLs. Pt. deficits include decreased balance and limited R ROM.*

Transfer: Stand pivot transfer bed to w/c to L side SBA. Min A with transfers w/c to toilet using grab bar.

Mobility: Client rolled supine to R side SBA with VCs to flex trunk. Client supine to sit SBA; sit to stand min A; independent with w/c mobility.

Dressing: Client donned shirt independently.

    Client donned bra min A with VCs while standing.

    Client donned socks and shoes independently.

    Client donned underwear and pants with min A and VCs to stand with walker.

    Client needs set-up for dressing activities.

    UE ROM: L UE—WFL; R UE—decreased range in shoulder flexion.

Static Standing: Client used walker for B UE support with CGA.

Dynamic Standing: SBA with walker for balance.

A: *Deficits noted in R UE coordination, B UE strength, and dynamic standing balance. Client independent in dressing EOB, but is min A in dressing when standing with a walker. L UE AROM is WFL, but R UE has deficits noted in shoulder flexion. Client needs SBA in bed mobility when rolling to unaffected side and min A in sit to stand 2° decreased UE strength. Client needs SBA for transfer to unaffected side in pivot transfer bed to w/c and min A w/c to toilet. Client would benefit from skilled OT to continue UE strengthening and coordination exercise and to increase dynamic standing balance using walker to increase independence in ADLs.*

P: *Client to be seen 30 minutes bid for 2 weeks to continue work on dynamic standing balance during ADLs.*

What suggestions do you have for improving this note?

WORKSHEET 11-4

Revising a Note

This worksheet will help you apply the principles of SOAP note writing described in Chapters 8 through 11. Jenna is a preschool child who is receiving occupational therapy twice weekly to increase her tolerance for sensory input for improved success with ADLs and play skills. As you read through each section of the note, make a bulleted list of ways to improve that section. Then rewrite the entire note.

S: *Grandma came in and stated, "Jenna was excited this morning to come see you girls." She also commented that Jenna tolerated a few seconds of tooth brushing this morning. Throughout session, Jenna stated several times, "wipe my hands" or "wipe my arms" when foam got on them for too long. She also cried out and yelled "stop" when she had enough of the oral ranging exercise.*

Revisions for S:
-
-
-

O: *Child was seen in the clinic to decrease oral defensiveness.*

Proprioception/Deep Pressure: *The therapist began the session with a variety of proprioception and deep pressure activities to allow Jenna to have a better sense of her position in space. Jenna chose to bounce on the big therapy ball first, needing CGA. Jenna then began jumping and sliding, which added a vestibular element. These activities prepped her to engage attentively to the remainder of the session.*

Sensory: *The therapist presented Jenna with foam, water, and foam stick-ups to play with. Jenna was hesitant to play with or touch any of the objects, but after prompting, Jenna actually touched the foam but immediately wanted her hands wiped off. Touching this texture is the beginning of a desensitization process that will assist her to be more tolerant of different textures for the purpose of feeding and hygiene.*

Oral Motor: *The therapist introduced the idea of Jenna feeding the babies food in hopes of imitation. However, when Jenna put the spoon to her own mouth, she began spitting. The therapist followed up this activity with completing oral resistive exercises of elongating and protruding the lips as well as stretching the cheek muscles. The intention is to increase muscle length and range for feeding. Jenna had an adverse reaction to this.*

Revisions for O:
-
-
-
-
-

WORKSHEET 11-4 (CONTINUED)

Revising a Note

A: *Child has increased tolerance for proprioception activities, which has led to an increased ability for her to concentrate on one activity at a time. However, her unwillingness to engage in sensory activities with wet and semi-wet media is still a concern in relation to eating. Hopefully with continued desensitization and oral resistive exercise, Jenna will have decreased oral/tactile defensiveness.*

Revisions for A:
-
-
-

P: *Continue plan of care.*

Revisions for P:
-
-
-

Revised SOAP Note:

S:

O:

A:

P:

Chapter 12

Intervention Planning

Now that you know the basics of writing a SOAP note, I will back up a little and give some attention to the intervention planning on which your notes are based. You may recall from Chapter 1 that the *Occupational Therapy Practice Framework: Domain and Process, Fourth Edition* (*OTPF-4*; American Occupational Therapy Association [AOTA], 2020), describes both the domain and the process of occupational therapy. The first part of the occupational therapy process involves a thorough evaluation, including development of an occupational profile, analysis of occupational performance, and synthesis of all evaluation data to determine client values and priorities, collaboratively set goals with the client, and identify targeted outcomes.

The next step in the occupational therapy process is documenting the intervention plan to guide practitioners involved in the client's care. According to the *OTPF-4*, "the intervention plan is developed collaboratively with clients or their proxies and is directed by

- Client goals, values, beliefs, and occupational needs and
- Client health and well-being,
  as well as by the practitioner's evaluation of
- Client occupational performance needs;
- Collective influence of the contexts, occupational or activity demands, and client factors on the client;
- Client performance skills and performance patterns;
- Context of service delivery in which the intervention is provided; and
- Best available evidence" (AOTA, 2020, p. 25)

As explained in Chapter 11, the intervention plan is part of the "P" section of an evaluation note. Chapter 15 will discuss additional requirements related to evaluation documentation. This chapter will focus specifically on the goals, objectives, and intervention strategies contained in the intervention plan.

The *OTPF-4* explains that interventions may be developed for a person, group, or population (AOTA, 2020). For purposes of learning, this manual will focus only on interventions targeted at individuals. However, the techniques described in this manual can be adapted for occupational therapy practitioners who serve groups and populations.

Gateley, C. A. *Documentation Manual for Occupational Therapy, Fifth Edition* (pp. 161-176). © 2024 Taylor & Francis Group.

THE INTERVENTION PLANNING PROCESS

From the moment a referral is received, an occupational therapist begins intervention planning. The client's age, primary diagnosis and comorbidities, and reason for referral should stimulate an occupational therapist to begin reviewing in their mind the areas of occupation likely to be assessed, the areas of deficit that might be found, and the possible interventions that will benefit the client. The mental preparation for *"Clyde C, age 68, L CVA, evaluate and treat"* takes a therapist on a professional reasoning journey along one road of thought, whereas *"Brooke J, age 4, ADHD, evaluate and treat"* takes the therapist down a different professional reasoning pathway. From day one, a good therapist also begins discharge planning based on the client's occupational profile, prior level of performance, and probable discharge placement.

The initial evaluation and intervention plan are written in whatever format the facility uses, and this varies greatly depending on practice setting. In earlier chapters, you learned how to write functional problem statements and how to address those problems by writing long-term goals (LTGs) and short-term goals (STGs), also known as *objectives*. Now I will discuss how to select intervention approaches and specific strategies to address the identified problems and to assist the client in meeting the established goals.

APPROACHES TO INTERVENTION

According to the *OTPF-4*, "approaches to intervention are specific strategies selected to direct the evaluation and intervention processes on the basis of the client's desired outcomes, evaluation data, and research evidence" (AOTA, 2020, p. 63). The *OTPF-4* defines the following approaches to intervention:

1. **Create or promote**—This approach focuses on creating experiences and enriching contexts to enhance occupational performance.
2. **Establish or restore**—This approach focuses on development of new skills or remediation/restoration of impaired skills or abilities.
3. **Maintain**—This approach focuses on preserving performance capabilities, assuming that performance would decline without intervention.
4. **Modify**—This approach focuses on revising the context or activity through adaptation or compensatory techniques.
5. **Prevent**—This approach focuses on the prevention of occupational performance problems or barriers for people with or without a disability.

As discussed in Chapter 5, the word "maintain" can be a red flag to reviewers. Although the 2013 *Jimmo v Sebelius* Supreme Court ruling clarified that the potential for improvement is not required for Medicare reimbursement (Centers for Medicare & Medicaid Services, 2021), your documentation must clearly demonstrate that the skills of an occupational therapy practitioner were required to prevent further functional decline.

TYPES OF OCCUPATIONAL THERAPY INTERVENTIONS

The approach to intervention that you use will help determine which specific occupational therapy interventions you will select to meet your client's goals. Table 12-1 summarizes the types of occupational therapy interventions described in the *OTPF-4* (AOTA, 2020). "Occupational therapy interventions facilitate engagement in occupation to enable persons, groups, and populations to achieve health, well-being, and participation in life" (AOTA, 2020, p. 59).

Table 12-1

TYPES OF OCCUPATIONAL THERAPY INTERVENTIONS

TYPES OF OCCUPATIONAL THERAPY INTERVENTIONS	DESCRIPTION	EXAMPLES
Occupations and Activities	"Occupations are broad and specific daily life events that are personalized and meaningful to the client" (AOTA, 2020, p. 59). "Activities are components of occupations that are objective and separate from the client's engagement or contexts. Activities as interventions are selected and designed to support the development of performance skills and performance patterns to enhance occupational engagement" (AOTA, 2020, p. 59).	**Occupations:** • Completing morning dressing routine • Going through school lunch line to obtain lunch tray and transporting it to a table to eat lunch with peers **Activities:** • Practicing clothing fasteners with a button hook/zipper pull in preparation for dressing • Completing a simulated bill-paying activity
Interventions to Support Occupations	These interventions are used as a means of preparing the client for or supporting the client during occupational performance. They should be part of a broader intervention plan and should not be used exclusively.	• Physical agent modalities (PAMs) such as electrical stimulation, paraffin, and iontophoresis • Mechanical modalities such as manual lymphatic drainage for lymphedema • Orthotics and prosthetics • Assistive technology • Environmental modifications • Wheeled mobility • Self-regulation approaches such as sensory environments
Education and Training	Education focuses on imparting knowledge, whereas training is focused on the acquisition of concrete skills. "Training is differentiated from education by its goal of enhanced performance as opposed to enhanced understanding," but they often are used in conjunction with each other (AOTA, 2020, p. 61).	**Education:** • Educating a client regarding IADL completion following post-surgical precautions • Giving a parent a list of home activity ideas to support infant development **Training:** • Showing a client how to don a post-surgical back brace and then having the client demonstrate the skill • Showing a caregiver how to apply a resting hand splint and then having the caregiver demonstrate the skill

(continued)

Table 12-1 (continued)

TYPES OF OCCUPATIONAL THERAPY INTERVENTIONS

TYPES OF OCCUPATIONAL THERAPY INTERVENTIONS	DESCRIPTION	EXAMPLES
Advocacy	Advocacy involves "efforts directed toward promoting occupational justice and empowering clients to seek and obtain resources to support health, well-being, and occupational participation" (AOTA, 2020, p. 61). This includes efforts by the occupational therapy practitioner or self-advocacy by the client.	**Advocacy:** • Occupational therapy practitioner writes letter to local agency requesting funding for adaptive equipment for client's home • Occupational therapy practitioner provides recommendations to school staff for increased inclusion of student in annual school musical performance **Self-Advocacy:** • Client contacts campus disability center to request learning accommodations • Client contacts local independent living center to inquire about support for building a wheelchair ramp
Group Interventions	Group interventions involve two or more clients working on similar activities or focused on similar topics.	• Residents in a memory care unit participating in reminiscence group • Individuals in a long-term inpatient psychiatric hospital discussing coping skills needed for community re-entry
Virtual Interventions	Virtual interventions involve the use of telehealth or smart phone technology to provide occupational therapy services.	• Telehealth visit with a client in a rural area • Visit via smart phone video chat with an early intervention client and family during a pandemic when in-person visits are not possible or discouraged

Data source: American Occupational Therapy Association, 2020.

OTHER CONSIDERATIONS IN INTERVENTION PLANNING

In addition to being aware of the different intervention approaches and techniques, there are other factors that must be considered when setting goals and selecting interventions to meet those goals.

Estimating Rehab Potential

Rehab potential should always be stated as good or excellent for the goals you and the client have selected. If your client's rehab potential is not good or excellent for the stated goals, you may need to select smaller, more incremental goals. It is not helpful to set and work toward goals that the client does not have a good chance of accomplishing. Estimating rehab potential as *poor*, *fair*, or *guarded* is a red flag to reviewers, and they may be reluctant to set aside health care dollars for someone who is unlikely to benefit from your intervention.

Note: "Rehab potential" does not mean "independence." It means potential to reach the goals you have set or potential for the client to make significant change. For example, you may set a goal that reads:

Client will complete all dressing tasks seated in chair with min A from caregiver by November 15th.

In this case, the expectation is not that the client will be independent but you believe the client has good potential to progress to a level sufficient that the caregiver can provide the level of assistance needed in order to return home.

Selecting Meaningful Intervention Strategies

To an inexperienced therapist, it can seem like reinventing the wheel to select different strategies and treatment media for each individual client. One of the striking differences between occupational therapy and other disciplines is the way in which strategies and media are selected to meet the client's goals. Occupational therapy is a client-centered profession, and the selected interventions should be meaningful to each individual client (Ikiugu et al., 2019). Occupational therapy is a process of creative problem solving with each client in each area of occupation. What is meaningful to one client may not be meaningful to another.

Even the most basic task such as dressing may not seem meaningful to some clients. For example, a person with tetraplegia who has a personal attendant will never be able to complete self-dressing without assistance and may consider it an enormous waste of time to be required to learn to do so. However, they may be very motivated to learn how to use a power wheelchair operated with head controls to be independent with mobility needed to re-engage in social participation with their friends. Some clients will not need to do laundry because family helps with that chore, while others may not be able to return to living independently without this skill. The difference between competent and exceptional occupational therapy may lie in the ability to find meaningful activities, and design these into intervention strategies. The occupational therapist asks questions such as:

- What do you want to be able to do?
- What keeps you from being able to do that?
- What are the possible options for making that happen?

The options for intervention strategies may include teaching new skills or performance patterns, working to increase client factors (ROM, strength, endurance), or modifying the activity or the environment (context) to improve occupational performance. Occupational therapists use their creativity in intervention planning. How many ways are there to get light into a room if the client can no longer manage a light switch? How many activities that require wrist extension could be adapted as interventions to work toward a LTG of returning to an assembly line position that requires increased AROM of the wrist? Would any of these activities qualify as meaningful to this client?

The treatment media used in occupational therapy is also different from that used by other disciplines. Occupational therapists often use common household objects to accomplish tasks or activities related to occupational performance. For example, the client's own clothing is a common treatment media. The clothes may be used for dressing to teach the client to don clothing, for folding to have the client perform a meaningful activity while increasing standing tolerance, or for hanging in a closet to help the client increase AROM at the shoulder. The approach would depend on what the client will need to do in the setting to which they will be discharged. An experienced occupational therapist can find many different uses for common household objects. The same sponge that is used to wash dishes may be used for squeezing to develop grip strength or for throwing to develop AROM in the UEs.

"Bottom-Up" Versus "Top-Down" Approaches

The concepts of "bottom-up" and "top-down" approaches for evaluation and intervention have received considerable attention in the recent occupational therapy literature (Boone, 2018; Ikiugu et al., 2019; Ko et al., 2017; Skubik et al., 2021). Bottom-up approaches use interventions that address foundational deficits related to occupations such as ROM, fine motor coordination, and attention skills. Top-down approaches involve the use of meaningful occupations and activities as a means of addressing underlying client deficits. Examples include engagement in dressing tasks, opening a toothpaste cap, opening a food package, and engagement in higher-level cognitive processes such as self-awareness of stress levels during social interaction. Although both approaches have merit, top-down approaches or top-down approaches combined with bottom-up approaches are believed to result in better carryover and generalization of skills than bottom-up approaches used in isolation. Occupational therapy practitioners should ensure that they are not using only bottom-up approaches in their intervention plans. Effort should be made to focus on top-down approaches as well.

Theoretical Basis of Intervention

Throughout your occupational therapy curriculum, you will be introduced to several theories, conceptual models, and frames of reference that guide occupational therapy practice. Cole and Tufano (2020) explained that these terms often are used interchangeably. However, they clarified that a model is "an organizing technique designed to assist in categorizing ideas and structuring approaches to thinking about complex problems" (Cole & Tufano, 2020, p. 91). Models explain how the person, environment, and occupation interact and can be applied across most occupational therapy practice settings. In contrast, a frame of reference guides evaluation and intervention for specific types of clients or practice settings. As you are developing an intervention plan, you should be able to relate your planned interventions back to one or more frames of reference. It is common practice for occupational therapists to use a combination of approaches.

Note: Students and new practitioners need to be very intentional in connecting theoretical foundations to clinical decisions regarding intervention. However, as occupational therapists gain experience, they rarely articulate or document the theoretical basis underlying specific strategies in their intervention plans. It is beyond the scope of this textbook to review the numerous frames of reference that guide occupational therapy intervention.

Orthopedic Post-Surgical Protocols

I have been an occupational therapist for nearly 3 decades. Few areas of occupational therapy practice have changed more drastically in that time than the rehabilitation approach for individuals who have had an elective orthopedic surgery. Years ago, patients who had a hip or knee replacement would be hospitalized for 1 to 2 weeks, or perhaps even longer. The average length of stay steadily decreased over time, and now it is common for people to discharge home just 1 or 2 days after surgery (Mundi et al., 2020). If a patient is not able to discharge home in a short amount of time, the interprofessional care team begins exploring options for post-acute care, such as a SNF or inpatient rehabilitation facility.

Previous editions of this textbook included examples of clinical pathways after orthopedic surgery that detailed what the occupational therapy practitioner should do each day of the patient's hospital stay. "Clinical pathways provide hospitals with a consistent template for patient care by creating a predetermined standardized approach to care" (Duggal et al., 2020, p. 437). Clinical pathways help optimize quality and efficiency of care by providing expected outcomes for the client and standardized orders for nursing and therapy practitioners. Clinical pathways originally "were designed to improve the patient experience focusing primarily on improvements in pain management and post-operative physical rehabilitation" (Duggal et al., 2020, p. 437). By the late 2000s, in response to advances in surgical procedures and pressures from payers for increased efficiency, pathways were modified "to help reduce length of stay to accommodate a large increase in the volume of these procedures in the setting of a fixed bed capacity" (Duggal et al., 2020, p. 438).

It is now common practice for most patients who have undergone elective hip or knee arthroplasty to receive physical and occupational therapy on the day of surgery for early mobilization and education regarding any relevant post-surgical precautions. Rather than specifying a particular day on which other interventions should occur, post-surgical protocols often include a list of precautions, interventions, and patient expectations, with the assumption that each intervention and outcome should be targeted as quickly as the patient tolerates. See Table 12-2 for examples of orthopedic post-surgical protocols. In many cases, occupational therapy practitioners must address all these issues in only one or two sessions. The client's medical status certainly plays a role in length of stay as medical providers and nurses address pain management, incision healing, removal of post-surgical drains, discontinuation of intravenous fluids and medications, and any management of any pre-existing or new comorbidities. Clients are discharged as soon as they are medically stable and have either achieved all expected outcomes to return home or an alternative post-acute placement has been arranged by the care team.

Table 12-2

EXAMPLES OF ORTHOPEDIC POST-SURGICAL PROTOCOLS

TYPE OF SURGERY	POST-SURGICAL PROTOCOL
Total Hip or Knee Arthroplasty	• Day-of surgery evaluation to include transfer bed to chair or BSC as able and education regarding applicable WB and hip/knee precautions; see specific surgeon orders for details • Continue functional transfers and mobility each session in the context of ADL performance • Educate re: applicable positioning restrictions; see specific surgeon orders for details (e.g., abductor wedge for THA, no pillows under knees for TKA) • Ongoing skilled instruction in all precautions; provide handouts; review each session and have pt. and caregivers verbalize and demonstrate adherence • Assess adaptive equipment needs for dressing, bathing, toileting; procure via hospital procedures or educate pt./caregiver regarding other available resources • Practice dressing, toileting, bathing, and grooming in stand at sink; check physician orders re: bathing restrictions • Educate regarding car transfer; must demonstrate before discharge if returning home or family transporting to post-acute facility • Provide home safety education regarding ADLs and IADLs

Spinal Surgery	• Post-op Day 1 eval to include, at minimum, transfer bed to chair or BSC; mobility in room during ADLs as able
	• Educate re: log roll technique for supine to/from sit (PT also does this)
	• Educate re: back precautions (no "BLT")
	  ◦ No bending
	  ◦ No lifting (amount varies by physician protocol, check orders)
	  ◦ No twisting
	• Educate re: any applicable sitting restrictions (varies by physician protocol, check orders)
	• Train pt./caregiver to don back brace or cervical collar, if applicable (varies by surgeon and specific procedure)
	  ◦ Check orders re: whether brace/collar must be donned supine or EOB
	  ◦ Check orders re: whether brace/collar can be off in bed or recliner
	• Continue functional transfers and mobility each session in the context of ADL performance
	• Ongoing skilled instruction in all precautions; provide handouts; review each session and have pt. and caregivers verbalize and demonstrate adherence
	• Practice dressing, toileting, bathing, and grooming in stand at sink; check physician orders re: bathing restrictions
	• Educate regarding car transfer; must demonstrate before discharge if returning home or family transporting to post-acute facility
	• Provide home safety education regarding ADLs and IADLs

(continued)

Table 12-2

Examples of Orthopedic Post-Surgical Protocols

TYPE OF SURGERY	POST-SURGICAL PROTOCOL

Shoulder Arthroplasty	• Post-op Day 1 eval to include, at minimum, transfer bed to chair or BSC; mobility in room during ADLs as able
	• Educate re: shoulder precautions (check physician orders for details)
	  ○ No lifting arm away from body (shoulder flexion or abduction)
	  ○ No reaching behind head or back (shoulder IR or ER)
	  ○ No lifting anything heavier than a coffee cup
	  ○ No pushing/holding body weight up with arm during transfers and mobility
	  ○ No sudden or jerky movements
	• Train pt./caregiver re: don/doff sling or brace and wearing schedule
	• Train pt./caregiver re: placing pillow under elbow of operated arm to prevent shoulder extension beyond neutral, particularly in supine
	• Assess adaptive equipment needs for dressing, bathing, toileting; procure via hospital procedures or educate pt./caregiver regarding other available resources
	• Practice dressing, toileting, bathing, and grooming in stand at sink; check physician orders re: bathing restrictions
	• Teach pendulum exercises (check physician orders; varies by physician and procedure)
	• AROM of elbow, wrist, and hand of operated UE

Data sources: Orthopedic Specialists of North Carolina, 2022; St. Elizabeth's Medical Center, 2022; and author's personal experience.

Please note that the protocols in Table 12-2 are written in terms of the interventions that the **therapist** will carry out. Your goals still need to be written in terms of the occupational performance that the **client** will demonstrate. We do not just want the client to repeat their precautions to us. We want them to follow those precautions during occupational performance. In many cases, "while adhering to post-surgical precautions" becomes a portion of the "S" part of your COAST goal:

Example: *Client will don pants with SBA using reacher and walker, adhering to all post-surgical hip precautions, by discharge in 2 days.*

Sample Intervention Plan

Client Name: *Norma H*   **Age:** *85*   **1° Dx:** *L CVA*   **2° Dx:** *DM*

Setting: *SNF*   **Frequency/Duration:** *5x/wk for 4 weeks*

Occupational Profile: *Mrs. H is a widow who lives with her daughter and grandson in a one-story house in a small town. Mrs. H was independent in all ADL and IADL tasks before her CVA. She has never worked outside her home. She raised 7 children in the town where she now resides and takes pride in her ability to do homemaking tasks such as cooking, sewing, and decorating. She drives in her own small town but is not comfortable driving long distances. She intends to return to the home she shares with her daughter and grandson and hopes to return to her PLOF.*

Problem: *Client requires mod A in self-care due to inability to spontaneously use R UE due to L CVA.*

Long-Term Goal: *Client will complete all ADL and IADL activities independently with adaptive equipment within 4 weeks.*

STG (OBJECTIVE)	INTERVENTION	TYPE OF INTERVENTION
STG #1: *Client will complete grooming tasks with set-up using R UE spontaneously as a functional assist within 1 week.*	1. *Normalize tone through weight bearing on R UE with facilitated weight shifting.* 2. *Therapy putty exercises to improve hand and finger strength.* 3. *Neuromuscular electrical stimulation to strengthen R wrist extensors.* 4. *Facilitate grasp/release for use of prehension; facilitate reach patterns through handling, joint approximation, guided resistance, and muscle stretch.* 5. *Provide activities that require use of R UE as an assist (stabilizing tablet or clipboard while writing).* 6. *Complete morning grooming routine involving stabilizing toothpaste while removing lid and applying body lotion.*	1. *Intervention to support occupation* 2. *Intervention to support occupation* 3. *Intervention to support occupation* 4. *Intervention to support occupation* 5. *Activity* 6. *Occupation*
STG #2: *Client will dress self with min A within 2 weeks using R UE as a functional assist.*	1. *UE ergometer ("arm bike") for increased R UE strengthening.* 2. *Instruct in adaptive dressing techniques and adaptive equipment as needed: long shoehorn, elastic laces, reacher, button hook.* 3. *UE exercise group with other SNF clients with similar deficits in strength.* 4. *Facilitate trunk control and balance in weight shifts forward and backward, side to side, and in rotational patterns while engaged in reaching.* 5. *Practice use of button hook to fasten buttons on shirt.* 6. *Complete morning dressing routine using R UE to hold bra while hooking in front, assist in pulling up pants, and stabilize shirt while buttoning.*	1. *Intervention to support occupation* 2. *Education and training* 3. *Group intervention* 4. *Intervention to support occupation* 5. *Activity* 6. *Occupation*
STG #3: *Client will complete light meal prep and clean-up using wheeled walker with SBA for safety within 3 weeks.*	1. *In collaboration with client and family, make recommendations for environmental modifications to adapt kitchen for safe accessibility and mobility.* 2. *Provide family with contact info for local equipment consortium to explore equipment that can be borrowed for free.* 3. *Select and instruct in use of adaptive equipment for one-handedness as needed to peel and chop vegetables, open cans and jars.* 4. *Remove/replace items from kitchen cabinet.* 5. *Practice item transport in kitchen using a wheeled walker and rolling cart.* 6. *Plan a hypothetical meal with attention to money management, organization, and sequencing.* 7. *Bake brownies in preparation for family visit.*	1. *Education* 2. *Advocacy* 3. *Education and training* 4. *Activity* 5. *Activity* 6. *Activity* 7. *Occupation*

Note that the interventions planned for Mrs. H include a variety of intervention types with a progression toward activity and occupation. In an actual intervention plan, you would not need to specify the type of intervention. That column is included here to encourage you to think beyond supportive interventions such as modalities and exercises and to move toward occupation-based goals and interventions. Note also that the planned interventions are based on multiple frames of reference including biomechanical, rehabilitative, and motor learning.

COMMON ERRORS IN WRITING INTERVENTION PLANS

Problem Identification

- Problems identified in the Assessment are not addressed in the Plan.
- Problems are not stated in terms of behavioral manifestations, areas of occupation, and contributing factors.
- The number of visits requested does not match the severity of the documented problems.

Goals

- Goals are not functional or do not focus on the reason for referral to occupational therapy.
- Intervention plan does not focus on specific rehabilitation goals that will increase a client's ability to engage in meaningful occupation in the probable discharge environment.
- Goals focus on the client participating in or cooperating with treatment (unless the client is in the habit of refusing treatment; more acceptable in behavioral health settings).
- Goals are not measurable or do not have a target date for completion.

Intervention Strategies

- Interventions do not focus on increasing functional behaviors to return the client to the least restrictive environment.
- Interventions do not consider the age, gender, and interests of the client or are not meaningful to the client.
- Acquired skills are not transferred into more functional contexts in the client's life.
- Intervention strategies focus too heavily on preparatory supportive approaches without progression toward purposeful activities and occupation-based interventions.

Client Involvement

- The client is not involved in the treatment planning process. In many settings, you will be required to ask the client what their goal is and document that goal in your evaluation or intervention plan.
- Intervention plan does not reflect the client's strengths, desires, and preferences.

"Canned" Plans

- "Canned" intervention plans reflect the exact same goals, objectives, and interventions for each client based on the diagnosis and services available rather than on client need. Even clinical pathways need to be individualized to fit the client.

REFERENCES

American Occupational Therapy Association. (2020). Occupational therapy practice framework: Domain and process (4th ed.). *American Journal of Occupational Therapy, 74*(Suppl. 2), 7412410010. https://doi.org/10.5014.ajot.2020.74S2001

Boone, A. (2018). Feasibility of combining virtual reality motor rehabilitation with cognitive strategy use for people with stroke. *American Journal of Occupational Therapy, 72*(4_Suppl_1), 7211515276p1. https://doi.org/10.5014/ajot.2018.72S1-PO6046

Centers for Medicare & Medicaid Services. (2021). *Jimmo settlement.* https://www.cms.gov/

Cole, M. B., & Tufano, R. (2020). *Applied theories in occupational therapy: A practical approach* (2nd ed.). SLACK Incorporated.

Duggal, S., Flics, S., Kujawa, K., & Cornell, C. N. (2020). Introduction of clinical pathways in orthopedic surgical care: The experience of the hospital for special surgery. In C. MacKenzie, C. Cornell, & S. Memtsoudis (Eds.), *Perioperative care of the orthopedic patient* (pp. 437-443). Springer. https://doi.org/10.1007/978-3-030-35570-8_35

Ikiugu, M. N., Lucas-Molitor, W., Feldhacker, D., Gebhart, C., Spier, M., Kappels, L., Arnold, R., & Gaikowski, R. (2019). Guidelines for occupational therapy interventions based on meaningful and psychologically rewarding occupations. *Journal of Happiness Studies, 20*(7), 2027-2053. https://doi.org/10.1007/s10902-018-0030-z

Ko, S. B., Kim, J. H., Kim, M. Y., & Park, H. Y. (2017). Interventions for neglect with stroke: A systematic review. *American Journal of Occupational Therapy, 71*(4_Suppl_1), 7111505110p1. https://doi.org/10.5014/ajot.2017.71S1-PO3050

Mundi, R., Axelrod, D. E., Najafabadi, B. T., Chamas, B., Chaudhry, H., & Bhandari, M. (2020). Early discharge after total hip and knee arthroplasty—An observational cohort study evaluating safety in 330,000 patients. *Journal of Arthroplasty, 35*(12), 3482-3486.

Orthopedic Specialists of North Carolina. (2022). *Orthopedic rehabilitation protocols.* https://orthonc.com/your-health/postoperative-rehabilitation-protocols

Skubik, C., Hight, J., & Rushing-Carr, C. (2021). What improves handwriting: Occupation-based or handwriting interventions? *American Journal of Occupational Therapy, 75*(Suppl. 2), 7512515348p1. https://doi.org/10.5014/ajot.2021.75S2-RP348

St. Elizabeth's Medical Center. (2022). *Patient resources and rehabilitation protocols.* https://www.semc.org/services-directory/orthopedics/patient-information/rehabilitation-protocols

WORKSHEET 12-1

Choosing Intervention Strategies

Intervention strategies do not stand alone. Strategies must be based on problems and LTGs, and they must be purposeful to the client to be useful. However, for purposes of learning to generate possible strategies, we will suspend that requirement and think of as many ways as possible to meet a treatment objective. Consider the following example:

STG (OBJECTIVE)	INTERVENTION	TYPE OF INTERVENTION
With SBA, client will complete ADL or IADL tasks while standing for 5-minute increments, taking rest breaks as needed, by discharge date of January 10th.	1. Have client complete 5 minutes on UE exercises ("arm bike") while standing. 2. Set up task to make coffee while standing at counter in the ADL kitchen. 3. Have client stand at the bathroom sink to complete face washing and tooth brushing. 4. Have client stand at a table to play a card game. 5. Have client stand while watering plants in windowsill of rehab dining room. 6. Have client stand to retrieve clothing from closet when dressing in the AM. 7. Have client stand to fill rehab bird feeder that her family placed outside her SNF window like the one she has at home.	1. Intervention to support occupation 2. Activity 3. Occupation 4. Activity 5. Activity (may be an occupation if plant care is important to her and she did it at home) 6. Occupation 7. Occupation

Using the STG below, think of as many intervention strategies as possible that would help the client meet this goal. Try to use a mix of intervention types as described in the *OTPF-4*.

STG (OBJECTIVE)	INTERVENTION	TYPE OF INTERVENTION
Client will manage finances independently within 3 weeks.		

WORKSHEET 12-2

Writing the Assessment and Intervention Plan—The Case of Georgia S

Name: *Georgia S*   **Age:** *87*   **Dx:** *L SDH on 8/10/23; hx. of HTN, hearing loss*
Date of Evaluation: *8-15-2023*

Background Data and Beginning Occupational Profile: *Prior to her stroke, Georgia had been living for the past 10 years with her unmarried daughter, Janice, who is 60 years old and works full-time. They live in a two-story house with the only bathroom on the second floor. Georgia was in acute care and has just been transferred to a rehabilitation center. She expresses a desire to return to her daughter's home. Her daughter has concerns about being able to care for her mother at home. Georgia has Medicare as her only insurance coverage.*

S: *Client expressed frustration trying to brush her teeth with her affected dominant R hand. Client c/o back pain 2/10 when standing for grooming. Client's daughter said that client was independent in self-care prior to her stroke but has not cooked or done housework for years; also stated that client has hearing loss but no hearing aids.*

O: *Client participated in 45-minute OT session in room for initial evaluation. Pt. presents with R UE weakness, decreased coordination, and decreased dynamic standing balance.*

Dressing/Grooming: *Client stood with CGA for 5 min while brushing teeth after set-up and 2 verbal cues. SBA in donning/doffing socks with extra time. Attempted to don R sock using same technique over and over for several minutes before being successful; did not attempt an alternative technique. Client donned/doffed gown with mod A, pulling the robe around her back and threading R UE into the sleeve. Client required four 30-second rest breaks during dressing activity due to fatigue.*

Functional Mobility: *Sit to stand SBA with wheeled walker; mod A needed for standing balance while managing clothing during bedside commode transfer. Ambulated 3 ft. w/c to sink using walker with CGA.*

UE ROM and Strength: *All UE AROM WNL except B shoulder abduction and flexion which were WFL. B UE strength 5/5 overall except 3/5 in B shoulder flex. and abd.*

Grip Strength: *L 37#, R 29#*   **Lateral Pinch:** *L 9#; R 7.5#*   **Tripod Pinch:** *L 7#; R 4#*

Sensation: *B light touch and sharp/dull discrimination intact. Client correctly identified 1 of 4 objects in R stereognosis test.*

Coordination (9 Hole Peg Test): *Placing pegs: L 37 secs, R 52 secs*
                                    Removal: L 14 secs, R 26 secs

Write the "A" and "P" as you learned in Chapters 10 and 11. Turn your problems into correctly worded problem statements. Identify the rehab potential you see for Georgia. On the intervention plan, you will include some of these items as "strengths."

A:

P:

Strengths:

WORKSHEET 12-2 (CONTINUED)

Writing the Assessment and Intervention Plan—The Case of Georgia S

For space consideration, this worksheet does not include the column asking you to identify the type of intervention. However, be sure to include a mix of intervention types as described in the *OTPF-4* as you develop Georgia's intervention plan.

Functional Problem Statement #1:

LTG #1:

STG (OBJECTIVE)	INTERVENTION
STG #1:	
STG #2:	

Functional Problem Statement #2:

LTG #2:

STG (OBJECTIVE)	INTERVENTION
STG #1:	
STG #2:	

Discharge Plan:

Worksheet **12-3**

Planning Interventions Using Groups—Complex Mental Health Needs

In some practice settings, clients are seen primarily in groups rather than individually. This strategy has the advantage of using peer feedback and support as part of the treatment process. It also provides challenges for the therapist in finding ways to structure the group to meet the needs of all the clients attending. Below is a description of a client who is being treated in a psychiatric unit where intervention strategies generally take place in groups. After you read about this client, choose intervention strategies to use for her in each of the groups she attends.

Heather S is a 40-year-old, unemployed woman with major depressive disorder who recently separated from her husband. She is on disability due to her psychiatric condition and has not worked in several years. She has two children, a daughter age 22 and a son age 18. Heather was admitted through the emergency department after ingestion of an overdose of psychiatric medications. She was lavaged and admitted briefly to a medical unit, where she was stabilized in 8 hours and transferred to the inpatient psychiatric unit.

Heather was sexually abused from the ages of 10 to 13 years by an uncle who lived in the home where she was one of five children. Her estranged husband abuses alcohol and is emotionally abusive to Heather when he has been drinking. Heather married him when she was 18 years old and pregnant with their first child. They have been married 22 years.

Heather reports that she has trouble with expression of anger. She does not always know she is getting angry, and then "explodes" in ways that are destructive to herself, others, and property. She also says she is having a lot of trouble making decisions, and that her husband has traditionally made decisions for her. She says that she "just can't think" and has difficulty paying attention to anything for more than a few minutes. For example, she is unable to complete a magazine article she is reading. Her appearance is disheveled, and her hair is uncombed. She picks at her clothing while she talks to you, looking at the floor and making little eye contact.

The problem areas identified by the treatment team include anger, decision making, and poor self-esteem with suicidal ideation. Heather's anticipated length of stay is 4 days. The psychiatric unit provides an array of individual and group treatment sessions. In addition to the medication group and the individual sessions with the psychiatrist, there is group therapy facilitated by a psychologist and an evening wrap-up group provided by nursing. Occupational therapy provides three groups per day:

- Goals group ½ hour each morning
- Stress management group 1 hour daily
- IADL group 1 hour daily

The IADL group covers topics such as money management, parenting, assertion skills, and other IADL skills depending on the needs and issues that are common to the current clients. For example, if several clients have difficulty expressing anger in useful ways, you could use IADL group time to address anger management.

In a psychiatric unit, the treatment plan is usually interdisciplinary, meaning that all team members work together to identify areas of concern, goals, and interventions. Because we are working with a 4-day length of stay and an interdisciplinary treatment plan, we will not write objectives for each of Heather's goals. Heather will be seen in occupational therapy groups every day while she is in the hospital. In this worksheet, you will decide how to use the group time to Heather's best advantage in meeting her established goals. Keep in mind that your interventions will include not only the activities you plan to use but also your therapeutic use of self with Heather—the ways you might plan to interact with her and the behaviors you want to model.

WORKSHEET **12-3** (CONTINUED)

Planning Interventions Using Groups—Complex Mental Health Needs

Problem #1: *Exacerbation of depressive symptoms resulting in a suicide attempt.*

LTG #1: *By anticipated discharge in 4 days, Heather will verbally identify strengths, care for her appearance, make eye contact when interacting with others, and develop a plan for coping with suicidal thoughts, all as evidence of improved self-esteem.*

GROUP	INTERVENTION
Goals Group	
Stress Management Group	
IADL Group	

Problem #2: *Stress related to recent role changes results in Heather's inability to concentrate and make decisions for her daily life.*

LTG #2: *Heather will apply a decision-making strategy to her two most important current life decisions by discharge in 4 days.*

GROUP	INTERVENTION
Goals Group	
Stress Management Group	
IADL Group	

Problem #3: *Inability to manage anger constructively resulting in behaviors that damage self, relationships, and property.*

LTG #3: *By anticipated discharge in 4 days, Heather independently will identify potential anger triggers, identify her physical reactions to being angry, and develop a plan to prevent escalation and destructive behaviors.*

GROUP	INTERVENTION
Goals Group	
Stress Management Group	
IADL Group	

Chapter 13

Documentation in Different Practice Settings

In this chapter, I will examine documentation in several different practice situations. Each of these practice settings has some requirements that are specific to the setting or the primary payment source. Documentation in these settings is different in some ways from the examples you have learned so far.

DOCUMENTATION IN PSYCHOSOCIAL PRACTICE SETTINGS

Although the occupational therapy profession has historical roots in mental health (MacRae, 2019c), only about 2% of occupational therapy practitioners currently report working primarily in a mental health setting (American Occupational Therapy Association [AOTA], 2019a). AOTA has been actively engaged in federal-level advocacy for occupational therapy practitioners to be able to provide, bill, and be reimbursed for mental health services. "AOTA has also engaged in significant advocacy, in conjunction with state associations, to remove barriers keeping occupational therapy practitioners from providing mental health services at the state level and promoting the value of OT in mental and behavioral health settings" (Parsons, 2022, para. 14). Despite these ongoing challenges, occupational therapy is offered in a variety of psychosocial settings, which can be divided into the following levels of service (AOTA, 2016):

- **Tier 1 includes universal services** provided to individuals with and without behavioral health concerns. At this level, occupational therapy is focused on promotion and prevention.
- **Tier 2 includes targeted services** provided to individuals at risk of developing behavioral health challenges due to "emotional experiences (e.g., trauma, abuse), situational stressors (e.g., physical disability, bullying, social isolation, obesity), or genetic factors (e.g., family history of mental illness)" (AOTA, 2016, p. 3).
- **Tier 3 includes intensive interventions** "for individuals with identified mental, emotional, or behavioral disorders that limit daily functioning, interpersonal relationships, feelings of emotional well-being, and the ability to cope with challenges in daily life" (AOTA, 2016, p. 2).

If you transition from a job in a rehabilitation center to one in a psychosocial practice setting, you might think that nothing you have learned about documentation applies. Problems, goals, and interventions are often interdisciplinary or transdisciplinary in nature and may be written in a different format from what you have learned. Professional roles often overlap, and there is often a blurring of professional identities. The language used in documentation may seem less specific than in other settings, and intervention is often provided in groups. Although not all-inclusive, Tables 13-1 through 13-3 will provide you with some terminology you may find helpful when documenting in psychosocial practice settings.

Gateley, C. A. *Documentation Manual for Occupational Therapy, Fifth Edition* (pp. 177-187). © 2024 Taylor & Francis Group.

Table 13-1

POTENTIAL FOCUS AREAS FOR PSYCHOSOCIAL INTERVENTION

Addiction recovery	Eating disorders	Job skills
Anger management	Educational skills	Legal issues and resources
Anxiety management	Emotional expression	Life transitions
Basic living skills	Establishing routines	Medication management
Behavioral problems	Financial management	Social relationships
Body image issues	Grief management	Substance use
Community reintegration	Health maintenance	Symptom management
Community resources	Health promotion	Transportation access
Coping with trauma	Home maintenance	Vocational skills
Depression management	Housing procurement	Wellness

Data sources: AOTA, 2016; MacRae 2019a, 2019b, 2019c, 2019d; MacRae & Smith, 2019; Parsons, 2022; Sutton, 2015.

Table 13-2

WORDS AND PHRASES TO DESCRIBE PSYCHOSOCIAL SYMPTOMS AND OTHER OBSERVATIONS

Acting out	Disengaged	Hypervigilance	Perseveration
Aggressive	Disheveled appearance	Impatient	Pessimistic
Agitated	Disinhibited	Impulsivity	Phobia
Akathisia	Disoriented	Inability to concentrate	Poor boundaries
Alogia	Disregard for others	Inappropriate	Poor hygiene
Aloof	Dissociation	Incoherent	Pressured speech
Angry	Distractibility	Inconsistent	Psychosis
Annoyed	Distraught	Indifference	Racing thoughts
Anxious	Dominating conversation	Insomnia	Restless
Antagonistic	Echolalia	Intoxication	Risky behaviors
Apathy	Euphoric	Irrational thought	Sedated
Avoidant	Executive dysfunction	Irritable	Self-destructive behavior
Avolition	Fatigued	Isolated	Self-injurious behavior
Belligerent	Fearful	Labile	Self-mutilation
Blunted affect	Flat affect	Lack of energy	Sleep disruption
Catatonic	Flight of thought	Lack of engagement	Social withdrawal
Circumstantial speech	Frustrated	Lack of eye contact	Suicidal ideation
Cluttered	Grandiosity	Lethargic	Suspicious
Combative	Guarded	Loosening of associations	Tangential thinking
Compulsions	Hallucination	Loss of appetite	Tics
Concrete thinking	Hesitant	Manic	Truancy
Confused	Hoarding	Mood fluctuations	Unkempt appearance
Delirium	Hopelessness	Negative thoughts	Unpredictable
Delusions	Hostile	Obsessions	Vengeful
Denial	Hyperactivity	Overwhelmed	Vindictive
Depressed	Hypersexuality	Panic attack	Withdrawal symptoms
Despondent	Hypersomnia	Paranoid	Worthlessness

Data sources: AOTA, 2016; MacRae 2019a, 2019b, 2019c, 2019d; MacRae & Smith, 2019; Parsons, 2022; Sutton, 2015.

Table 13-3

WORDS AND PHRASES FOR WRITING GOALS AND DESCRIBING THERAPEUTIC INTERVENTIONS

Acknowledged	Environmental supports	Quality of performance
Active engagement	Exhibit	Reality testing
Active listening	Explore	Recommended
Adapting	Express	Reflection
Advice	Following through	Reframing
Assertiveness	Formulated	Reinforcement
Attendance	Frustration tolerance	Relaxation techniques
Attention span	Generated	Replacing destructive habits
Brainstormed	Goal setting	Requesting assistance
Clarification	Grading	Response to authority
Coaching	Identifying interests	Response to feedback
Cognitive flexibility	Implement	Role model
Communicate effectively	Impulse control	Role play
Concentration	Insight	Self-confidence
Conflict management	Interacting with others	Self-control
Confrontation	Judgment	Self-esteem
Cooperative	Managed	Sequencing
Coping	Mediated	Setting limits
Correcting misinformation	Memory strategies	Skill development
Created	Mentoring	Socialization
Crisis stabilization	Modeled	Strengths-based approach
Cueing	Modifying	Taking responsibility
De-escalated	Motivational interviewing	Task initiation
Direction following	Occupational storytelling	Thought blocking
Discharge planning	Orientation strategies	Time management
Educational techniques	Organizational skills	Trained
Emotional regulation	Peer support	Trauma-informed approach
Empathy	Persisting	Trust building
Empowerment	Planning	Use of time
Encouragement	Problem solving	Validation
Engagement	Processes	Well-groomed
Endurance	Prompting	Work appearance
Energy level	Provide opportunities	Work behaviors
Environmental modification	Punctuality	Working with others

Data sources: AOTA, 2016; MacRae 2019a, 2019b, 2019c, 2019d; MacRae & Smith, 2019; Parsons, 2022; Sutton, 2015.

DOCUMENTATION IN SCHOOL-BASED PRACTICE

The goal of occupational therapy in school-based practice is to "help children fulfill their roles as students. Overall, occupational therapy practitioners work to promote positive behaviors and skills necessary for academic and non-academic success" (AOTA, 2019b, p. 1). Although this list is not all-inclusive, occupational therapy practitioners may focus on (AOTA, 2017, 2019b; Heffron, 2022):

- Academics including math, reading, and writing
- Play and leisure
- Behavior management
- Social participation
- Handwriting and keyboarding skills
- Inappropriate sensory responses
- Self-regulation
- Visual or perceptual deficits
- Cognitive processing
- Mental health concerns
- Self-care skills needed in the school environment
- Motor skills for participation in classroom (e.g., cutting, grasping utensils)
- Technology access and use
- Difficulty staying on task
- Disorganization
- Difficulty navigating the school environment
- Seating and positioning supports
- Transition/work skills

Occupational therapy practitioners may work with individual children in special education or with students in general education as part of classroom-wide, school-wide, or district-wide efforts such as identifying and providing services for struggling learners, bullying prevention, and promoting mental health and positive behaviors (AOTA 2017, 2019b; Heffron, 2022). Children who qualify for special education have an **Individualized Education Program (IEP)**, and occupational therapy is recognized as a related service under the Individuals with Disabilities Education Act (IDEA; U.S. Department of Education, 2019). Although the format of IEPs will differ among school districts, all IEPs must include the following:

- Present level of academic and functional performance
- Measurable annual goals
- Special education and related services to be provided
- Description of anticipated participation with nondisabled children
- Description of anticipated participation in state and district-wide tests
- Dates and places for service provision
- How progress will be measured
  Older students' IEPs must also contain the following:
- At age 14 (or younger if appropriate), a statement of transition service needs, including courses needed to reach post-school goals
- At age 16 (or younger if appropriate), a statement of the needed transition services to help prepare the student for leaving school, such as resources for vocational training, independent living, and community participation
- At least 1 year before the child reaches the age of majority (as defined by each state), a statement that the student has been told rights will transfer to the student if state law requires such transfer of rights

The IEP is developed by a team consisting of the student's parents or guardians, general education teacher/s, special education teacher/s, related services personnel (including occupational therapists), a school district representative who can approve school resources (often a Special Education Coordinator), a translator if needed, and the student if appropriate. Rather than writing separate occupational therapy goals, the occupational therapist should contribute to the development of the overall IEP. You can locate numerous IEP examples online. Since an IEP can be quite lengthy, the one provided here has been condensed to show only the aspects that are most pertinent to occupational therapy.

Individualized Education Program (IEP) Example

Name: *Truman T*   **Age:** *5 yrs, 11 mos*   **Grade Level:** *Kindergarten*

Present Level of Academic Achievement and Functional Performance:

Truman will be 6 years old in just a few days. He was diagnosed with autism spectrum disorder at age 2. He attended the Early Childhood Special Education program for 2 years and is currently enrolled in a full-day Kindergarten. The decision has been made by the IEP team to retain Truman in Kindergarten for the upcoming school year. Truman's parents are in agreement with this decision and hope that another year in Kindergarten will allow him to improve his academic performance and social skills prior to advancing to 1st grade. Truman does not qualify for Extended School Year services at this time.

Truman spends the majority of his day in the general education classroom with a paraprofessional present for support with classroom participation. He spends 60 minutes daily in the special education classroom for additional 1:1 and small group instruction in reading and writing skills. He also participates in adaptive physical education twice weekly for 45 minutes.

Truman's verbal skills are delayed in comparison to same-age peers, although he has demonstrated considerable improvement over the past year. He is now able to communicate in three- to five-word sentences consistently. He also utilizes a Picture Exchange Communication System (PECS) to supplement his verbal communication.

Truman is easily distracted by auditory and visual stimuli in and near the classroom and has difficulty remaining in his seat for more than 5 minutes at a time. He has difficulty with transitions between activities and locations, but this has improved following implementation of a visual schedule. Truman sometimes responds with negative behaviors (yelling, hitting, pinching) when classmates inadvertently touch or bump into him during classroom activities.

Truman is hesitant to engage in play activities with his peers. He prefers to play alone and does not initiate interactions with peers. Toward the end of last school year, he was beginning to participate in some simple ball activities with others during recess with significant support from his paraprofessional. He will continue participation in a weekly after-school peer communication group led by the elementary school counselor.

Truman is able to recognize all letters of the alphabet, but he does not yet read any words. He can copy the letters of his name when provided with a visual model, but legibility is inconsistent. His ability to copy other letters of the alphabet remains very inconsistent. Truman has difficulty achieving a tripod grasp on writing utensils and staying on the lines of standard writing paper. He also has difficulty with consistent letter size and spacing. His writing performance improves with the use of adaptive writing paper and rubber pencil grip. He does consistently copy basic shapes including circle, square, and cross.

Truman requires assistance to obtain and carry his tray in the lunchroom. He is easily upset by the noise in the lunchroom and often needs to be taken to a quieter room to finish lunch. Truman consistently indicates when he needs to use the restroom, but continues to have difficulty managing the button and zipper on his jeans. He needs hand-over-hand assistance to complete hand washing because he prefers to play in the water. Truman is now able to take his coat on and off independently. He can also manage Velcro tennis shoes independently.

TYPE OF SERVICE	ANTICIPATED FREQUENCY	AMOUNT OF TIME	LOCATION OF SERVICE
Special Education *Special education teacher will provide intensive reading and writing instruction in both 1:1 and small group formats.*	*Daily*	*60 minutes*	*Special Education Classroom*
Supplementary Aids and Services *Truman will have a paraprofessional present throughout the school day except when with the special education teacher.*	*Daily*	*340 minutes*	*General Education Classroom and Across Settings*
Program Modifications *Adaptive PE*	*Weekly*	*90 minutes*	*Indoor/Outdoor PE Settings*
Accommodations for Assessments *Truman will be allowed additional time for completion of classroom, district, and state assessments.*	*Weekly*	*60 minutes*	*General and Special Education Classrooms*
Related Services *Occupational Therapy*	*Weekly*	*30 minutes*	*General and Special Education Classrooms and Across Settings*
Related Services *Speech-Language Pathology*	*Weekly*	*90 minutes*	*General and Special Education Classrooms and Across Settings*

Annual Goal #1: *Using compensatory strategies, Truman will demonstrate legible handwriting in the classroom with appropriate baseline orientation, letter size, and spacing with 80% accuracy.*

Evaluation Methods:
- ☐ Curriculum-Based Assessment
- ☐ State Assessments
- ☑ Data Collection Chart
- ☑ Work Samples
- ☐ Other:

Primary Implementers:
- ☑ General Education Teacher
- ☑ Special Education Teacher
- ☐ Physical Therapy
- ☑ Occupational Therapy
- ☐ Speech-Language Pathology
- ☐ Other:

Measurable Benchmarks/Objectives:

1. Truman will demonstrate tripod grasp on writing utensils using adaptive pencil grip with 80% accuracy.
2. Truman will write his first name on adaptive paper without a visual model, demonstrating appropriate letter formation, size, and line orientation on 4 of 5 consecutive days.
3. Truman will copy 22/26 lowercase letters onto adaptive paper using a visual model, demonstrating appropriate letter formation, size, and line orientation on 4 of 5 consecutive days.

Date of Mastery:

1.

2.

3.

Annual Goal #2: *Truman will demonstrate improved attention and work behaviors during classroom activities with no more than three sensory breaks per hour throughout the day on 4 of 5 consecutive days.*

Evaluation Methods:	**Primary Implementers:**
☐ Curriculum-Based Assessment	☑ General Education Teacher
☐ State Assessments	☑ Special Education Teacher
☑ Data Collection Chart	☐ Physical Therapy
☐ Work Samples	☑ Occupational Therapy
☐ Other:	☐ Speech-Language Pathology
	☐ Other:

Measurable Benchmarks/Objectives:	**Date of Mastery:**
1. Truman will remain seated at his desk or during circle time for 15 minutes with minimal verbal cues and no more than one sensory break.	1.
2. Truman will transition between classroom activities with minimal verbal cues using a visual schedule and without demonstrating negative behaviors (yelling, hitting, etc.) toward peers and staff on 4 of 5 consecutive days.	2.
3. Truman will tolerate unexpected touch from classmates without demonstrating negative behaviors (yelling, hitting, etc.) on 4 of 5 consecutive days.	3.

Annual Goal #3: *Truman will demonstrate school-related self-care skills using adaptive strategies with no more than minimal assistance on 4 of 5 consecutive days.*

Evaluation Methods:	**Primary Implementers:**
☐ Curriculum-Based Assessment	☐ General Education Teacher
☐ State Assessments	☐ Special Education Teacher
☑ Data Collection Chart	☐ Physical Therapy
☐ Work Samples	☑ Occupational Therapy
☐ Other:	☐ Speech-Language Pathology
	☑ Other: Paraprofessional

Measurable Benchmarks/Objectives:	**Date of Mastery:**
1. Truman will complete toileting without assistance to manage clothing fasteners on 4 of 5 consecutive days.	1.
2. Truman will wash hands following a visual schedule with minimal verbal cues on 4 of 5 consecutive days.	2.
3. Truman will obtain/transport his lunch tray and remain seated in the cafeteria for the duration of the lunch period with minimal verbal cues on 4 of 5 consecutive days.	3.

DOCUMENTATION IN EARLY INTERVENTION

Part C of IDEA requires that early intervention services be provided in natural environments such as home or community settings in which typically developing peers of a comparable age would participate (Center for Parent Information & Resources, 2021). Children receiving early intervention services will have a document called the **Individualized Family Service Plan (IFSP)**. Although each state will have a specific format for the IFSP, there are certain elements that must be contained in the document, including the following (U.S. Department of Education, 2017):

- Information about the child's status, including present level of:
  ○ Physical development (including vision, hearing, and overall health status)
  ○ Cognitive development
  ○ Communication development
  ○ Social or emotional development
  ○ Adaptive development
- Family information including:
  ○ Resources
  ○ Priorities
  ○ Concerns
- Measurable results or outcomes expected to be achieved including:
  ○ Criteria and procedure for determining if outcome is met
  ○ Anticipated timeline
- Early intervention services to be provided:
  ○ Length, duration, frequency, intensity, and method of each service
  ○ A statement regarding provision of services in natural environments to the maximum extent possible, or a justification for why particular services will not be provided in natural environments

You can locate numerous IFSP and early intervention documentation examples online. A unique feature of early intervention services is that all documentation is written in plain language that is understandable to parents rather than in professional jargon common in other practice settings. Although the SOAP note format is not used, you can see that all the SOAP elements are still included:

> Kiara participated in a 30-minute OT session in her home with her mother and grandmother present. Focus this date was on self-feeding. Mother reports that Kiara has been feeding herself finger foods from the highchair tray but is not showing much interest in using a spoon. With Kiara seated in the highchair, mother showed how she helps her hold the spoon to scoop yogurt out of the container, but Kiara became fussy and threw the spoon down. Suggestion was made to place yogurt in small bowl to make scooping easier, and Kiara was then able to scoop 4 bites without help and needed only a little help from her mother to scoop 5 more bites. Recommendation also made for use of rubber mat (such as shelf liner) under bowl to keep it in place, and grandmother reports she will bring some from her house. Improved ability to feed herself with a spoon shows good progress toward expected outcome of Kiara feeding herself all meals without help. Plan to address drinking from sippy cup next session as mother has stated goal to "get her off the bottle."

CONSULTATION

Consulting work is another area of occupational therapy practice that may use a slightly different method or language for documentation. Occupational therapists consult on a wide variety of questions about which they have special expertise. For example, a psychiatric unit that relies on recreational therapists and activity aides for its activity therapy program might ask for an occupational therapy consult on a client who has both physical and psychiatric disabilities. A newborn nursery might ask for an occupational therapy consult on a high-risk infant. An occupational therapist may be asked to evaluate a work, home, or school setting to make recommendations regarding safety, adaptations for work simplification, ergonomics, energy conservation, or compliance with ADA standards. An occupational therapy consultant might be used to peer review charts for quality improvement monitoring or for reimbursement issues.

A consultant gives a professional assessment of what needs to be done, rather than actually doing it. Two of the most common requests for occupational therapy consultations are for consultation on individual consumers and for consultation on the context in which the consumer works or resides.

Individual Consumers

A consult on an individual consumer is written in the consumer's health record, just as any occupational therapy note would be. In a problem-oriented medical record, the note is written in chronological order in the progress note section in a SOAP format. In a source-oriented record, the consult would more likely be written in a different format and would be found in the section of the record marked "consults." It might be in the form of a letter or memo, or it might be written on a form that the consulting occupational therapist uses routinely. The following note documents a consultation provided for a community-based psychiatric client who had positioning needs and is written in SOAP format.

Occupational Therapy—Positioning Consultation

S: *Consumer reports that he is not able to find a comfortable position in his wheelchair, and that he is not able to propel it in a straight line around his home or in the community due to a drag on one of the wheels.*

O: *At the request of Dr. Carter, consumer participated in consultation at community mental health center to assess his positioning needs. Consumer noted to be leaning to the R with increased pressure on the R elbow. Back of wheelchair noted to be hammocking badly. Arm rests do not provide a good position for functional use of arms. Gel cushion in chair seems to be working well as an anti-pressure device but transfers cold sensation to consumer. Upon inspection, wheel found to have hairs wound around the axle and is also in need of oiling.*

A: *Ill-fitting wheelchair limits client's independence with functional mobility and performance of ADLs and IADLs. Several changes in the wheelchair are needed to increase comfort and functional use. Client would benefit from the following:*

- *Add an anti-sling insert to the back of the chair to provide a more upright posture.*
- *Add a pad to the gel cushion to prevent cold transfer of gel to consumer and for ease of cleaning in case of incontinence.*
- *B arm bolsters are needed for wheelchair arm rests to bring consumer's arms closer to midline for increased functional use.*
- *Clean and oil wheels at axle.*

P: *The adaptations listed above have been ordered. Consumer to be re-evaluated after the wheelchair is repaired and adapted.*

Marisa B, OTR/L

Setting in Which the Consumer Works or Resides

If evaluating a client's home or workplace prior to discharge, a SOAP note might also be used. However, if an entire work setting was evaluated for ergonomic correctness or for ADA compliance rather than in relation to one specific client, a letter or standardized evaluation form would be more appropriate. The following letter documents a work site evaluation that was done on a consulting basis.

MEMO

To:	*Earl Y, RPh*
From:	*Charlet Q, OTR/L*
Re:	*Computer ergonomics in the pharmacy*

A visit was made to the 2nd floor pharmacy in response to your request to perform an ergonomic evaluation of the computer workstations located there. This was in response to multiple employee complaints of carpal tunnel pain and neck and shoulder discomfort. The following are my recommendations:

1. *Computer keyboards must be positioned low enough so that the shoulders can be relaxed during sustained usage and so that wrists can be maintained in neutral position rather than in extension or flexion. When the wrist is in extension or flexion, there is more stress on the median nerve that is compressed in the carpal tunnel and may cause pain.*

   The best position may be achieved by lowering some of the keyboards and/or angling them so the wrists can be kept neutral. Sometimes keeping the keyboards flat or even inclining them with the far end slightly down may help keep the wrists in neutral position. A wrist rest used in conjunction with the keyboard is helpful to some users.

   If an ergonomic keyboard is used to avoid wrist deviations, it still must be positioned so the wrists are not either flexed or extended. The correct position for each person will be slightly different since all body builds are different. It will be important for each user to know the correct body mechanics and be able to make some adjustments in the workstation to meet their needs.

2. *The chair should support the back well while maintaining the trunk in an upright position (not leaning back or forward). Thighs should be supported, and the entire foot should be supported while sitting in a chair at a computer station. Foot support may be either the floor or a footrest (flat or angled) as needed to support the feet. The rungs attached to the high stools do not allow adequate foot support and may tend to disrupt back alignment. Adjustable-height chairs are recommended to meet individual needs.*

3. *The monitor needs to be placed directly in front of the viewer, so it is not necessary to maintain a rotated position of the neck and trunk. Several monitors were angled to the side, requiring the user to maintain asymmetrical posture, causing neck and back strain. The height of the monitor should be adjusted so the eyes of the viewer look directly forward onto the upper one-third of the screen. This prevents neck strain, which can occur if the viewer is having to look up for sustained periods of time.*

4. *If the mouse is to be used with any frequency, it should be positioned near the keyboard rather than requiring a forward reach. A wrist rest attached to the mouse pad is preferred to remove stress from the heel of the hand.*

5. *Ideally, it seems that the computer workstations should be lowered from high counters to normal table or desk work-height. Tabletop should ideally be 26" from floor and the distance eye to screen should be 26" to 30". However, it is possible to manage the existing problems with the correct chairs, footrests, monitor positioning, and keyboard/mouse positioning.*

6. *Taking a break every 30 minutes to do some active movement and stretching exercises is recommended. A copy of sample exercises was left in the pharmacy.*

If you plan to purchase chairs, footrests, etc., it would be best to actually go to an office supply vendor to try out specific pieces of furniture or arrange to have the items on loan so the potential users can check the fit. I hope this is helpful. Please let me know if I can be of further assistance.

Charlet Q, OTR/L

DOCUMENTATION IN PALLIATIVE CARE

Occupational therapists who work in hospice settings or in other practice settings where clients have terminal illnesses often provide palliative care rather than rehabilitation. Palliative care provides comfort, relief from symptoms, and quality of life as clients prepare for death. In this situation, there is no expectation that the client will make progress in physical functioning. Goals often center around pain control, energy conservation, maintaining independence in areas of occupation that are meaningful to the client, obtaining adaptive equipment, and family/caregiver education. Relaxation, active listening, and complementary and alternative therapies are often used with hospice clients. The following note shows one of the complementary/alternative therapies (Tai Chi) being used to increase relaxation and social participation and to maintain activity tolerance, balance, functional mobility, and satisfaction with quality of life.

Jean is a 48-year-old woman whose throat cancer was diagnosed late and has now metastasized to the brain. She is a single woman who has devoted her life to her career in one of the health professions. She understands her prognosis and has entered a home-based hospice program where she receives occupational therapy as a part of her care. Jean wants to maintain her social participation and her independence in basic and instrumental ADL activities as long as possible. She has always been physically active, but many of the physical activities she has enjoyed doing with friends are too strenuous for her limited energy.

S: Client states, "I feel so much better after doing Tai Chi with you ladies, even on days when I think I'm too tired or just don't feel like I'm able to do anything."

O: Client participated in 45-minute session in her home with 2 friends present to increase social participation, decrease risk of falling, and incorporate energy conservation techniques taught last week into everyday tasks. Five minutes of warm-up exercises focused on breath awareness and relaxation were followed by 15 minutes of modified therapeutic Tai Chi with one 5-minute rest period. Client touched chair back as needed for stability during movements requiring weight shift and balance on one foot. Gentle push hands activity was used to challenge balance and to provide physical contact and social engagement during movement activities. Friends remained for short visit and refreshments on the deck, and plans were made to repeat the activity as tolerated in 1 week. Home instruction sheets and a Tai Chi video with relaxation music were provided for use as desired over the next week.

A: Client's homebound status, decreased balance, and variable energy levels limit her social participation and IADL activities. Her perception of increased energy and activity tolerance following the Tai Chi activity allows her to continue to engage in occupation she values. Using furniture as props allows client to practice weight shifting and balance in a safe environment. Physical contact and social exchange during push hands reduced social isolation and distress of "not being able to do anything." Client would benefit from continued Tai Chi activities to address energy conservation, balance, and safety concerns through breathing and relaxation activities done in a social setting.

P: Client to be seen in her home weekly for 45 minutes or as tolerated for 3 more weeks for instruction in mobility, balance, energy conservation techniques to maintain functional mobility, IADL tasks, and valued role as a friend in a modified home exercise energy conservation program.

Sandy M, PhD, OTR/L

REFERENCES

American Occupational Therapy Association. (2016). *Occupational therapy's distinct value: Mental health promotion, prevention and intervention across the lifespan.* https://www.aota.org/

American Occupational Therapy Association. (2017). *What is the role of the school-based occupational therapy practitioner?* https://www.aota.org/

American Occupational Therapy Association. (2019a). *AOTA 2019 workforce & salary survey.* https://www.aota.org/

American Occupational Therapy Association. (2019b). *Occupational therapy's role in schools.* https://www.aota.org/

Center for Parent Information & Resources. (2021). *Providing early intervention services in natural environments.* https://www.parentcenterhub.org/

Heffron, C. (2022, January 4). *What is school based occupational therapy?* The Inspired Treehouse. https://theinspiredtreehouse.com/

MacRae, A. (2019a). Consultation and program development. In A. MacRae (Ed.), *Cara and MacRae's psychosocial occupational therapy: An evolving practice* (4th ed., pp. 73-91). SLACK Incorporated.

MacRae, A. (2019b). Direct service provision In A. MacRae (Ed.), *Cara and MacRae's psychosocial occupational therapy: An evolving practice* (4th ed., pp. 49-71). SLACK Incorporated.

MacRae, A. (2019c). Philosophical worldviews of mental health. In A. MacRae (Ed.), *Cara and MacRae's psychosocial occupational therapy: An evolving practice* (4th ed., pp. 3-17). SLACK Incorporated.

MacRae, A. (2019d). Psychiatric institutions and hospitals. In A. MacRae (Ed.), *Cara and MacRae's psychosocial occupational therapy: An evolving practice* (4th ed., pp. 19-31). SLACK Incorporated.

MacRae, A., & Smith, J. (2019). Community behavioral health services. In A. MacRae (Ed.), *Cara and MacRae's psychosocial occupational therapy: An evolving practice* (4th ed., pp. 33-48). SLACK Incorporated.

Parsons, H. (2022, August 1). *OT in mental health: 10 years of congressional advocacy.* American Occupational Therapy Association. https://www.aota.org/

Sutton, R. (2015). *The counselor's STEPs for progress notes: A guide to clinical language and documentation* (2nd ed.). Amazon Publishing Agency.

U.S. Department of Education. (2017). *Sec. 303.344—Content of an IFSP.* https://sites.ed.gov/

U.S. Department of Education. (2019). *A guide to the Individualized Education Program.* https://www2.ed.gov/

Chapter 14

Electronic Documentation

Electronic health records (EHRs), also known as *electronic medical records* (EMRs), are used in nearly all occupational therapy practice settings. With the prevalence of electronic documentation software, students often question the relevance of learning the SOAP note format. I strongly believe that learning the SOAP note format teaches students and entry-level practitioners to use professional reasoning in documenting a client's background information, performance, and response to therapeutic interventions. Furthermore, electronic documentation software typically contains all the elements found in a SOAP note, although they may be presented in a different order or format. Some software programs specifically use a SOAP note format.

Each time you start a new fieldwork placement or new job, you likely will have to learn a new EHR system. If you stay at any particular job for long enough, you likely will experience the transition from one EHR system to another as companies occasionally make such changes based on cost and efficiency of the software product. If you are in a management position within your company, you may even find yourself in charge of or contributing to the decision of which product to purchase and implement for your company and then training employees in its use. Beyond the obvious issue of cost, below is a list of several other things to consider when exploring various documentation software products (My School Therapy, 2021; PracticePro, 2022):

- Availability of pre-existing templates that contain information relevant to your practice setting
- Ability to modify existing templates and create new templates
- Inclusion of a goal bank or goal library that allows individualization of each goal based on client needs
- Integration of coding and billing requirements specific to your setting and funding sources
- Built-in scheduling and calendars
- Automatic reminders for re-evaluation or progress notes as required by setting or funding source
- Option to generate written or electronic reports that can be shared easily with referring providers, clients, and funding sources
- Analytic options such as tracking therapist productivity or reimbursement per payer source
- Ability to create customized home exercise or home activity programs for clients to support direct intervention
- Client portals that allow clients to complete registration paperwork, schedule appointments, and view documentation
- Ability to use the software on portable devices such as tablets and smart phones
- Security features
- Telehealth capacity
- Training and ongoing technical support

Gateley, C. A. *Documentation Manual for Occupational Therapy, Fifth Edition* (pp. 189-202).

> EHRs provide quick access to documentation if it is ever needed for reimbursement or legal issues. "Defensible documenta-
> tion can be the difference between a compliant, lucrative practice, and a practice that is audited and penalized from frequent
> regulatory mistakes that cannot be justified or otherwise explained" (PracticePro, 2020, para. 1).

As discussed briefly in Chapter 5, EHRs significantly reduce documentation time, and many systems allow for point-of-service documentation, which is completed while the therapist is working with the client. Perhaps the most critical issue to remember when using EHRs for point-of-service documentation is the importance of developing a rapport with your client and including the client throughout the documentation process. There is a temptation to interact solely with the computer in selecting goals, objectives, and intervention strategies. Always remember to set goals **with** your client rather than **for** your client. It can be helpful to simply explain to the client why you are documenting during the session. For example, "You will see me taking some notes while we work together today. This is so I can make sure everything I document is accurate while it is still fresh in my mind."

Some practice settings or client populations simply do not lend themselves to point-of-service documentation. For example, if you are working in an intensive care unit with a patient who needs maximum assistance for balance, transfers, and ADLs, you will not be able to document during the session. In another example, you might be working with a pediatric client in a home, outpatient, or school setting, and that client may require your undivided attention during the session. Whenever you cannot provide point-of-service documentation, you should complete your documentation as soon as possible for best accuracy. It is a good idea to jot a few notes down after the session to remind you of intervention strategies and assist levels when you are able to complete the documentation.

EXAMPLES OF ELECTRONIC DOCUMENTATION

The remainder of this chapter will provide several examples of electronic documentation from various practice settings. As you read through each example, try to identify the Subjective, Objective, Assessment, and Plan information that would have been present if the same data were presented in SOAP note format.

> Please note that electronic documentation samples contained in the software screenshots in this chapter may not follow the guidelines of this textbook precisely. Each practice setting has its own documentation guidelines and expectations. Additionally, all client names included in the screenshots are fictional and provided only for purposes of demonstrating the features of each software product.

Work Hardening Clinic Example

Figure 14-1 shows an example of electronic documentation that allows the occupational therapist to document the initial evaluation, plan of care, and discharge summary all in the same report. You will see that this form includes several tables for entering data common to a work hardening setting as well as the option to include a standardized description of the assessment tools that were used. You will also note some abbreviations not covered in this manual that are specific to the work hardening setting:

- CV: coefficients of variance
- PDC: physical demand characteristics
- PILE: progressive isoinertial lifting evaluation
- PRE: progressive resistive exercise

WORK HARDENING EVALUATION – SUMMARY REPORT
Initial Evaluation Date: 4/3/23
Exit Evaluation Date: 4/28/23

Name	Chet D.	
Age	40	
Height (inches) - **72**	**Weight** (lbs) - **250**	**Dominance** (L/R handed) – **R**
Physician: Dr. Lance Sawbones	Follow-up Physician Appointment: 5/1/23	
Diagnosis	s/p L4-5 Fusion	
Date of Injury	1/2/23	
Mechanism of Injury/Medical Tx (as reported by patient)	"Lifted a box at work and felt a pull in my back". Conservative tx for 2 weeks including PT, medications, and time off w/o relief. MRI (+) for large HNP. Fusion 2/1/23 & PT 2/22/23 to 3/15/23. Attempted return to work on 3/20/23 but unable to tolerate. Rx for Work Hardening written 3/27/23.	
Employer & Job Title	XYZ Corporation – Order Filler	
Insurance Carrier/Adjuster	Coverall Insurance/Sue Payer	
Case Manager	Nancy Nurse, RN, CCM	

Work Hardening Program Attendance:

Attended 18/18 visits for up to 7-hour days. No tardies.

Work Hardening Treatment Program:

Aerobic exercise, stretching/stabilization, PRE, functional tasks, and body mechanics education.

Work Hardening Exit Evaluation Performance Criteria Profile:

Consistency of Effort – CVs low. Cross validation in PILE v. Occasional lifts acceptable.
Quality of Effort – HR during evaluation >/= 25% variance. Acceptable kinesiophysical signs.
Non-Organic Signs – Subjective reports consistent with test behavior. Complaints specific.

Work Hardening Exit Evaluation Assessment:

Significant progress noted in program. He is currently meeting all return to work goals. See the work requirements/goals v. demonstrated physical tolerances on the following page. Feasibility for success at return to work is **GOOD** at this time.

Work Hardening Exit Evaluation Recommendation/Plan:

Pending physician f/u and exam, I recommend return to work at full duty at this time.

Chet D.   Page 1

Figure 14-1. (Reproduced with permission from Vic Zuccarello, OTR/L, C.E.A.S. II, ABDA—Former owner of BIO-ERGONOMICS, INC.) (*continued*)

Work Hardening Evaluation	Chet D.	Page Two

Demonstrated Physical Tolerances

Task	Initial Eval – 4/3/23	Exit Eval – 4/28/23	Job Description	Met? (yes/no)
Pain Level (0-10)	6/10	**3/10**	*Job Description Information (Goals to be Met) Provided By: Employer & Employee*	
Chief Complaints	Midline lumbar aching into R hip.	**Midline lumbar aching.**		
Material Handling Lifting in pounds unless stated otherwise/Push/Pull in Pounds of Force (Occ. = 0-33% of day, Freq. = 34-66%, Const. = > 66%) or (Occ. = 1-12/hr, Freq. = 13-60/hr, Const. = > 60/hr)				
Floor to Waist Lift	25# occasional	**75# occasional, 35# frequent**	**70# occasional, 25# frequent**	MET
Waist to Shoulder Lift	"	"	"	MET
Overhead Lift	"	**50# occasional, 25# frequent**	**40# occasional, 20# frequent**	MET
Carrying (50 feet)	"	**75# occasional, 35# frequent**	**70# occasional, 25# frequent**	MET
Pushing (Force)	55#	**100#**	Pallet jack, dolly	MET
Pulling (Force)	43#	**97#**	"	MET
Non-Material Handling Positions and movements in activities and associated tasks (Occ. = 0-33% of day, Freq. = 34-66%, Const. = > 66%) or (Occ. = 1-12/hr, Freq. = 13-60/hr, Const. = > 60/hr)				
Standing	Occasional	**Frequent**	**Frequent**	MET
Walking	"	"	"	MET
Squatting/Bending	"	"	"	MET
Kneeling/Crawling	"	**Occasional**	**Occasional**	MET
Reaching/Grasping	Frequent	**Constant**	**Constant**	MET
PDC Level (S,L,M,H,VH)	**MEDIUM**	**HEAVY**	**HEAVY**	MET
Perceived Disability	Oswestry – 44%	**Oswestry – 22%**		

Physical Demand Levels of Work *Dictionary of Occupational Titles (US Dept. of Labor, Fourth Edition, Revised 1991)*

PDC Level	Occasional (0-33% of day)	Frequent (34-66% of day)	Constant (>66% of day)
Sedentary	*1# to 10#* / Stand & Walk	*Negligible/* Sitting	*Negligible/* Sitting
Light	*11# to 20#*	*Up to 10#* / Stand & Walk *and/or* Standing pushing/pulling controls	*Negligible and/or* Seated & pushing/pulling arm/leg controls
Medium	*21# to 50#*	*11# to 25#*	*Up to 10#*
Heavy	*51# to 100#*	*26# to 50#*	*11# to 20#*
V-Heavy	*Over 100#*	*Over 50#*	*Over 20#*

END OF SUMMARY

Vic Z., OTR/L, C.E.A.S. II, ABDA

Chet D.   Page 2

Figure 14-1 (continued). (Reproduced with permission from Vic Zuccarello, OTR/L, C.E.A.S. II, ABDA—Former owner of BIO-ERGONOMICS, INC.) *(continued)*

Example of Work Hardening Evaluation Data Pages (from Chet's Initial Evaluation)

LUMBAR MUSCULOSKELETAL SCREEN

Resting HR	84 (min acceptable increase = 105)	Resting BP	124/66
Pre Pain Level	5/10	Description	Midline lumbar and R hip
Posture	increased lumbar lordosis, protruding abdomen, PSIS even, no shift.		
Gait	mild R antalgia	Palpation	increased muscle density lumbar PVM's

NEUROLOGICAL

	L	R	Comments
Knee Reflex (L4)	2+	2+	symmetrical
Ankle Reflex (S1)	"	"	"

WADDELL SIGNS
(+) = abnormal response to examination, or possible non-organic sign

TENDERNESS		SIMULATION		DISTRACTION		REGIONAL		OVER-REACTION
Superficial	-	Axial loading	-	L SLR +	R SLR -	Cogwheel	-	-
Non-anatomic	-	Simulated rotation	-	Sit 75	Sit 75	Numb	-	
				Supine 30	Supine 55	Weak	-	

RANGE OF MOTION
(Pre test AROM take 3 trials and calculate coefficient of variance; CV >15% = Inconsistent Test)

MOTION	PRE TEST (°)			AVERAGE (°)	CV%	POST TEST (°)	NORM
Lumbar flexion	35	30	35	33	7.1	30	60
Lumbar extension	10	10	12	11	8.8	15	25
L lateral flexion	20	22	22	21	4.4	15	25
R lateral flexion	20	25	25	23	10.1	25	25

STATIC STRENGTH

MOTION	TRIALS			AVERAGE	CV%	Manual Muscle Test
R knee flexion	34.4	36	40.1	36.8	6.5	4
L knee flexion	26	25	22	24.3	7.0	5
R knee extension	77.3	88	80.2	81.8	5.5	4
L knee extension	33	31	25	29.7	11.5	5
R plantarflexion	33.3	30	34	32.4	5.4	4
L plantarflexion	36.2	36	32	34.7	5.6	5
R dorsiflexion	22	24.4	18.6	21.7	11.0	4
L dorsiflexion	20	22.6	20.6	21.1	5.3	5

QUALITY OF MOVEMENT (Non-Material Handling) SCREEN (5x each)

Squatting	full, UE assist required	Overhead Reach	full, fluid, unguarded
Bending	50%	Finger Flexion	as above
Kneeling	full, UE assist	Opposition	as above
Crawling	symmetrical, guarded	Climbing	step to step, decreased RLE WB.
Comments	Guarding in lower-level postures.		
Post-Pain Level (0-10)	6/10 – no change in location of symptoms. Denies need for break, "let's go".		

Chet D.　　　　　　　　　　　　　　　　　　　　　　　　　　　　Page 3

Figure 14-1 (continued). (Reproduced with permission from Vic Zuccarello, OTR/L, C.E.A.S. II, ABDA—Former owner of BIO-ERGONOMICS, INC.) (*continued*)

Work Hardening Evaluation	Chet D.	Page Four

Material Handling Test

Description of lift/carry test: This test format is based on other commercial lifting tests and utilizes a lifting box and weights. The worker is instructed in proper body mechanics, the therapist demonstrates proper procedure, and the worker is then allowed to perform a preferred number of practice trials. After each successful lift, weight is added in progressive fashion and the worker is asked if the load is "light, medium, or heavy". The worker is also asked if they feel safe to perform the lift with heavier weight. If the worker answers with a "yes" response and the form on the previous load was safe, weight is added (5-10# for a 'heavy' response, 10-15# for a 'medium' response, and 15-20# for a 'light' response) until one of three termination criteria are met: physiological (ie heart rate, perspiration, flushed complexion); kinesiophysical (ie recruitment of surrounding body parts, substitution, counterbalancing, muscle tremor)); or psychophysical (ie desire to stop because of 'heaviness' of load, perceived pain, or perceived cardiopulmonary exertion). During the test, these aspects of performance are observed and utilized to determine if the worker provided acceptable effort, and if the worker's subjective reports are in proportion with test behavior. Maximum safe effort is solicited and encouraged. The worker is never forced to perform a task they feel is unsafe.

- ☐ 50-foot Carrying is assessed by first testing with the max load achieved in the waist to shoulder lift and progressing as in the above procedure.
- ☐ Upon reaching the end-point, the load is decreased by 50% and 10 repetitions are performed to determine the frequent carrying load.

Description of push/pull test: Static testing is performed to assess for level of participation in testing as well as to elicit a measure of pushing/pulling strength. The worker is instructed in safe technique (including by not limited to avoidance of jerking or holding the breath, etc.), the therapist demonstrates proper procedure, and a preferred number of practice trials are performed. The worker then performs 6-second trails at their own preferred safe-maximum force. A maximum rest period of 15 seconds is given between 3 trials. Therapist observes for physiological (heart rate, flushed complexion, perspiration); kinesiophysical (substitution, recruitment, tremor, counterbalancing); and psychophysical (pain level, heart rate v. rate of perceived exertion) indicators. Maximum safe effort is solicited/encouraged, but subject is not coerced into providing higher force than they feel is safe.

Pre-test Heart Rate	90	Pre-test Pain Level	5/10

Test	Load (#)	Heart Rate	Rate of Perceived Exertion (6-20)	Pain Level (0-10+)	Kinesiophysical Indicators
Floor to waist lift	25	114	14-15/20	6	Counterbalance and recruitment
Waist to shoulder	25	114	13-14/20	6	"
Overhead Lift		110	14-15/20	6	"
███████████					
* Carrying Max	25	110	15-16/20	6	"
███████████					
Pushing (force)	55	115	11-12/20	6	"
Pulling (force)	43	122	"	6	"

Comments: Body mechanics were safe and steady. HR and kinesiophysical signs suggest acceptable effort.

END OF EVALUATION

Chet D.   Page 4

Figure 14-1 (continued). (Reproduced with permission from Vic Zuccarello, OTR/L, C.E.A.S. II, ABDA—Former owner of BIO-ERGONOMICS, INC.)

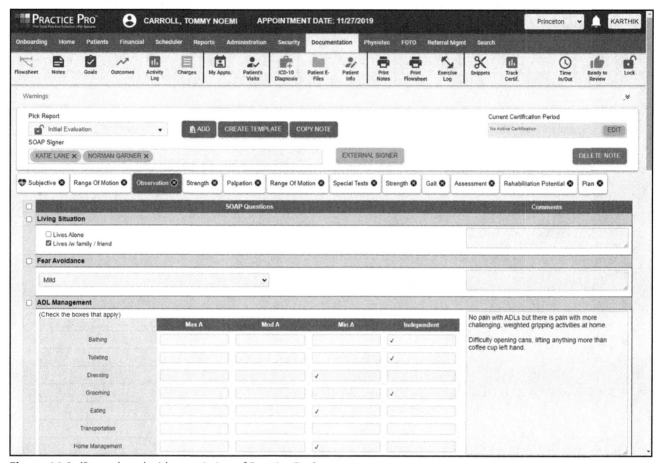

Figure 14-2. (Reproduced with permission of Practice Pro.)

Outpatient Hand Therapy Clinic Example

- The software featured in Figure 14-2 is structured much like common office software programs, presenting a dashboard with various tabs and windows that enable the user to move efficiently through different screens such as scheduling, notes, goals, outcomes, and charges.
- This software has integrated ICD-10 diagnosis coding, as discussed in Chapter 3.
- The Snippets tab at the top of the screen allows the occupational therapy practitioner to establish word prediction or shortcuts for commonly used words, phrases, or paragraphs. For example, you could type "FL" and the software would automatically change it to "functional limitations." Or you may have an entire paragraph description of a particular assessment or intervention strategy that you can pull into your documentation by typing one word or a simple abbreviation.
- In the middle of the screen, you can see another navigation tab that follows a SOAP note format:
  - There is a specific Subjective tab where the therapist would document the client's report and any relevant background information.
  - The next several tabs (Range of Motion, Strength, Palpation, Special Tests, etc.) allow the therapist to select and document only the sections that are relevant for a particular client. These represent the Objective portion of documentation.
  - Next the therapist would document under the Assessment and Rehabilitation Potential tabs.
  - Finally, the therapist would document goals and interventions under the Plan tab.
- The ADL Management section at the bottom of the screen allows the therapist to quickly assign an assist level to each area. Note that there is also a free text box to the right where the therapist can make additional comments.

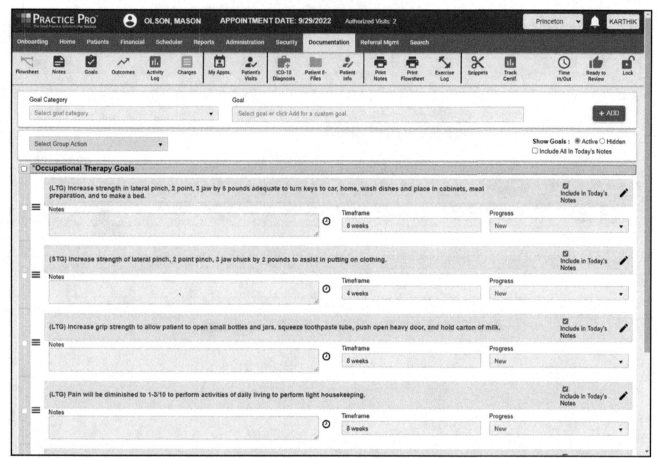

Figure 14-3. (Reproduced with permission of Practice Pro.)

- Figure 14-3 shows the section of the software where the therapist would document new goals for the client and/ or progress toward established goals.
- There is a free text box in the Notes section where the therapist can provide additional details about goal criteria or progress toward the goal.
- Note that the therapist can choose to include any or all of the goals in a daily note by selecting them individually or selecting the Include in Today's Notes option.
- To add a new goal for the client, the therapist would either select a pre-established goal from the Goal Category tab or click the + Add button near the top right of the screen to add a customized goal.

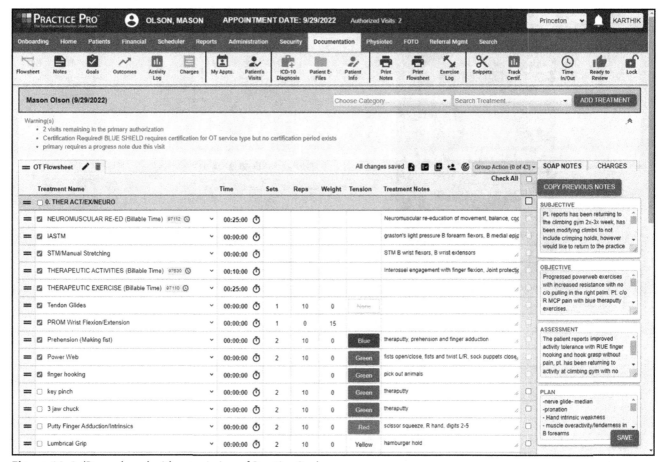

Figure 14-4. (Reproduced with permission of Practice Pro.)

- Figure 14-4 shows a flowsheet screen that allows the therapist to document in considerable detail while the client is completing various strengthening and neuromuscular re-education exercises.
- This therapist has pulled forward a note from a previous session with a list of exercises that were completed last time using the Copy Previous Notes button on the right side of the screen. This feature allows the therapist to select relevant exercises for this session and easily change the sets, repetitions, weight, and tension to show the client's progress between sessions.
- CPT codes are built into this documentation software. The therapist documents the time spent on each activity, and the software will calculate the number of units billed for each code.
- The Treatment Notes column provides free text boxes for the therapist to document additional details as needed.
- The SOAP note boxes to the right of the screen also allow the therapist to provide free text for a more thorough note.
- Note that there are automatic reminders that pop up regarding this client so the therapist is aware that only two visits remain under the current insurance authorization, the client's insurance requires a certification for all occupational therapy services, and the primary care physician needs a progress note after this visit.

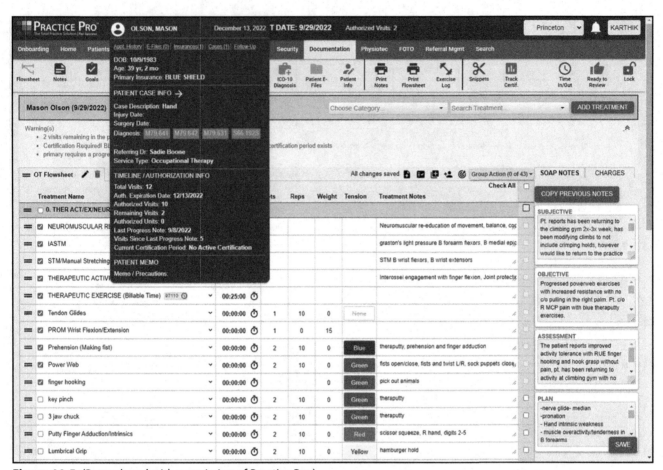

Figure 14-5. (Reproduced with permission of Practice Pro.)

- Figure 14-5 shows that the therapist can easily check all of the client's relevant information from the flowsheet, or any other screen, simply by clicking the client's name at the top of the screen to open up a dropdown menu.
- This option pulls up the client's date of birth, age, and insurance.
- The Patient Case Info section of this dropdown window allows the therapist or scheduler to enter information such as date of injury, surgery date (if applicable), ICD-10 diagnosis codes, referring physician, and service type (occupational therapy, physical therapy, etc.).
- The Timeline/Authorization Info section of this dropdown window shows the total number of authorized visits, the authorization expiration date, how many visits have been used, how many visits remain, and when the last progress note was completed.
- The Patient Memo section of this dropdown window allows the therapist to enter additional information about precautions or other important client information. This feature is particularly important if the client is seen by multiple occupational therapy practitioners during the course of treatment.
- Figure 14-6 shows that this software can quickly print or create an electronic report to provide to the client, referring physician, or insurance company.
- This report can be created by selecting the Print Notes tab at the top of the screen in Figures 14-2 through 14-5.

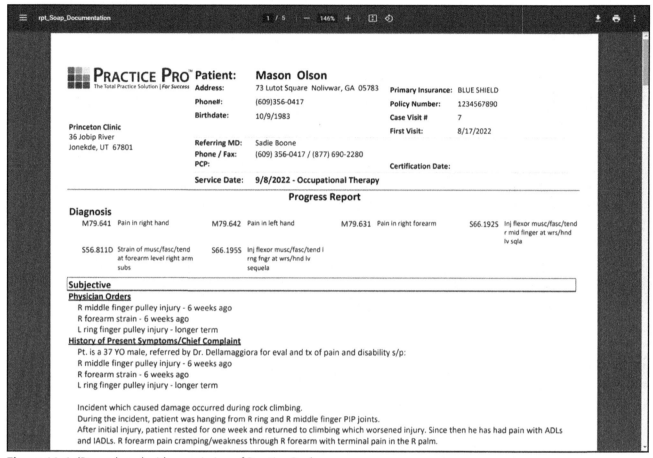

Figure 14-6. (Reproduced with permission of Practice Pro.)

School-Based Occupational Therapy Example

- Figure 14-7 shows an electronic software program that has been designed specifically for school-based occupational therapists, physical therapists, speech-language pathologists, and other school providers.

- Much like the previous examples from an outpatient hand therapy clinic, this software has multiple navigation tabs so the therapist can easily click between Student Records, Session Notes, etc.

- This Student Record screen allows the therapist to access any available information about the student including Contacts, Student Schedule, Session and Progress Notes, and AT [Assistive Technology]/Equipment checked out to the student.

- The Student Records tab also has a Documents sub-tab that shows when a student's triennial evaluation is due and allows the therapist to access existing PDF documents such as previous evaluations.

- Note that this program also has a place to store a prescription ("script") and a letter of medical necessity, both of which may be required if Medicaid is helping to pay for school-based services (Centers for Medicare & Medicaid Services, 2022; Gorman & Rodriguez, 2018).

- Figure 14-8 shows the Session Notes section where the therapist enters details about each session's activities and the student's progress toward goals.

- This screen also allows the therapist to enter the date and exact time of the session as well as any mileage units if applicable based on the contract agreement between the school and therapist.

- This software also has ICD-10 and CPT codes built in.

- At midscreen, the therapist can document a Focus area for this particular session and enter additional information in the free text area of the Contact Note box.

- On the left side of the screen, the therapist selects a relevant Goal/Objective from the student's IEP and then describes any Activities used to address that goal.

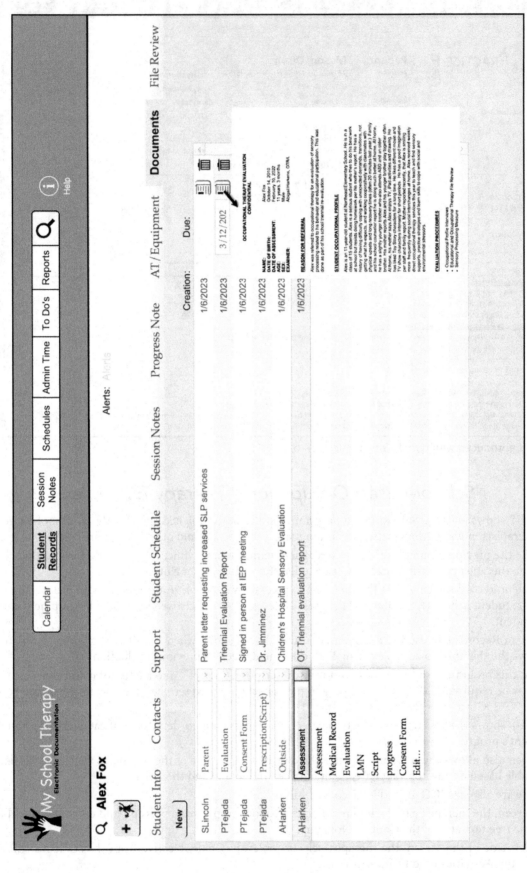

Figure 14-7. (Reproduced with permission of My School Therapy©.)

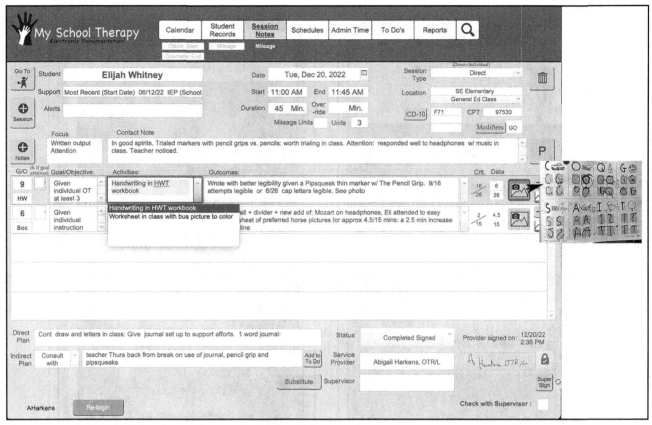

Figure 14-8. (Reproduced with permission of My School Therapy©.)

- The Outcomes box allows free text so the therapist can type details about the child's performance.
- Each time the therapist enters a comment in the Activities or Outcomes section, the software saves the comment. The next time the therapist documents on that student, a list of previous comments is available to carry forward so the therapist can make minor edits without retyping the entire sentence or paragraph.
- To the right of the Outcomes section are columns for goal Criteria and performance Data so the therapist can easily track a student's progress toward a particular goal.
- Note that there is a camera button on the right that allows the therapist to take a picture of the student's work related to this goal. For example, the therapist may want to upload a picture of a handwriting sample or a cutting activity.
- At the bottom of the screen is an option to enter Direct Plan and Indirect Plan information. In this example, the therapist makes notes of activities for future sessions and documents a reminder to consult with the teacher regarding activities that can be incorporated into the classroom for greater carry over.
- At the bottom right, there is an option for both a therapy provider and a supervisor to sign off on the note. This is particularly helpful in situations where an occupational therapist may need to review and co-sign notes by an occupational therapy assistant or student.
- Figures 14-9 and 14-10 show that this school-based electronic documentation system can also be used on a smart phone to allow for point-of-service documentation when a desktop or laptop is not feasible for the setting.
- Figure 14-9 shows the main menu screen, allowing the therapist to Find Session, add a New Session, view a Student File, see a list of To Do items, and view Daily Time or a weekly or monthly Calendar.
- Figure 14-10 shows how the therapist can locate sessions by Session Type, Status, Therapist, Supervisor, or Student.

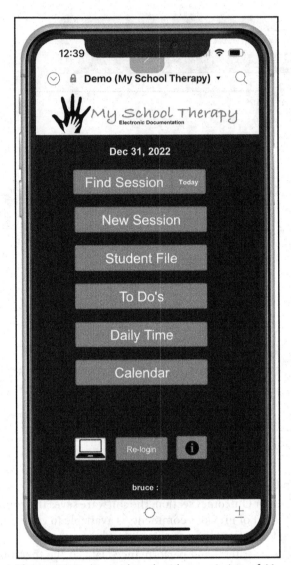

Figure 14-9. (Reproduced with permission of My School Therapy©.)

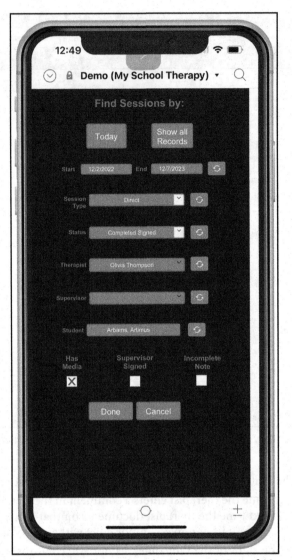

Figure 14-10. (Reproduced with permission of My School Therapy©.)

REFERENCES

Centers for Medicare & Medicaid Services. (2022). *CMCS informational bulletin: Information on school-based services in Medicaid—Funding, documentation, and expanding services.* https://www.medicaid.gov/

Gorman, A., & Rodriguez, C. H. (2018, March 9). *How Medicaid became a go-to funder for schools.* KFF Health News. https://khn.org/news/how-medicaid-became-a-go-to-funder-for-schools/

My School Therapy. (2021). *School-based therapist documentation software: Save time, document, and organize your school therapy notes with ease.* https://myschooltherapy.org/

PracticePro. (2020). *Making your documentation more defensible through an EMR.* https://ptpracticepro.com/blog/making-your-documentation-more-defensible/

PracticePro. (2022). *Physical therapy documentation software: Document the way you want with the templates and flexibility you need.* https://ptpracticepro.com/features/physical-therapy-documentation/

Examples of Notes Across Various Stages of Occupational Therapy Service Delivery

This chapter provides examples of notes from all stages of treatment and from a variety of practice settings. **The specific format and content of some notes will vary from the guidelines provided throughout this textbook.** They are provided here as examples of the wide variety of documentation that you may encounter across occupational therapy practice settings. In each note, regardless of format, you should be able to identify elements of Subjective, Objective, Assessment, and Plan that you would see in a SOAP note.

CHAPTER CONTENTS

Gateley, C. A. *Documentation Manual for Occupational Therapy, Fifth Edition* (pp. 203-237). © 2024 Taylor & Francis Group.

REQUIRED ELEMENTS OF
DOCUMENTATION ACROSS STAGES OF SERVICE DELIVERY

You may recall from Chapter 5 that there are several elements that are essential to all types of documentation (American Occupational Therapy Association [AOTA], 2018):

- Name, date of birth, gender, and case or health record number (if applicable)
- Date and type of occupational therapy contact
- Terminology, acronyms, and abbreviations acceptable to the setting
- Clear rationale for provision of skilled occupational therapy services
- Professional signature including name and credentials
- Co-signature and credentials if required by supervision guidelines, payer policy, state or federal laws, or facility standards
- Errors noted and initialed or signed
- Adherence to state and federal regulations, payer and facility requirements, practice guidelines, and confidentiality requirements for documentation storage and disposal

In addition to the required elements listed above, there are additional requirements for each stage of service delivery. See Table 15-1 for a list of these requirements. The AOTA (2018) *Guidelines for Documentation of Occupational Therapy* provides a thorough explanation of each of these elements. Finally, across all stages of service delivery, occupational therapy practitioners should ensure that client information including current health status, diagnoses, precautions, and contraindications are readily available in the client's health record. Depending on your practice setting, the client information may be repeated in each note you write, or it may be in a separate location in the client's health record. Most settings you will encounter in fieldwork and entry-level practice will have an established format for documentation that includes all required elements. **Please note that for space consideration, the example notes provided in this chapter may not contain all required elements in each note,** such as client information and referral source, with the assumption that required information would be located elsewhere in the client's health record. Most example notes also will not have a date listed. In practice, you would date every entry in the health record.

Table 15-1

REQUIRED ELEMENTS OF DOCUMENTATION ACROSS STAGES OF SERVICE DELIVERY

TYPE OF DOCUMENTATION	REQUIRED ELEMENTS
Screening Report	• Referral information • Occupational profile • Assessments used, if applicable, and results • Recommendations
Evaluation Report	• Referral information • Occupational profile • Assessments used and results • Analysis of occupational performance • Interpretation and summary • Codes of client performance, only if required by setting or funding source (e.g., Section GG codes required in post-acute settings) • Recommendations
Re-Evaluation Report	• Referral information • Occupational profile • Re-evaluation results • Analysis of occupational performance • Interpretation and summary • Recommendations
Intervention Plan	• Intervention goals • Intervention approaches and types of intervention • Service delivery mechanisms (e.g., location, frequency, duration) • Plan for discharge • Outcome measures
Contact Note	• Therapy log (e.g., client report, description of services provided, response to intervention, current level of functional performance)
Progress Report	• Goals addressed • Summary of services provided • Current level of client performance • Recommendations
Transition Plan	• Current level of client performance • Transition plan • Recommendations
Discharge Report	• Summary of the intervention process and progress toward goals • Recommendations

Data source: American Occupational Therapy Association, 2018.

SCREENING REPORTS

An occupational therapy screening involves a brief review of client information, observation, and potential administration of a screening instrument to determine whether a full occupational therapy evaluation is appropriate (AOTA, 2020). "Screening provides occupational therapy practitioners with a glimpse of a person's or population's potential needs, strengths, limitations, and contexts; however, screening does not inform treatment planning and indicates only whether additional formal evaluation is required" (Boone et al., 2022, p. 1).

Screening Report: Neonatal ICU Follow-Up Outpatient Clinic

Name: *Maverick D*   **Age:** *11 months*   **Primary Dx:** *R/O developmental delay*

Pertinent History: *Maverick is an 11-month, 11-day-old male child whose adjusted age for prematurity is 9 months, 27 days. He was initially discharged from hospital at chronological age 1 month, 2 weeks; adjusted age 2 weeks. Since discharge, Maverick has been seen twice for medical evaluation at the hospital at 3 months adjusted age and 6 months adjusted age. He is being seen today for his first OT developmental screening as a part of the Outpatient Neonatal Follow-Up Program. His mother is present at the evaluation.*

S: *Child is not yet old enough to use language to communicate, but makes sounds ("ba, da, ma," etc.) WFL for adjusted age. Client also makes frequent eye contact with parents and points/reaches toward desired items.*

O: *Today's screening reveals:*
- *Atypical patterns of posture and movement (persistent primitive reflexes, presence of tonic reflexes, moderate increase in muscle tone, limited repertoire of movement, and postural asymmetry).*
- *Possible visual difficulties (immature visual tracking and intermittent malalignment (one/both eyes drift inward).*
- *Delayed milestones (child exhibits skills clustering around the 4- to 6-month developmental level).*
- *Raw score of 24 on the Alberta Infant Motor Scale (AIMS) indicating motor performance below the 5th percentile in comparison to peers of the same adjusted age.*

A: *The findings of this screening indicate that Maverick is experiencing developmental delays, atypical patterns of motor development, and possible visual difficulties, all of which limit his success in play and emerging self-care skills. Maverick would benefit from referral to the State Early Intervention Program to initiate comprehensive evaluation for OT and other therapy services.*

P: *Maverick's mother has been informed of the results of the evaluation and is in agreement with the following plan:*
- *OT will contact the Neonatal Follow-Up Clinic physician regarding vision concerns.*
- *Referral made to State Early Intervention Program to initiate OT services.*
- *Maverick scheduled to return to Neonatal Follow-Up Clinic in 3 months.*

Emma A, OTR/L

Screening Report: Primary Care Clinic

Name: *Kathy T*   **Age:** *83*   **Primary Dx:** *R/O dementia*

Pertinent History: *Client is an 83-year-old female with an unremarkable medical history. She has had no significant medical concerns up to this point, and her only medication is a daily multi-vitamin. After living independently in a very rural area for several years after her husband's death, her family convinced her 3 years ago to move to a small house in town just two doors down from her daughter and son-in-law, who now check on her daily. She has been independent in completing her basic self-care and IADLs, including financial management and driving. Family members requested visit with primary care physician this date due to concerns of recent decline in memory function and inability to figure out bank and credit card statements. They also note concerns about patient's safety with driving. Physician requested OT to complete a brief cognitive screen to determine need for more comprehensive evaluation.*

S: Pt. reports, "I'm fine. I don't know what all this fuss is about." Pt. noted to have difficulty coming up with family member's names when OT asked pt. to introduce them.

O: Pt. participated in brief screening as part of primary care visit to determine present cognitive level and ability to complete IADL tasks.

Mini-Cog: Pt. scored 1 of 5 points possible (1 of 3 words recalled, 0 of 2 points on clock drawing for duplicate numbers and incorrect positioning); score is consistent with dementia.

Bill-Paying Task: Pt. required max verbal cues to locate amount and date due on simulated utility bill statement.

Form Completion Task: Pt. incorrect on both address and phone number on simulated client information intake form. Handwriting was only minimally legible, and daughter reports this is a recent change.

Road Sign Test: Pt. correctly identified 2 of 8 road signs presented and was dismissive of her errors, claiming that her small town does not have those signs.

A: Cognitive deficits including decreased STM, inability to identify payment information, and difficulty identifying common road signs result in significant concern for pt. to be driving and managing her financial affairs. Family's awareness of deficits and willingness to provide additional support with financial management and transportation are good indications that pt. may be able to remain in independent living situation for the immediate future. Client would benefit from thorough evaluation by a neuropsychologist to determine extent of cognitive deficits. Client would also benefit from outpatient OT services to establish compensatory measures to maintain independent living status as long as possible. Finally, client would benefit from a thorough driving skills evaluation by an OT Driving Rehabilitation Specialist.

P: Reviewed results of screening and recommendations with patient, family members, and primary care physician. Provided written and online resources for patient and family in dealing with cognitive deficits. Also provided contact information for OT Driving Rehabilitation Specialists within a 2-hour radius of pt.'s hometown. This OT will follow up only if requested by physician during future primary care visits.

Abigail B, OTR/L

EVALUATION REPORTS

After a referral for occupational therapy is received for a client, you begin gathering information about the client's occupational history as well as other factors that impact engagement in occupation. This is the beginning of the occupational profile, which will tell you what the client needs and wants from occupational therapy. The *AOTA Occupational Profile Template* (2022) is based on the *Occupational Therapy Practice Framework: Domain and Process, Fourth Edition*, and is easily accessible on the AOTA website. It is a great tool for students and new practitioners who need some guidance in gathering and organizing client information.

In an evaluation, first you collect data from the client, the family, the chart, and any other pertinent sources. Then you select and administer any standardized tests or survey instruments that will help you determine more specifically what contributing factors support or hinder participation in occupations. You also use your clinical observation skills to analyze occupational performance. Finally, you compile all your data into a comprehensive report.

Evaluation Report: Inpatient Rehabilitation

Name: Rosa S   *Age:* 68   *Physician:* Dr. Boyce
1° Dx: R CVA   *2° Dx:* DM, HTN, CAD, recurrent UTI

Occupational Profile: Client was admitted after a stroke resulting in confusion and left-sided weakness. Prior to admission, she was living alone in a one-story home and was independent in all ADLs. Client is a retired librarian and states she values her independence and fully intends to return to her own home. Hobbies include mostly sedentary activities such as sewing, reading, and playing cards with friends. Only recent fall was being found down on floor by family with this CVA. Daughter works during the day, lives two blocks away, and is willing to visit daily and assist with transportation but cannot provide 24-hr. supervision.

S: Client stated, "I'll work hard in rehab. I need to get home."

O: Client participated in 60-minute evaluation in room and shower room for Mini-Mental Status Examination (MMSE), and evaluation of ADLs, functional mobility, and contributing factors (MMT, AROM). Pt. presents with L UE weakness, decreased balance, and limited activity tolerance.

SECTION GG ITEM	DESCRIPTION	SECTION GG SCORE ADMISSION PERFORMANCE
Eating	Assist required for set-up, opening packages, clean-up.	5
Oral Hygiene	Supervision required due to L inattention and sequencing deficits.	4
Toileting	Mod A to obtain tissue, perform perineal hygiene, and manage clothing; verbal cues to flush.	3
Showering	Completed seated on shower chair; assist required for B LEs, peri-area, buttocks, and R UE.	2
Upper Body Dressing	Mod A to fasten and adjust bra; cues needed to use front-fasten method after repeated failures to fasten in back. Mod A to get shirt overhead and adjusted in back. Min verbal cues needed for sequencing and orientation.	3
Lower Body Dressing	Max A to thread feet into underwear and pants and to stand with wheeled walker to pull up over hips.	2
Put On/Take Off Footwear	Dependent to don socks and slip-on shoes.	1

Functional Mobility: Supine to/from sit with min A; sit to stand from EOB with wheeled walker CGA with verbal cues for safety/proper arm placement; mod A from low surfaces. Min A stand pivot transfer bed to chair with wheeled walker. Ambulation in room with wheeled walker during ADLs min A initially, progressed to needing mod A as became fatigued.

Functional Endurance: Required rest break after less than 10 minutes of ADLs.

Motor Planning/Perception: WFL.

Cognition: Score of 17/20 on MMSE. Sequencing problems during dressing tasks noted.

Sensation: R UE intact; L UE light touch, pain, temperature intact; stereognosis 3 of 5.

UE AROM: WFL for all B UE movements, except ¾ range L shoulder flex/abd against gravity.

MMT: R UE 4+/5 throughout; L UE 3+/5 throughout

Strength:

	LEFT HAND	RIGHT HAND
Grip	21 lbs	42 lbs
Lateral Pinch	6 lbs	14 lbs
Tripod Pinch	5 lbs	12 lbs
Tip Pinch	2 lbs	8 lbs

A: Poor problem-solving skills (needing cues to sequence activity and inability to initiate alternative way to don bra) and need for verbal cues to initiate some ADL tasks limit her ability to manage ADLs and IADLs independently. Decreased AROM and strength in L UE along with slow response to cognitive tasks, decreased ability to sequence tasks, and decreased short-term memory raise safety concerns in returning to independent living. Client motivation and available family support indicate good potential for returning home with intermittent family assistance for bathing and IADLs. Client would benefit from environmental cues to orient her to environment, facilitation of problem solving, sequencing activities, and activities to increase strength in L UE for improved ADL and IADL performance.

P: Client will receive OT for 60-minute sessions 5x/wk for 2 weeks to work toward increased independence with ADLs, with focus on improving sequencing, problem solving, L UE strength, and endurance for functional activities. Calendar will be placed in client's room to increase orientation to month, day, and season. Client's ability to respond to emergency household situations will be assessed during next session.

Section GG Discharge Goals:

- Eating—6
- Oral Hygiene—6
- Toileting—6
- Showering—5
- Upper Body Dressing—6
- Lower Body Dressing—6
- Put On/Take Off Footwear—6

Grace B, OTR/L

Evaluation Report: Skilled Nursing Facility

Name: Anna J   **Age:** 80   **1° Dx:** L hip fx   **2° Dx:** Early-stage dementia

Brief Occupational Profile: Ms. J reports living alone and being I in all ADLs prior to admission. She had gone upstairs to use the bathroom since there was none on the first floor. She became light-headed, fell down the stairs, and broke her hip. She spent 3 days in acute care and was admitted to SNF yesterday. She wants to return home. Her family lives out of town and cannot stay with her long term, but daughter plans to stay a few weeks upon return home from SNF. Ms. J has supportive neighbors and lives in a small town where she is retired from her position as a second-grade teacher. She lives across the street from the elementary school and is in the habit of visiting with the children and some of their families when school is out each day. She is also active in her church.

S: Client stated that she would like to "get this leg well" and go home to "live a regular life." Client rates current pain at surgical site as 6 out of 10. Client recalled 2 of 3 hip precautions from acute care hospitalization.

O: Client participated in 45-minute ADL eval. in room to assess capabilities following L THR to repair hip fx. Supine in bed upon therapist's arrival; required min A for supine to sit to move L LE to side of bed while adhering to hip precautions. During ADL evaluation, client was observed flexing hips beyond 90° and required 4 verbal cues to remain at or below 90° during the 45-minute session. Other 2 hip precautions were followed.

Upper Extremity Function: B UE ROM and strength WFL.

Bathing: Upper body sponge bath seated at sink with set-up; lower body sponge bath with long-handled sponge and mod A to stand for bathing peri-area and buttocks.

Dressing: Upper body dressing with set-up. Lower body dressing with mod A using reacher, sock aid, and long shoehorn.

Grooming: Independent from w/c level.

Following verbal reinforcement of hip precautions, client demonstrated good problem solving by trying different body positions to perform ADLs while adhering to hip precautions and correct use of adaptive equipment. Client demonstrated decreased activity tolerance as she required four 2-minute rest breaks during dressing tasks.

A: Decreased endurance, decreased balance, and inconsistent compliance with hip precautions present safety concerns during lower body dressing and bathing. Client's motivation, problem-solving skills, and understanding of equipment use indicate good rehab potential to return home with intermittent check-ins from family and neighbors. Upper body strength and AROM WFL are beneficial to learning adaptive techniques for self-care and functional mobility. Client would benefit from skilled instruction on hip precautions and use of adaptive equipment with ADL performance, therapeutic activities that facilitate dynamic standing balance, and increased ADL activity tolerance. Exploration of interim living arrangement or possible continued home visits and home equipment procurement will be needed if progress warrants discharge to home.

P: Client to be seen 6x/wk for 3 weeks to increase independence in self-care tasks through instruction on hip precautions and use of adaptive equipment, with tasks to increase activity tolerance and dynamic balance needed for ADLs and IADLs.

LTG: *By anticipated discharge in 3 weeks, client will:*

- *Complete lower body dressing independently utilizing adaptive equipment with 100% adherence to hip precautions.*
- *Complete toileting independently using adaptive equipment (walker and bedside commode).*
- *Complete light meal prep with supervision using wheeled walker to navigate around kitchen.*

Tamaya C, OTR/L

Evaluation Report: Seating and Mobility Consultation (Independent Vendor Format)

Name: *Hallie C*   **Age:** *17*   **Primary Dx:** *Incomplete C6 SCI due to MVA*
                                                       Secondary Dx: *Depression*

Medical History and Occupational Profile: *Hallie is a 17-year-old young woman with a diagnosis of incomplete C6 SCI resulting from a motor vehicle accident (MVA) on her prom night. Her boyfriend was killed in the MVA, and Hallie continues to deal with depression related to that event and her residual functional deficits. Hallie had no significant medical history prior to the MVA. She will be a senior in high school this fall and enjoys photography and playing piano. She lives at home with her parents and 15-year-old brother. Hallie has undergone 6 weeks of intensive inpatient rehabilitation. She is being evaluated for a power wheelchair in preparation for discharge home. Hallie, her mother, and the rehab facility OT attended this evaluation.*

Current Seating/Mobility: *For the last 2 weeks of her rehabilitation stay, Hallie has utilized a loaner tilt-in-space power wheelchair on a trial basis. Per client, family, and staff report, Hallie has been independent with mobility in her hospital room and throughout the facility.*

Home Environment *(based on report from rehab facility OT): Home is a large one-level ranch with an open floor plan. Family has already made considerable modification to the home including installation of ramp to enter front door, widening of doorways, and renovation of bathroom for w/c accessibility. Hallie completed a home visit with the facility OT 1 week ago and reportedly was able to access the bedroom, living room, kitchen, dining room, bathroom, and patio using the power w/c. Mother reports that an anonymous member from their church has donated a van with a w/c lift.*

Cognitive/Visual Status: *Rehab OT, speech therapist, and neuropsychologist report Hallie's cognitive and visual perceptual function as WNL.*

ADL Status: *Hallie completes upper body dressing and bathing with set-up. She requires mod A with lower body dressing and bathing using adaptive equipment. She currently requires max A for bowel program and catheter management, although rehab team is addressing client and caregiver training this week to increase Hallie's independence with these tasks.*

UE Function: *Hallie has 4/5 strength throughout her dominant R UE. She has 3+/5 strength in her L UE shoulder and elbow, and no active movement in her L wrist or hand.*

Sensation: *Sensation intact R UE; absent in distal L UE. Impaired R trunk and LE; absent L trunk and LE.*

Transfers/Mobility: *Hallie requires minimal assist for bed mobility with a rail, including supine to sit. Hallie completes squat pivot transfers from bed to w/c or toilet with mod A. She is independent in maneuvering a power w/c using a standard joystick. She operates the tilt-in-space option independently for pressure relief.*

Assessment: *Hallie is non-ambulatory due to motor impairments resulting from incomplete C6 SCI. She is unable to propel a manual w/c independently due to significant impairments of L UE AROM and strength as well as decreased strength in R UE. Hallie is not a candidate for a scooter as she would not be able to transfer safely into a scooter seating system or operate the tiller driving system effectively. Therefore, the use of a power w/c is necessary to improve Hallie's ability to participate in mobility-related ADLs. Tilt-in-space and air cushion are necessary as Hallie sits in the w/c for 10+ hours daily and is therefore at high risk for development of pressure ulcers. Hallie is unable to perform a functional weight shift and unable to transfer independently to the bed for pressure relief.*

Without this device, Hallie would be at risk for decreased ability to participate in mobility-related ADLs such as accessing the bathroom for bathing and toileting and accessing the dining room for family meals. She would have no independent, safe, or effective means of mobility or function within her home, school, or community. Additionally, she would be at significant risk for development of pressure sores, postural deformity, and pain.

Recommendation: *Recommend purchase of the following to accommodate Hallie's body dimensions, postural alignment, and pressure relief needs:*

- *18" X 16" power wheelchair with power tilt-in-space*
- *Push-button lap belt*
- *Desk-length flip-up height-adjustable armrests with standard joystick mounted on right armrest*
- *Removable headrest*
- *Rear anti-tippers for stability during tilt of wheelchair*
- *Ankle straps and heel loops to maintain feet on footplates*
- *Air cushion with incontinence cover to prevent pressure ulcers*
- *Lap board for UE support during feeding and school activities*
- *Standard tires and casters with flat free inserts.*

Plan: *Hallie will discharge home using existing loaner wheelchair from this company. Upon insurance approval of the above recommendations, equipment will be delivered to Hallie's home for fitting and training in safe and effective use. Follow-up appointments will be conducted as needed for modification of equipment.*

Matt C, OTR/L, ATP, RTS

Evaluation Report: Outpatient Assistive Technology Center (Facility Format for Funding Request)

Occupational therapists are often members of an assistive technology team when assessing clients for augmentative and alternative communication (AAC) devices or other assistive technology equipment. The following note was co-written by an occupational therapist and a speech-language pathologist. It is not in SOAP format because it is being sent to a local agency for funding of recommended equipment.

Name: *Alyssa F*   ***Age:*** *13*   ***Dx:*** *Muscular dystrophy*   ***Funding:*** *County Agency*

Alyssa participated in a consultative appointment at assistive technology clinic to determine effective hardware and software adaptations for independence in computer use.

Subjective: *Alyssa states, "I want to be able to use the computer for school stuff, email, and social media without my mother helping me." Mother reports that client currently navigates the internet by telling her mother what to click.*

Hearing: *WNL.*

Vision: *Alyssa presented with decreased visual acuity but demonstrated compensation using high contrast, enlarged computer screen, and a large high-contrast cursor.*

Speech and Language: *The client's receptive skills were commensurate with her expressive language skills. She was able to process and follow complex verbal directions for her age. Due to decreased air volume, speaking becomes fatiguing after just a few minutes of conversation.*

Mobility: *Alyssa uses a power wheelchair with a mini proportional joystick for mobility independently in a familiar spacious environment.*

Neuromuscular Skills: *Alyssa presents with progressive quadriparesis throughout her body. Due to the nature of her diagnosis, she fatigues very quickly.*

Visual Skills: *The client presents with good visual scanning skills to scan keys on a keyboard and good visual tracking to follow a cursor.*

Sensory Processing: *Alyssa demonstrates good cause/effect understanding and functional attention to access a computer. She demonstrates high motivation to access a computer and the internet.*

Results of Assistive Technology Assessment: *Alyssa is physically unable to use a standard keyboard or mouse but likes to navigate the internet by telling her mother what to click. Alyssa was unable to use a joystick mouse, trackball mouse, or glide point. She demonstrated good use of a mini proportional joystick to drive her wheelchair. She does not have Bluetooth capabilities in the electronics of her wheelchair. After observing her use of the mini proportional joystick, Alyssa was presented with an ABC Joystick and an XYZ Mini-Joystick, ABC and XYZ onscreen keyboards, USB switch interface, and an ultralight switch. Alyssa demonstrated the ability to move the highly sensitive ABC Joystick and spell on both onscreen keyboards, but preferred the letter contrast and simplicity of XYZ keyboard using small movements of her right index finger and thumb. She clicked on choices using her left hand and the ultralight switch. She was highly successful with this combination and independent to navigate the internet and spell out messages using a word processing document. She also demonstrated the ability to check her email and social networking accounts with the above-mentioned adapted computer equipment. She was unable to move as accurately or quickly with the XYZ Mini-Joystick. Alyssa also presents with low vision related to the above diagnosis. It was felt during the evaluation that Alyssa would benefit from Text Enlargement Software, which would provide screen reading as well as magnification as needed.*

Recommendations: *As a result of the assistive technology evaluation, it has been determined that Alyssa is an excellent candidate for adaptive software/hardware to allow her improved access to her computer and internet. It is recommended that she receive an ABC Joystick USB, a USB switch interface, XYZ Keyboard, Text Enlargement Software, and an ultralight switch to increase her independence on the computer and internet. It is also recommended that Alyssa receive an updated computer system to increase her independence with written communication needs.*

Shawna D, MLS, OTR/L, ATP   Michelle W, MS, CCC-SLP

Evaluation Report: Outpatient Pediatric Clinic (Facility Format)

This note is not done in a SOAP format because it is designed to be sent to the school rather than written in the child's health record. This note also provides an example of a note that is done by a student co-signed by the supervising occupational therapist.

Name: *Reagan L*   ***Chronological Age:*** *5 years, 2 months*

Reagan is a 5-year, 2-month-old girl who is being seen today upon request of her family and the UMC Kindergarten Program. Reagan was an active, healthy child until April of this year, at which time she developed Haemophilus influenzae *type-B meningitis. Reagan was hospitalized for 10 days and had a "long recovery" by the family's report. Although Reagan's parents believe she has now made a full recovery, they are concerned that this illness slowed her previously fast progress and that she may not be ready for kindergarten this fall. The parents and the UMC Kindergarten Program are requesting an evaluation to assess her readiness for kindergarten.*

Assessment Results: *Three subtests of the Peabody Developmental Motor Scales, Second Edition, were administered to Reagan. The PDMS-2 is a standardized norm-referenced evaluation designed to assess fine and gross motor skills in children birth to 71 months of age. Today's evaluation of Reagan (at chronological age 5 years, 2 months) reveals:*

SUBTEST	*STANDARD SCORE	PERCENTILE RANK	AGE EQUIVALENT
Object Manipulation	11	63rd	5 years, 11 months
Grasping	10	50th	5 years, 3 months
Visual Motor Integration	11	63rd	5 years, 8 months
*Standard scores are based on a mean of 10 and a standard deviation of 3.			

Reagan's combined performance on the grasping and visual motor integration subtests resulted in a Fine Motor Quotient (FMQ) of 103 (mean of 100, standard deviation of 15), placing her in the 58th percentile for overall fine motor skills.

Reagan was alert and cooperative throughout the 25-minute evaluation. She exhibited a right-hand dominance, utilizing the right upper extremity as the main initiator of activity and the left upper extremity as an assist and stabilizer. Posture, muscle tone, strength, and endurance all appeared to be within normal limits for chronological age. Response to auditory stimuli in the environment was appropriate. The parents do not report any hearing or vision concerns. During the evaluation, the child did not squint, rub eyes, nor exhibit any difficulties with visual regard/tracking.

Summary: *Results of the three subtests of the PDMS-2 indicate that Reagan is functioning slightly above the mean in fine motor skills for her chronological age. Motor coordination and response to environmental stimuli appear to be within normal limits for chronological age. Although Reagan was recently hospitalized with a serious illness, she currently exhibits adequate fine motor abilities to perform kindergarten activities.*

Actions Taken: *Evaluation results were discussed with Reagan's parents, who attended the evaluation session today. A copy of this report will be sent to the family and to the UMC Kindergarten Program as requested by the family.*

Plan: *Re-evaluation upon request.*

Sydney C, OTS
Emily C, OTR/L

Evaluation Report: Community Living Consultation for Adaptive Equipment Recommendations

Background Information: *Ashley is a 20-year-old female with spastic quadriplegic cerebral palsy. Client has lived at home with her family her entire life, with her mother providing maximum to dependent assistance for all basic self-care tasks. Client's mother was recently diagnosed with multiple sclerosis and is no longer able to provide the level of physical assistance that Ashley requires. Client will be transitioning into a group home for adults with developmental disabilities at the end of this month. County Agency has requested an OT consult to determine adaptive equipment necessary for group home staff to provide care for Ashley.*

S: *Client is nonverbal but did communicate through facial gestures and by touching a yes/no response system mounted to her manual w/c. Client's parents provided information about how they had previously assisted Ashley with ADLs at home.*

O: *Pt., family, and group home staff participated in a consultation at Ashley's future group home to determine adaptive equipment necessary to provide care for Ashley. Client presents in manual tilt-in-space w/c with lateral trunk supports, seatbelt, headrest, and footplate straps to maintain positioning. Per observation and family report, client has limited functional use of all extremities. Her parents have been completing total lift transfers between bed and w/c. The group home already has a ceiling track lift system installed in Ashley's future bedroom. Group home staff demonstrated lift system transfer w/c to/from bed with Ashley, who smiled and vocalized throughout process. Concern was raised by group home staff regarding bathing. Ashley's family previously lifted her into the bathtub but in recent months have been completing sponge baths at the bed level as it has become more difficult for Ashley's mother to lift her. Group home has a zero-entry shower stall with hand-held shower hose and a simple shower/commode transport chair. OT and group home staff attempted to transfer Ashley bed to shower chair using the ceiling lift system. However, due to significant deficits in trunk control and spasticity in all extremities, Ashley was not able to maintain upright positioning in the chair.*

A: *Limited trunk control and spasticity of B UEs and B LEs limits client's ability to maintain upright positioning and perform functional transfers during ADLs. Ashley's positive response to use of ceiling track lift system is a good indication that she will transition well to her new home environment. Client would benefit from purchase of a reclining, rolling shower/commode with head support, lateral trunk supports, and straps for positioning pelvis, trunk, and LEs during transport and bathing.*

P: *Reviewed equipment recommendations with Ashley, group home staff, and family. Specifications for recommended shower chair sent to County Agency who will coordinate funding and procurement. No further recommendations at this time. This OT is available for future consults as needed should new concerns arise with Ashley's transition to her new home.*

Lindsay F, OTR/L

RE-EVALUATION REPORTS

In some practice settings, clients must be re-evaluated at certain intervals, such as monthly or quarterly. In other settings, re-evaluation is done as needed. The frequency of re-evaluation depends on the setting, the funding source, and the progress of the client. Assessments that were used initially are re-administered. You want to provide a thorough comparison of assessment results and functional performance between the initial evaluation and the client's current level to determine the effectiveness of the treatment being provided. Goals and planned intervention are revised, and new timelines are projected.

Re-Evaluation Report: Outpatient Hand Therapy Clinic

Name: *Leanna G*   **Dx:** *Osteoarthritis of B CMC joints*   **Precautions/Contraindications:** *None*

Reason for Referral: *Client is 1-month post-surgery (LRTI) to the L CMC joint and carpal tunnel release.*

Occupational Profile: *Leanna is a 41-year-old female who works as an administrative assistant in the University English Department. She lives alone in a small, two-story farmhouse 7 miles outside of town. The house is heated with wood that Leanna cuts and stacks in the summer. Leanna plants a large vegetable garden each year, in addition to holding both a full-time job at the University and a part-time job in a department store. She began experiencing pain in the CMC joints of both hands approximately 3 years ago. She intends to continue her present living arrangement and both of her jobs. She was originally admitted to the outpatient hand clinic 1-month post-surgery for hand rehabilitation following a successful ligament reconstruction and tendon interposition (LRTI) of the L CMC joint and L carpal tunnel release. She is being re-evaluated today to determine whether further OT services are needed.*

S: *Client initially reported continuous pain at a level of 3/10 in L hand and pain on overexertion at a level of 5/10 in L hand, resulting in irritability and difficulty performing bilateral work and daily living tasks, as well as some tasks requiring L hand use. On this date, she reports no continuous pain and pain at a level of 1/10 when typing for more than 45 minutes without rest breaks.*

Initial ability to engage in work/ADL/IADL tasks (by client report):

- *Unable to use keyboard with all fingers of L hand. Typed with one finger on standard keyboard.*
- *Unable to grasp cylindrical objects smaller than 1½ inches (broom handle, toothpaste tube) due to decreased AROM.*
- *Unable to wear watch or rings on L hand due to swelling.*
- *Unable to turn door knob with L hand to enter house when R hand is full.*
- *Unable to lift laundry basket and other items requiring B UE use. Unable to lift purse or other items needed for IADL tasks with L hand.*

Current ability to engage in work/ADL/IADL tasks (by client report):

- *Able to use new ergonomic keyboard for primary work task using all fingers.*
- *Able to sweep floors with a regular broom.*
- *Able to fold laundry using B hands.*
- *Able to grasp small items needed for ADL and IADL tasks (toothpaste tube, key, lids) with L hand, but not at PLOF.*
- *Able to turn doorknob with L hand if door is unlocked.*
- *Able to hang clothes on clothesline, including carrying basket and holding garments with L hand.*

O: *Client has participated in three 45-minute visits in outpatient hand clinic since admission. AROM and PROM exercises have been performed and taught to client, and home program has been modified as she progressed. Heat has been used to relieve pain, and client has purchased a home paraffin unit. Electrical stimulation has been used to elicit specific motion and facilitate strengthening of the flexor pollicis longus. A strengthening program has been added to the HEP, and client is able to demonstrate all HEP exercises correctly. Client educated on structure and use of the hand, common features of CMC arthritis, ergonomics of the workstation, energy conservation, use of heat for pain relief, and adapted techniques for ADL activities. Client provided with written material covering the same content and reports implementing recommendations into both home and work activities.*

A: Increase in L grip strength of 7# shows good progress in strength needed to perform functional tasks. Improved thumb AROM (WFL) and wrist AROM (80% of average) now allow client to perform most work and ADL tasks independently in ways that do not damage the joint. Change to an ergonomic keyboard and understanding and correct self-administration of HEP indicate good potential to continue improvement without further OT services. Client would benefit from continuation of daily HEP.

P: Plan to discontinue OT services at this time as results of re-evaluation indicate no further need for OT services unless new problems arise. Client to call hand clinic if questions arise and follow the home program of heat, exercise, and adapted techniques.

Brad E, OTR/L, CHT

Re-Evaluation Report: Outpatient Work Hardening Clinic
(Facility Format)

Note: This example contains terminology and abbreviations specific to a work hardening setting that are not listed in Chapter 5.

Worker: *Joe Fireman*   **Age:** *33*   **Job Title:** *Firefighter/Paramedic*

Physician: *Dr. Pain*   **Dx:** *s/p L shoulder reconstruction*   **Attendance:** *5/5 sessions*

Subjective Complaints: *Pain level was rated as 3-4/10 pre-test and post-test. He described sharp pain near the left acromioclavicular (AC) joint, with aching in the anterior/posterior deltoid and into the left upper trapezius musculature.*

Work Plan: *Return to his usual and customary job when able.*

Perceived Disability: *Worker scored 14/70 on the Pain Disability Index, which indicates a low level of self-perceived disability. This represents a moderate improvement from 39/70 upon initial evaluation.*

Musculoskeletal Screen

Musculoskeletal Deficit Changes Since Last Evaluation: *In comparison to the unaffected right shoulder, slight ROM gains are noted with the L UE, while still remaining below expected AMA norms. Left shoulder strength is 5/5 within the given range (exception for external rotation 4+/5), while R UE strength is 5/5 in all planes. Occasional sustained forward/overhead reaching task continues to be completed at an above competitive proficiency level.*

Quality of Movement Changes: *Functional overhead reaching and internal/external rotation with the L UE has improved, but remains decreased vs. R UE. Mild decreased control was noted with the L UE with maximum load handling at all levels. Mild compensation patterns were observed with use of L UE when crawling and climbing ladders.*

Summary of Demonstrated Abilities:

MATERIAL HANDLING	MAX. OCCASIONAL (LBS)			EMPLOYER-REPORTED JOB REQUIREMENTS
	ENTRANCE (5/03/23)	*RE-EVAL (5/17/23)*	*RE-EVAL (6/07/23)*	
Floor—Waist Lift	55	60	70	*May lift >100 lbs from floor to chest or shoulder height in emergency scenarios (occas.); may handle tools up to 45 lbs lifting floor to overhead (up to frequent as needed)*
Waist—Shoulder Lift	20	45	55	
Shoulder—Overhead Lift	15	35	40	
Bilateral Carry	60	60	70	
Unilateral Lift/Carry (L/R)	30/55	55/55	55/55	
Pushing (Force) (L/R)	73 (31/42)	57 (31/31)	89 (39/51)	*Up to 70 lbs (hands in front); up to 35 lbs overhead push/pull with pike pole*
Pulling (Force) (L/R)	70 (33/37)	57 (35/25)	80 (41/39)	

(continued)

NON-MATERIAL HANDLING	FREQUENCY DISPLAYED			JOB REQUIREMENTS
Sitting	Unrestricted	Unrestricted	Unrestricted	Occasional
Standing	Unrestricted	Unrestricted	Unrestricted	Frequent
Walking	Unrestricted	Unrestricted	Unrestricted	Frequent
Climbing	Limited	Improved	Frequent	Frequent
Bending	Unrestricted	Unrestricted	Unrestricted	Frequent
Reaching (Forward/Overhead)	Occasional/ Limited	Occasional/ Limited	Frequent	Frequent
Squatting/Kneeling	Unrestricted	Unrestricted	Unrestricted	Frequent
Crawling	Occasional	Occasional	Up to Frequent	Occasional

Consistency and Quality of Effort: *Client continues to provide good and consistent effort with testing, based upon positive HR response to activity, low coefficients of variation (CV) values with ROM/static strength tests, and the presence of external effort indicators. Please see chart below for description of criteria.*

Global Effort Rating: Consistency and Quality of Effort Indicators:

CRITERION	RESULTS	COMMENTS
Pain Diagram: Reports of circumferential pain, glove or stocking presentation would in most cases be supported in the literature as inconsistent with the diagnosis.	Expected	No unusual markings for given diagnosis.
Pain Behavior and Function: High pain ratings should be consistent with altered movement patterns and range of motion. Alteration of movement patterns should be consistent in associated tasks/transitional movement patterns vs. direct measurement. A patient's behavior should consistently reflect distress, and not only during performance of evaluation tasks.	Expected	Pain level was rated as 3-4/10 pre-test, up to 5/10 with testing, and as 3-4/10 post-test. Subjective reports were consistent with displayed function.
Perceived Disability Score: In the absence of organic findings, high-perceived disability may compromise recovery from injury.	Expected	Client's score on the Pain Disability Index (14/70) indicates a low level of self-perceived disability currently.
Coefficients of Variation: Repeated test trials must be low to indicate consistent effort.	Expected	Worker displayed high CV values during 0 of 10 ROM tests and 0 of 6 static strength tests.
5-Position Grip (Bell Curve): Deviation from bell curves may indicate sub-maximal effort, especially when performed on non-hand diagnoses.	Expected	Worker displayed modified bell-shaped distribution on right/left.
Cross-Reference Validity Check: Tests repeated at intervals with full volitional effort with >20% variation may be indicator of sub-maximal effort.	Expected	Variance between results for position 2 on standard grip test and Maximum Modified Voluntary Effort (MMVE) test was 12.1% to 18.8%.
Static Force Curve Analysis: Force curves during static trials should follow a predictable pattern. Delayed and/or erratic force curves may indicate that maximal effort was not achieved during that test.	Expected	During static strength testing, delayed peak contractions and erratic force curves were noted during 0 of 18 trials.
HR and RPE Correlation: A patient's report of physical exertion (RPE) should correlate with a corresponding increase in working heart rate.	Expected	Working HR and corresponding RPE values were proportionate in all instances.

Impression:

- *Client has provided high levels of effort while attending 5 scheduled sessions on the most recent prescription, resulting in additional gains with heavy load handling, pushing/pulling ability, and tolerance for sustained work-simulated activities. He continues to wear his turn-out gear during sessions to simulate completing essential job functions.*

- *Mr. Fireman has displayed safe function in at least the Medium work demand level, with some function into the Heavy demand level, up to the above-listed tolerances. The abilities displayed with testing this date do not meet the employer-reported essential job demands. The main factors limiting return to work continue to be decreased tolerance for the required work demand level, decreased load handling ability, decreased push/pull tolerances, decreased tolerance for sustained work tasks involving the L UE (reaching, tool use), decreased AROM for overhead job tasks, and his subjective pain complaints at this time.*

Plan: *Mr. Fireman has a follow-up appointment with physician 7/08/23. We will await your recommendations.*

Shelia T, OTR/L, CHT, CEAS

Re-Evaluation Report: Outpatient Driver Rehabilitation

Name: *James S*   ***Age:*** *71*   ***Dx:*** *Multiple TIAs*

S: *Client reports successful completion of 6-week Mature Driver Improvement Course recommended during initial evaluation 2 months ago. "I do okay during the day, but I'm afraid to drive at night. I just don't see that well." Client declined opportunity to drive on 4-lane highway during on-road assessment, indicating that he only drives short distances in his small community and relies on family for longer distance transportation.*

O: *Client participated in driving re-evaluation this date to determine safety and independence with community mobility. Previous evaluation 2 months ago revealed minor hearing deficits, decreased reaction times, mild left inattention, and impaired ability to recognize and understand road signs.*

*   ***In-Clinic Evaluation:*** *Visual acuity WFL with bifocal lenses; depth perception WFL. No left inattention observed. Client scored WFL on brake reaction time test. Client correctly identified meaning of 29 of 30 road signs (missed side road intersection sign).*

*   ***On-Road Evaluation:*** *Client completed 20 minutes driving in car in residential and commercial areas of a suburban area. Results are as follows:*

- *Client demonstrated proper use of mirrors and over-the-shoulder checks; observed and responded to turn signals of other drivers by slowing down and obeyed all road signs and traffic control devices. Client demonstrated adequate visual scanning when entering the roadway and at all intersections.*

- *Client correctly used turn signals at appropriate times and activated horn, headlights, and emergency flashers when instructed to do so.*

- *Client observed posted speed limits and made appropriate adjustments to speed related to intersections, traffic flow, and roadway surfaces. Client demonstrated proper vehicle positioning while moving forward in traffic and before, during, and after all turns.*

- *Client demonstrated appropriate time and space judgment when changing lanes and negotiating intersections. Client demonstrated adequate brake, accelerator, and steering control when driving forward, backing up, merging, and parking.*

A: *Improvements in visual perception, reaction time, cognition (understanding road signs), and functional driving performance as compared to initial evaluation 2 months ago indicate enhanced ability to operate a motor vehicle safely in residential and commercial environments. Decreased night vision and comfort level with driving on busy highways pose safety concerns for driving in those situations. Client would benefit from continued family assistance for night-time or long-distance transportation.*

P: *It is recommended that client's driving be restricted to daylight hours in rural and small-town areas. Client should not drive at night or on large, busy highways. Recommendations have been discussed with client and family. They voice understanding that the results of this evaluation are indicative only of the client's functional driving ability on this date. Any changes in health or cognition that would impact driving should be addressed through follow-up with client's physician for potential referral to a Certified Driving Rehabilitation Specialist (CDRS).*

Myles H, OTR/L, CDRS

Adapted from content in Shipp & Havard, 2006.

INTERVENTION PLANS

Intervention Plan: Inpatient Rehabilitation

Functional Problem Statement #1: *Decreased L UE AROM, activity tolerance, and ability to sequence results in need for max A to complete dressing tasks.*

LTG #1: *Client will complete all dressing tasks independently within 2 weeks.*

STG (OBJECTIVE)	INTERVENTIONS
STG #1: *Client will don bra independently using adapted technique within 3 days.*	1. *Teach adaptive techniques.* 2. *Post picture of how to don bra by fastening in front.* 3. *Reinforce correct responses.* 4. *Teach strengthening program for L UE.*
STG #2: *Client will don shoes and socks independently using adapted technique and long shoehorn within 5 days.*	1. *Provide long shoehorn and instruct in use.* 2. *Instruct in adapted techniques for donning shoes and socks.* 3. *Post picture of adapted technique using long shoehorn.* 4. *Instruct in use of affected side as a functional assist in dressing.* 5. *Expand exercise program to include AROM.*
STG #3: *Client will complete dressing tasks with no verbal cues for sequencing for 3 consecutive sessions within 10 days.*	1. *Verbalize steps before beginning to dress.* 2. *Verbalize steps while dressing.* 3. *Post list of steps for client to follow.* 4. *Take rest breaks as needed for activity tolerance.*

Functional Problem Statement #2: *Lack of orientation to environment and inability to problem solve raise safety concerns with ADLs and home management.*

LTG #2: *Client will correctly answer questions pertaining to time, date, schedule, and emergency situations using only environmental cues within 2 weeks.*

STG (OBJECTIVE)	INTERVENTIONS
STG #1: *Within 1 week, client will correctly identify time, date, and situation without verbal cues when asked on 3 of 3 attempts.*	1. *Post calendar, schedule, and emergency information near clock in client's room.* 2. *Instruct family, nursing staff, and other therapy staff to quiz client several times daily re: date, time, and situation and to reinforce correct responses.*
STG #2: *Client will follow her daily printed schedule with <2 verbal cues within 1 week.*	1. *Post daily schedule on wall near clock and review with client during ADL session each morning.* 2. *Cue client to look at schedule to determine what she should be doing at any given time.*
STG #3: *Client will correctly problem solve responses to emergency situations independently on 9 of 10 attempts within 2 weeks.*	1. *Provide situations for client to problem solve, progressing from easy to more complex.* 2. *Provide telephone directory or other props as needed for problem solving.*

Intervention Plan: Skilled Nursing Facility

Strengths: *UE strength and AROM WFL; intact cognition and motivation to return home.*

Functional Problem Statement #1: *Increased fatigue, decreased endurance for ADLs, and inconsistent compliance with hip precautions makes client unsafe in ADL tasks.*

LTG #1: *By anticipated discharge in 3 weeks, client will safely complete lower body dressing and bathing independently utilizing adaptive equipment with 100% adherence to hip precautions.*

STG (OBJECTIVE)	INTERVENTIONS
STG #1: *Within 1 week, client will don shoes and socks with supervision, using adapted techniques and devices with 100% adherence to hip precautions.*	1. *Instruct and have client verbalize 3/3 hip precautions.* 2. *Provide written handout of hip precautions.* 3. *Instruct in use of adaptive techniques/devices followed by demonstration of use in dressing activities.*
STG #2: *Within 2 weeks, client will complete all lower body dressing tasks with SBA using adaptive equipment with no more than one 30-second rest break.*	1. *Continue instruction in use of adaptive techniques/devices followed by demonstration of use in dressing activities.* 2. *Educate client and provide written instructions on energy conservation techniques. Evaluate understanding by her application during ADL task; ask about how she performs ADL tasks at home.*
STG #3: *Within 3 weeks, client will safely bathe her peri-area independently using adaptive techniques and devices with 100% adherence to hip precautions.*	1. *Instruct in use of adaptive techniques/devices followed by demonstration of use in bathing activities.* 2. *Instruct in manipulation of clothing and bathing items while standing with walker at sink without violating hip precautions.* 3. *Assess for home equipment needs and continued home services if progress warrants discharge to home.*

Functional Problem Statement #2: *Decreased dynamic standing balance makes client unsafe during ADL tasks.*

LTG #2: *By anticipated discharge in 3 weeks, client will safely complete toileting independently using adaptive equipment (walker and bedside commode).*

STG (OBJECTIVE)	INTERVENTIONS
STG #1: *Within 1 week, client will complete toileting with SBA for sit to stand from bedside commode and manage clothing with no more than 2 verbal cues.*	1. *Instruct client in safe transfer techniques; reinforce compliance with total hip precautions.* 2. *Provide UE strengthening through reaching and weight-bearing activities at sink and closet for grooming and dressing items and pushing up from chair and bedside commode.*
STG #2: *Within 2 weeks, client will complete toileting with SBA using wheeled walker and commode frame over toilet.*	1. *Continue instruction in safe transfer techniques; reinforce compliance with total hip precautions.* 2. *Interview client regarding home environment; explore and discuss interim living arrangements or possible equipment use and placement in home; discuss support services needed if discharge home is warranted.*

Intervention Plan: Cancer Center Outpatient Clinic

Name: *Nicole G*   ***Age:*** *35*   ***Primary Dx:*** *Mastectomy 2° breast CA*

Strengths: *Prior to surgery, Nicole was in good physical condition and employed full-time. She has some social support from her sister who lives in another state.*

Functional Problem Statement: *Decreased self-esteem secondary to cosmetic alterations imposed by mastectomy results in avoidance of social outings, thus precluding ability to return to work.*

LTG #1: *Nicole will increase social interactions and activity to 6 outings/month within the next month, in preparation for return to work.*

STG (OBJECTIVE)	INTERVENTIONS
STG #1: *Nicole will identify one support group of interest to her within 1 week to increase willingness to be out in public for work and social activities.*	1. *Educate Nicole re: available support groups and peer visitation groups; their contact persons, telephone numbers, and social media information; and ask her whether she has made contact.* 2. *Ask if Nicole would like to have her contact information given to a volunteer from the hospital's peer mentor group.*
STG #2: *Nicole will attend one support group activity within 2 weeks to increase confidence in social and work situations.*	1. *Email, phone call, or text to remind Nicole of upcoming support group meetings.* 2. *Discuss with Nicole her experiences with the support groups.*
STG #3: *Nicole will initiate conversation with at least one other support group member during her first visit to the group to decrease negative impact of cosmetic alterations to body image.*	1. *Help Nicole identify a friend to accompany her into the community the first time she goes out.* 2. *Encourage participation in group discussion.*
STG #4: *Nicole will enroll in a women's exercise program to increase activity tolerance and positive body image.*	1. *Educate Nicole re: area exercise groups for post-mastectomy clients.* 2. *Follow-up phone call/email to ask if she has enrolled in an exercise program.*
STG #5: *Nicole will identify 5 assets she possesses other than physical to increase self-esteem and confidence in social and work situations.*	1. *Discuss Nicole's assets with her, encouraging her to think of as many as she can.* 2. *Educate Nicole regarding books and websites that address post-mastectomy concerns.*

Functional Problem Statement: *Nicole is unable to return to work 2° 3/4 AROM, 4-/5 muscle strength, decreased activity tolerance (fatigues after 1 hr.), and sensory changes.*

LTG #2: *Nicole will return to work part-time within 4 weeks.*

STG (OBJECTIVE)	INTERVENTIONS
STG #1: *Within 2 weeks, Nicole will complete 2 hours of work tasks with no more than one 15-minute rest break.*	1. *Scar massage and myofascial release to incision area along with client education on self-massage.* 2. *PROM to L shoulder—instruct in self-ranging program.* 3. *Work simulation tasks.*
STG #2: *Nicole will retrieve five items from overhead shelf independently using L UE in work simulation task within 3 weeks.*	1. *Active resistive ROM to L UE.* 2. *Resistive strengthening with thera-tubing, weights, and graded functional activities.* 3. *Work simulation tasks.*
STG #3: *Within 3 weeks, Nicole will transfer twenty 5# boxes from one table to another in <10 minutes using B UEs with reported pain level <2/10.*	1. *Work simulation with client education on energy conservation principles.* 2. *Provide home exercise program and modify as client progresses.*
STG #4: *Within 3 weeks, Nicole will use correct body mechanics independently in seated and active work tasks in order to have pain level of <2/10 while working.*	1. *Educate in ergonomics and posture to prevent pain.* 2. *Provide education on women's exercise groups.*
STG #5: *Nicole will implement sensory precautions independently in work and daily living tasks within 2 weeks.*	1. *Provide education on safety concerns with sensory loss.* 2. *IADL tasks and work simulation with sensory hazards to check application of safety techniques.*

CONTACT NOTES

Contact, visit, or treatment notes are used to document each visit or individual occupational therapy session. In some situations, contact notes are required in the health record each time a client is seen. In other cases, the occupational therapist keeps attendance records, logs, or informal contact notes, which will later be used for the purpose of writing a progress note. Contact notes are also written to document telephone or email contacts, meetings with others regarding the client, and cancellation of scheduled sessions.

Contact Note: Intensive Care Unit

S: *Client nonverbal and inconsistently made and maintained eye contact with OT and family members when spoken to.*

O: *Client participated in bedside OT session to work on initiating and attending to self-care tasks following TBI. Client presented with poor trunk control and limited attention span throughout session. Client demonstrated startle response with position change. When asked to point finger, client required multiple verbal cues and demonstrations, and demonstrated poor response time. Client required max A supine to sit EOB. Client required multiple verbal cues and hand-over-hand assist 75% of the time to initiate holding on to washcloth. Client able to bring washcloth to water with 1 verbal cue but required hand-over-hand assist to bring washcloth to face. Client attended to looking at self in mirror for ~1 minute. Client required hand-over-hand assist to initiate brushing hair. R shoulder AROM limited due to decreased tone.*

A: *Deficits in motor planning, task initiation, and attention limit client's participation in ADL tasks. Ability to attend for 1 minute indicates progress toward participation in ADL tasks. Client would benefit from ranging activities to increase shoulder elevation, as well as further interventions focusing on the skills of initiating and attending to task to complete ADL activities.*

P: *Client to continue OT 5x/wk to work on self-care activities and the underlying performance skills and client factors necessary to complete tasks. Recommend inpatient rehabilitation if patient demonstrates potential to tolerate 3 hours/day of therapy.*

Ashlyn L, OTR/L

Contact Note: Acute Care

S: *Pt. reports, "I want to get out of this bed. It's been a long night."*

O: *Client participated in bedside OT session for instruction in ADL tasks and AROM in B UEs. Pt. presents with significant trunk and B LE weakness and moderate B UE weakness resulting from Guillain-Barré syndrome. Mod A supine to sit rolling to R sidelying and pushing up through R elbow. Upon sitting, O_2 saturation initially dropped to ~85% on 2 L O_2. Grooming, dressing, and UE AROM activities not completed due to low O_2 levels. Client returned to supine with min A to bring B LEs up onto bed. After ~2 minutes, O_2 levels returned to ~95%. Client washed face after set-up in supine but declined further activity, citing fatigue. Nurse notified of pt.'s change in O_2 saturation during activity.*

A: *Ability to transition supine to sit indicates improved activity tolerance from yesterday when pt. was unable to tolerate this. Expressed interest for out-of-bed activity is a good indication for improving strength and function. Decreased activity tolerance related to drop in O_2 saturation with exertion limits ability to participate in self-care tasks. Client would benefit from instruction in energy conservation as well as correct positioning to decrease exertion and increase activity tolerance for ADL tasks. At this time, pt. does not have the ability to tolerate 3 hours daily therapy required for rehab unit stay; however, pt. would benefit from continued therapy at SNF level once medically stable.*

P: *Continue skilled OT 3-5x/wk to increase activity tolerance and independence in ADL tasks.*

Morgan M, OTR/L

Contact Note: Inpatient Rehabilitation—Prosthetic Adaptation

S: Client expressed pleasure with adaptations to prosthetic leg fasteners made this date, stating "this will work."

O: Client participated in OT session in rehab gym for adaptations necessary to don/doff prosthesis. Sit to stand with supervision from w/c keeping one hand on walker for support. Client positioned prosthetic leg and attempted to fasten straps. Mod A required to fasten straps, independent to unfasten straps to doff prosthesis. Adaptations of prosthetic leg harness completed this date.

A: Inability to don prosthesis without assistance limits independence with dressing, toileting, and functional mobility for IADLs. Ability to position prosthesis correctly and fasten straps indicates good progress toward stated goals. Client would benefit from additional skilled instruction in use of pulley-like fasteners installed this date on prosthesis to allow one-handed closure.

P: Pt. to be seen one more session prior to discharge home tomorrow to reinforce skilled instruction in donning prosthesis.

David W, OTR/L

Contact Note: Home Assessment During Inpatient Rehabilitation Stay

S: Client stated numerous times how nice it was to be home during this home assessment. Client verbalized more in this setting than at the facility.

O: Prior to admission, client lived at home alone with support from family, home health nurse, and housekeeping aide and was independent with all ADLs. Today, pt. participated in home assessment in preparation for discharge home next week. Pt. was transported by family in private vehicle, with OT meeting family at the home. The following are the results of a home evaluation:

- **Entry:** 2½" step, 4" door jam. Uneven grass to step. Concrete broken and no railings present.
- **Kitchen:** 26" area around table in center of kitchen, 27" between snack bar and fridge, 30" high snack bar located on outskirt of kitchen. Little room to maneuver safely. Needs utensils and appliances within reach.
- **Hallway:** 22" wide from dining room to bedroom with bathroom between inaccessible for walker. Remainder of entries adequate to accommodate walker.
- **Bathroom:** 17" floor to tub top, 18" floor to toilet seat. Bathroom small, but can accommodate wheeled walker.
- **Other:** Throw rugs in all rooms. Chair blocks bedroom access with wheeled walker. End tables block access to living room from dining room with wheeled walker.

A: With the following modifications and recommendations, home will be safe for client to return to after discharge:

- Remove all throw rugs to decrease falls; remove excess furniture to increase walking area and increase safety.
- Adaptive equipment needed:
  - Raised toilet seat with safety rails, shower chair with back support, grab bars, and hand-held shower.
  - Add railing to hallway to increase safety without walker.
  - Add railing and repair concrete to outside entry.
- Remove kitchen table and utilize snack bar or dining table to increase mobility in kitchen.
- Lower telephone by back door to improve reach.

P: Resident and family will implement the preceding recommendations and changes to allow discharge from facility to return home safely.

Lani M, OTR/L

Contact Note: Inpatient Mental Health—Multiple Groups

S: *Client reported she is currently not volunteering and has not worked for the past 4 years due to her disability status. Regarding volunteering, she says, "I need the structure," and further states that she wants to be productive. Currently, client reports she sleeps "too much" and is having relationship problems.*

O: *Client was admitted yesterday and attended 4/4 group sessions today. During expressive therapy group, client participated in baking with the rest of the group but did not eat anything. When each group member identified current emotions, client identified hers as miserable, angry, very anxious, overstimulated, frustrated, frightened, and alienated. During skills group, client identified a possible problem she may encounter upon discharge to be lack of organization, with her "red flags" being oversleeping and agitation. Client welcomed suggestions from others restructuring her use of time.*

A: *Refusal to eat with the group indicates continued appetite disturbance. Ability to identify emotions indicates good insight into current limitations. Client's participation in all 4 group sessions today indicates good rehab potential. Client would benefit from information about eating disorders. She would also benefit from continued group participation, with emphasis on increasing self-esteem and time management skills.*

P: *Client will continue to attend all daily group sessions while on the acute unit to work on increasing self-esteem and ability to structure her time.*

Rylie N, OTR/L

Contact Note: Inpatient Mental Health—One Group

The previous note summarized a client's participation in several groups on one day. Some mental health settings, particularly inpatient settings with short lengths of stay, require a note to be written for each group that the client attends. The following note illustrates this type of documentation.

S: *Client reports unhealthy self-esteem in the form of negative thoughts about herself. She describes feeling "stupid" and "ugly," particularly when she is under stress.*

O: *Client participated in 1-hr. self-esteem group in dayroom. Group session was designed to educate participants regarding healthy and unhealthy self-esteem and to instruct on goal setting and other ways to improve self-esteem. Client demonstrated active participation in all group discussions and activities. With encouragement from other group members and facilitator, client set goal for this week to decrease her negative thoughts and to plan for discharge. She independently identified a compensatory strategy to use when she recognizes negative thoughts; her plan is to replace negative thoughts with something more positive such as thinking about how much she enjoys being around her children. Client initiated discussion about setting up appointments for aftercare following discharge.*

A: *Focus on negative thoughts during periods of stress limits client's ability to complete IADL tasks, including caring for her children. Ability to set goals and identify steps to achieving those goals indicates excellent progress this date. Client has great potential to return to independent living. Client would benefit from continued practice in this area and assistance with identifying and replacing negative thoughts.*

P: *Client to attend self-esteem group daily for 3 days to address self-esteem issues that inhibit IADL performance. Sessions to include group discussions, role play, and written discharge plan development, as well as facilitation of setting up aftercare appointments.*

Cameron O, OTR/L

Contact Note: Community Living Mental Health

Name: Owen T   **Length of Session:** 75 minutes   **Goals Addressed:** 2, 4, and 5

S: Owen states that having a bank account instead of keeping all his money in cash in an envelope is very confusing to him, and he is never sure any more how much money he has. He also reported some continuing confusion regarding his medication.

O: Owen participated in home visit to review his grocery needs and for verbal cues to fill his medication organizer correctly. Skilled instruction provided in meal planning and calculating probable food costs. He was then taken to the bank to withdraw some money and to a local grocery store to purchase food. At the bank, the teller provided Owen an updated account balance following his cash withdrawal, which confused him. Skilled instruction provided in calculating a bank balance. At the grocery store, Owen purchased canned fruits and vegetables, ground beef, fresh lettuce, and a loaf of bread. Upon returning home, he put the lettuce and meat in the refrigerator independently and consulted his weekly menu planner to determine what he had planned for lunch. Owen needed 2 verbal cues to fill his medication organizer with correct doses of all medications.

A: Limited understanding of bank account management results in need for supervision in managing finances. Decreased number of cues required to fill medication organizer correctly indicates progress from 4 cues required last week. Independent choice of canned fruits and vegetables and the addition of lettuce to his sandwiches indicates progress toward healthier eating habits. Owen would benefit from continued skilled instruction in ADL skills such as independent management of medication, food, and money in order to be able to live independently in the community without the support of a professional caregiver.

P: Owen will continue to be seen weekly in his home and community settings in order to work toward independence in meeting his daily needs.

Alayna M, OTR/L

Contact Note: Assisted Living

S: Resident reports decreased activity tolerance and increased shortness of breath with exertion. Reports feeling ok about asking nursing for assistance with dressing, but has urgent incontinence and cannot always wait for assistance to manage O_2 tubing to toilet.

O: Resident participated in OT session in room to assess safety during toileting.
Cognition: WFL; no deficits.
Functional Mobility: Resident uses walker, has difficulty managing O_2 tubing, requires SBA for safety.
Upper Extremity Strength: WNL but fatigues quickly with use of B UEs.
ADLs: CGA for clothing management during toileting. Min A for O_2 tubing management and safety for mobility during toileting and dressing. Mod A for dressing due to decreased activity tolerance, needing rest after 5 minutes.

A: Inability to manage O_2 cord during functional mobility to toilet places client at risk for falls. Intact cognition is good indication for potential to incorporate adaptive strategies into ADL routines. Resident would benefit from adaptive equipment and techniques to toilet with increased independence as well as instruction in energy conservation techniques and increased activity tolerance for ADL tasks.

P: Resident will be seen 3x/wk for 1 week to improve independence and safety in toileting.

Hannah P, OTR/L

Contact Note: Skilled Nursing Facility

S: *Client reports she hopes to return home independently within 1 month. Client reports difficulty fastening her back brace "because I can't remember if I'm supposed to fasten the Velcro first and then pull the side strings tight or the other way around." Able to verbalize 2 of 3 back precautions (no bending, no lifting), but unable to recall 3rd precaution (no twisting).*

O: *Client participated in 45-minute session in her room to address increased independence with ADLs following recent lumbar laminectomy and fusion. She presented supine in bed upon OT's arrival; required min verbal cues for correct log roll technique to complete supine to sit transition.*

Upper Body Dressing: Donned bra and undershirt with set-up and required min A to sequence steps of positioning and fastening corset-style back brace. Donned oversized button-up shirt over brace with SBA.

Lower Body Dressing: Donned underwear and pants using reacher with SBA; min A required to don socks using sock aid as she originally had device positioned incorrectly to thread sock on it.

Grooming: Sit to/from stand with SBA and ambulated to sink CGA without assistive device; completed grooming tasks standing at sink with min verbal cues to avoid bending and twisting when reaching for grooming items. Received instruction to remember the "BLT" mnemonic: No Bending, No Lifting, No Twisting.

A: *Decreased ability to remember and adhere to back precautions and corset application limits resident's independence with dressing and grooming tasks. Ability to recall 2 of 3 back precautions from previous session indicates good progress toward goals. Client would benefit from visual reminders of back precautions and corset-donning sequence.*

P: *Client will continue to receive OT services 5x/wk for 3 weeks to address independence with ADLs in preparation for discharge back to home environment. OT will post visual reminders of back precautions and corset instructions in resident's room. Plan progression to IADLs within 1 week.*

Rachel R, OTR/L

Contact Note: Home Health

S: *Client stated that he was "shaky" from his shower earlier in the AM. Client's daughter reported that client showered and dressed with min A for balance and coordination to manage fasteners. Client reported that he has not consistently been following his HEP.*

O: *Client participated in home visit to assess current status in balance, coordination, level of compliance and independence with HEP, and to introduce new hand strengthening exercises. OT and OTA both present for collaboration and update to intervention plan. Client required mod verbal cues to initiate and complete pre-existing HEP.*

New hand-strengthening exercises added—finger spread with rubber bands of various sizes; intrinsic muscle coordination worksheet (e.g., pen rolling).

Client and daughter participated in discussion about planning treatment activities to complement client's interests. Gun repair projects and small woodworking activities were suggested for coordination and strength in hands. Client demonstrated good static sitting balance throughout the session but needed CGA for balance to stand safely from chair.

A: *Decreased dynamic balance places client at risk for falls during ADLs, IADLs, and leisure activities. Need for verbal cues to initiate HEP raises continued concerns about ongoing compliance to improve functional hand strength. Ability to tolerate increased resistance with Theraband exercises with decreased fatigue since initial eval. indicates progress in functional endurance. Ability to handle 1" items such as pajama buttons indicates good potential for ADL independence. Client would benefit from continued skilled OT to further instruct in energy conservation techniques, safety, and to modify HEP as client continues to progress.*

P: *Client to be seen 2x/wk for 2 more weeks to continue work on increasing independence with self-care, with focus on showering and dressing.*

Mihret T, COTA/L   Delaney M, OTR/L

Contact Note: Outpatient Hand Therapy Clinic

S: Client reports pain @ the ulnar styloid with forearm supination. Client reports she is still unable to start her car with R hand but can now use it to turn a doorknob.

O: Client participated in hand clinic visit for functional range of motion in UE to improve independence with IADLs. Moist heat applied to R hand and forearm for 10 minutes prior to beginning treatment.

A/PROM measurements for R hand and forearm:

Key: [Flexion/extension; ( ) PROM; -extension lag; +hyperextension]

R Hand	MP	PIP	DIP
Index	0/90	0/105	0/75
Long	0/90	0/105	0/80
Ring	0/90	0/105	0/80
Small	0/90	-14/105 (0/105)	0/79

R wrist: +45/40 composite (+60/50) composite +45/50 noncomposite

R forearm: supination 62 (78); pronation 90

Client performed the following R UE exercises: Isometric forearm supination x10, AAROM supination x5, AROM forearm supination x5. After exercise, client's supination increased to 77° AROM. HEP revised to include blue foam for flexion strengthening 2x to 3x day.

A: Decreased functional ROM and strength in dominant R hand limit client's ability to complete ADL and IADL tasks. Increased strength of R finger flexors, improved DIP flexion, increase in active pronation, and increased active wrist extension by 10° indicate progress toward goals. Client would benefit from continued skilled OT to regain functional AROM to complete IADLs and for general strengthening.

P: Client to be seen 2x/wk for 3 more weeks. Continue wrist exercises and modify treatment plan to include more supination stretching and strengthening with emphasis on ability to grasp, lift, and accurately place objects of various size and shape.

Bridget S, OTR/L, CHT

Contact Note: Outpatient Hand Therapy Clinic—Splint

S: Mr. J stated that the pain in his right wrist and thumb was "not as bad as it was 2 weeks ago." He reported that his splint is rubbing a calcium deposit on the dorsum of his hand and that he is not wearing the splint at work during the day. He also reported feeling pain during treatment with movement of the R thumb and that ice and iontophoresis decrease pain.

O: Mr. J arrived at clinic wearing R forearm-based thumb spica splint. Upon removal of splint, wrist appeared slightly swollen.

R UE AROM: Wrist flexion ~25%   Wrist extension <25%   Thumb flexion and extension ~25%

Mr. J tolerated ~3 minutes friction massage over abductor pollicis longus and extensor pollicis brevis tendons. Ice applied for 5 minutes; Mr. J instructed in using ice at home and at work to decrease pain by reducing inflammation of tendons. Splint reformed to eliminate rubbing on dorsum of hand, and Mr. J instructed in wearing schedule at work. HEP modified, and Mr. J demonstrated new procedures correctly.

A: Wrist and thumb AROM ~50% below normal due to pain limits ability to complete work-related tasks. Decreased swelling since last tx. session indicates good progress. Splint reconstruction results in potential for decreased pain and increased function. Mr. J would benefit from continued skilled OT to decrease pain, increase AROM, and increase ability to use R hand at work.

P: *Continue to see Mr. J 2x/wk for 3 weeks for the following skilled interventions to achieve goal of decreased pain in R wrist and hand for use in functional activity at work and home:*

- *Ice and iontophoresis to decrease pain in R hand and wrist.*
- *Friction massage to reduce inflammation and increase AROM in R wrist and thumb.*
- *Re-evaluation of splint for fit and use after reconstruction.*
- *Re-evaluation of effectiveness and compliance of HEP.*

Mark S, OTR/L

Contact Note: Outpatient Pediatrics—Cancellation

Received phone call from Lucia's mother canceling today's appointment due to schedule conflict. Mother was reminded of clinic attendance policy as child has now missed 3 of last 5 scheduled weekly appointments; mother voiced understanding that one more missed appointment may result in Lucia being discharged from OT services. Offered to change OT appointment to a more convenient time for family, mother declined this offer. Also reminded mother of 6-month meeting with therapy team and service coordinator from County Agency that is scheduled for August 24th; mother reports plan to attend that meeting and next OT visit on August 26th.

Hope S, OTR/L

Contact Note: Complementary/Alternative Therapy—Craniosacral

As occupational therapy practitioners increase their skills in the use of complementary and alternative therapy techniques, questions arise about how to document interventions that may be focused on client factors and that use nontraditional components such as energy work or chakra balancing. Many of these visits are done on a private pay basis because complementary therapy is often not reimbursable by either public or private insurance. It is best to report objectively on what was said, what was done, what impact the presenting problems have on the client's ability to engage in meaningful occupation, and what the plan is for continued services, just as you would for any service you might provide.

S: *Client reports decrease in functional mobility and increased pain since hip replacement surgery. He has adaptive equipment and recalls 3/3 hip precautions. He reports gains since last visit as follows:*

- *He was able to sleep 4/7 nights without medication and sleeps longer without waking.*
- *Headaches occur less often.*

O: *Client participated in 1-hr. craniosacral session in clinic to decrease pain and increase functional mobility needed for work and both personal and instrumental ADL activities. He arrived using quad cane in place of the walker he used last week. On evaluation, the craniosacral rhythm is asymmetrical, as is the body, with the left side cephalad and the head tilting right. The major restrictions identified are in the pelvis, which is treated first with a series of diaphragm holds, and release of the sacrum in supine. With increased symmetry to the pelvis, the Upledger cranial series ending with a long still-point is used to facilitate homeostatic healing activity in the body.*

A: *Improvement in sleep (decreased need for pain medication and increase in time asleep from 1 to 1½ hours), decrease in headaches, and graduation from walker to quad cane all indicate good progress in treatment, as does visual and palpable increase in pelvic symmetry after today's session. Client would benefit from continued work to the pelvis to alleviate cumulative trauma and residual restrictions from recent hip surgery, followed by work to more subtle restrictions that have resulted from a series of previous serious accidents.*

P: *Client to return in 1 week, at which time reassessment will determine the frequency, duration, and direction of treatment. As soon as pelvic symmetry is improved sufficiently to allow mobility WFL for work and IADL tasks, regional tissue release can be included to increase the mobility of the head and neck, which is contributing to the headaches.*

Sharon B, OTR/L, CST

Contact Note: Early Intervention

S: *McKenna said she wanted to play, but when the task was difficult for her, she said, "You do it. You fix it."*

O: *McKenna participated in an OT home visit to work on use of both arms to improve spontaneous use of hand as a functional assist, sitting balance while criss-cross sitting unsupported, and functional mobility, as a prerequisite to self-care and play skills. McKenna was engaged during ~90% of the session.*

Arm Use: McKenna required maximum assist to pull shirt over stuffed animal's arms with right hand while holding it with left hand. She spontaneously used left hand to assist with stabilizing stuffed animal while pulling sleeve over its arm and shoulder with right hand. McKenna initiated snapping shirt but needed maximum assist to use left hand to stabilize shirt while fastening snaps. Spontaneously used both hands used to hold stuffed animal steady during play.

Sitting Balance: McKenna required touch cues from stand to sit in walker and moderate assist from side sit to cross-legged sit. She demonstrated adequate sitting balance to play for 5 minutes, requiring touch cues twice to right herself from a side tilt.

A: *Improved coordination of both arms together and increased use of left hand as functional assist now ~60% of the time indicates progress since last week. Decreased postural control necessitates touch cues to maintain upright position when engrossed in an activity. She would benefit from continued skilled OT for activities that challenge postural support in order to gain protective responses, body righting, and vestibular integration in order to increase her independence during play.*

P: *McKenna will be seen weekly for 3 months to continue strengthening postural support in order to increase her independence in play activities, promote use of both hands, and improve use of left hand as a functional assist during ADL and play activities. Plan to re-evaluate in 3 months in prep for transition to early childhood special education program through local school district.*

Amara S, OTR/L

Contact Note: School

S: *Ezra did not use verbal language to communicate but did echo words spoken to him.*

O: *Ezra participated in OT session in classroom to work on fine motor skills to prepare for scissors use and improve prehension patterns for writing. After 5 minutes of facilitated sensory table exploration to decrease tactile sensitivity, Ezra practiced palmar pinch and tripod grasp prehension patterns using a Fruit Loop bracelet activity for 20 minutes. Ezra used tongs (in preparation for scissors use) to pull 15 Fruit Loops out of a cup one at a time. Then, using a palmar pinch, he placed each Fruit Loop over a pipe cleaner. Five verbal cues were required for task completion.*

A: *Delayed fine motor skill milestones limit client's success with classroom tasks. Improved manipulation and positioning of tongs this date is an indicator that proper scissors use will be attained soon. Good attention to task for entire 25 minutes demonstrates good progress toward being able to participate with peers without sensory breaks. Ezra would benefit from continued OT intervention to address educationally relevant fine motor skill development.*

P: *Continue prehension activities 2x/wk using a variety of media in 20- to 30-minute intervals until proper scissors use goal is achieved.*

Avrie T, OTR/L

PROGRESS REPORTS

Progress reports are written on a regularly scheduled basis (usually weekly or monthly), with the time frame determined by the facility. The facility policy is guided by accrediting agencies and funding sources in determining the time frame in which progress notes must be written. Rather than detailing a single session, a progress report provides a **summary of the intervention process over time** and documents the client's progress toward goals. It also includes recommendations for continuation/discontinuation of services and referral to other health care professionals if appropriate.

Progress Report: Inpatient Behavioral Health Center

Client: *Izabelle B*   **Dx:** *Depression*

S: *During first assertion group on 8/15, client talked about how her life had taken a "downward spiral" since early July, and she had become more passive and less proactive in getting her needs met, although she had not been aware of it at the time. She reported having "no energy or desire" to engage in daily activities. In recent days, she reports she feels "more like myself."*

O: *During first few days of admission last week, client attended only 2/8 groups with considerable prompting and arrived looking disheveled and unkempt. This week, client attended assertion group 2/2 times, communication group 1/1 time, and IADL group 3/5 times. She was on time to 4/6 groups without reminders, wearing clean clothing, makeup, and hair ties. In assertion group on 8/20, she shared without prompting 2 stories about her usual way of dealing with retail situations. In communication group on 8/21, she spontaneously answered one question addressed to the group as a whole, and in IADL group on 8/22, she offered to assist another client with his cooking activity.*

A: *Low energy level and lack of initiative limited client's participation in ADLs and IADLs at time of admission. More consistent group attendance, spontaneous actions in groups, and willingness to share verbally indicate an improved mood this week. Improved dress, hygiene, and makeup also indicate an improved mood from last week. Client would benefit from planning a structure for her days to prevent another "downward spiral" after discharge.*

Goals #1 (assertion) and #2 (communication) are met as of this date.

Goal #3 (leisure skills) is continued through planned discharge on 8/25 pending formulation of a plan.

Goal #4 (parenting skills) was discontinued on 8/17 as client's children will remain with grandparents for foreseeable future, and this goal is no longer relevant for acute care stay.

P: *Client to be seen in IADL group for 1 more day, with discharge anticipated tomorrow afternoon 8/25. IADL group will be used for preparing the structured plan for using her time. Will meet with client individually if needed to ensure that written plan is completed.*

Addison U, OTR/L

Progress Report: Community-Based Mental Health— Transitional Housing (Facility Format)

Client: *Marco P*   **1° Dx:** *Schizophrenia*   **2° Dx:** *Substance use disorder*

S: *Client reports feeling "very stressed" thinking about the upcoming holidays and "having to do what my family wants me to do. They think just because I have schizophrenia, I'm also stupid." Client also reports feeling "great" about his ability to maintain sobriety for 1 month.*

O: *Client completed first month at transitional housing facility. OT attendance, participation, and goals addressed are summarized below:*

GROUP PARTICIPATION		
Group Name	**Number Attended**	**Full Participation**
Cooking Club	2 of 3	2
Procovery	2 of 4	2
House Meeting	4 of 4	4
Health Class	2 of 3	3
Substance Abuse	3 of 4	2
Grocery Shopping	3 of 4	3
Leisure Trips	3 of 4	3

INDIVIDUAL SERVICE PARTICIPATION	
1-on-1 Appointments	**Number**
Completed	7
No Shows	0
Cancelled/Rescheduled	0
1-on-1 Hours	**Number**
Total Spent With OT	6 hrs.
Total Spent With OTS	2 hrs.

GOALS ADDRESSED DURING GROUPS AND INDIVIDUALIZED SERVICE MEETINGS									
Advocacy	X	Cooking	X	IADL Assessment		Mental Health Education	X	Substance Use	X
Anger/Emotional Management	X	Discharge Planning		Interpersonal Skills	X	Non-Grocery Shopping		Symptom Management	X
BADL Assessment and Training		Education/ GED		Laundry/ Clothing Care		Nutritional/ Meal Planning	X	Time Management	X
Budgeting/ Money Skills	X	Family Support		Leisure/ Social Skills		Problem Solving	X	Transportation	X
Bus Training		Goal Setting	X	Literacy		Routine and Schedule	X	Vocational/ Work	
Cleaning/ Home Care Skills		Grocery Shopping	X	Medical Health Management		Safety		Volunteering	
Computer Skills	X	Hygiene/ Self-Care		Medication Management		Self-Esteem	X	Other (Specify)	

Family Interactions: *Client set a plan for self-advocacy with family with max verbal cues. Following interpersonal skills training, client requested to contact family members to practice new skills. In two 30-minute visits, client demonstrated reciprocal conversation without outbursts, accusatory statements, or passive-aggressive behaviors.*

Sobriety: *Despite noted stressors, he independently was able to follow sobriety plan he created at admission.*

Internet Use: *Client able to access novel and routine websites of choice with min verbal cues (required mod A at admission) required for impulsivity and attention to task. Client has also established 2 social media accounts and posts thus far have been socially appropriate.*

IADLs: *Client completed grocery shopping with min verbal cues for item location and price comparison (required mod A at admission). Client declined to work on budgeting/savings plan this month due to spending all his income on the upcoming holidays. Client indicated desire to budget next month with intent to save $50 toward a TV for his room.*

A: *Stress related to family perceptions and expectations results in ineffective interactions with family members. Ability to participate in reciprocal conversation without negative interactions demonstrates progress toward goals. Sobriety for 1 month indicates great progress toward client's goal of refraining from drug and alcohol use. Impulsivity and decreased attention to task limit client's independent internet usage, but decreased need for verbal cues this month indicates progress. Continued need for assistance with budgeting and grocery shopping limit client's ability to transition to more independent living situation, but progress with grocery shopping indicates good potential for this goal. Client would benefit from continued group and individual service participation in this transitional housing facility to address limitations in social interaction, sobriety, internet usage, and independent living skills.*

P: *Client to attend all scheduled weekly groups and twice-weekly individual OT sessions to address social participation, sobriety, internet usage, and independent living skills. Plan to help client establish and follow monthly budget, increase social contact with family, maintain sobriety plan, and increase independence with internet usage.*

Stephanie S, OTR/L, QMHP

Progress Report: Early Intervention

Client: *Brooklyn M*   **Dx:** *Shaken baby syndrome*

Occupational Profile: *Brooklyn is a 2.5-year-old girl with a history of shaken baby syndrome from abuse by her biological mother's boyfriend at age 3 months. Brooklyn has been in foster care since her diagnosis, and her foster family recently received approval for adoption, which will become official in December. Brooklyn lives with her foster parents and 2 teenage siblings (biological children of her foster parents). She is home with her foster mother most of the time, although she does occasionally receive respite care services from the local County Family Support Agency so her foster mother can run errands and attend her older children's school events.*

S: Brooklyn's foster mother reports new skills in recent months, including putting simple shapes into a puzzle and scribbling with a crayon. Brooklyn has begun saying more single words during therapy sessions and occasionally puts 2 words together such as "More bubbles."

O: Brooklyn has participated in weekly Early Intervention sessions June through November in her foster home with foster parent and/or respite care provider present during each session. 22 of 26 sessions occurred as scheduled; 2 visits cancelled due to client illness, 1 for family schedule conflict, and 1 for Thanksgiving holiday. For this 6-month progress report, Brooklyn was reassessed using the fine motor subtests of the Peabody Developmental Motor Scales, Second Edition. See chart below for comparison of performance between May and November.

	MAY			NOVEMBER		
	STANDARD SCORE	*PERCENTILE RANK*	*AGE EQUIVALENT*	*STANDARD SCORE*	*PERCENTILE RANK*	*AGE EQUIVALENT*
Grasping	4	2nd	10 months	6	9th	13 months
Visual Motor Integration	3	1st	11 months	5	5th	19 months
	Total Fine Motor Quotient = 61 (<1st percentile)			*Total Fine Motor Quotient = 73 (3rd percentile)*		
Standard scores on the PDMS-2 have a mean of 10 and a standard deviation of 3. Total fine motor quotient scores have a mean of 100 and a standard deviation of 15.						

New skills observed during OT sessions in recent weeks include turning pages in a thick-page book, stacking 2 to 3 blocks, scribbling using a pronated grasp on crayon, and placing large stacking pegs into a pegboard. Brooklyn is also beginning to show interest in using a spoon to feed herself rather than relying only on finger feeding.

A: Delayed fine motor skills continue to impact Brooklyn's ability to participate in play and self-care activities. Improved standardized test scores indicate steady developmental progress. Brooklyn's recent increased interest in new fine motor activities indicates good potential for future improvements toward developmental milestones. Brooklyn would benefit from continued early intervention services once weekly for 6 months to address development of fine motor and self-skills in preparation for transition to Early Childhood Special Education (ECSE) services when she turns 3.

P: Client to receive OT once weekly in her home or family-selected community settings to address developmental deficits in play and self-care. Parent education in home program activities will be provided. Also plan to coordinate transition services with local Family County Support Agency and local public school district to ensure a smooth transition to ECSE services.

Alexandra A, OTR/L

Progress Report: Outpatient Balance and Vestibular Rehabilitation

Name: *Juanita S*   **Age:** *73*   **1° Dx:** *L peripheral vestibulopathy*   **2° Dx:** *OA, CAD, B cataracts*

S: Pt. reports continued feelings of spinning, blurred vision, and difficulty walking. She reports she has not completed the home exercises provided 2 weeks ago during evaluation because they make her feel dizzy and she gets scared. She also reports needing to hold onto the shower door for support when stepping in/out of the tub. No recent falls reported.

O: Client has participated in two 45-minute balance sessions in outpatient OT clinic to address balance deficits identified during initial eval. 2 weeks ago.

Initial Status: Client only able to perform 2 head turns with eyes focused on forward target before c/o severe dizziness and nausea. Unable to track target up/down.

Current Status: Client able to keep eyes forward on target and perform 10 reps of slow head turns with report of increased dizziness from 1 to 3 (0 = no symptoms, 10 = most extreme symptoms). Client able to follow visual target up and down with report of dizziness from 1 to 3 (same scale). With min verbal cues, client able to increase speed of head movements without further increase in reported dizziness.

Client Education: *Client was re-educated regarding the balance system, her dx, the reason for OT, and the importance of consistency with her home exercises for balance; client voiced understanding. HEP modified to accommodate client's comfort level with exercises, and she demonstrated ability to complete:*

- *Steady gaze with head turns*
- *Following visual target vertically, horizontally, diagonally during IADL task (putting away dishes)*

Pt. also instructed to have family member present for safety when showering; voiced understanding. Written recommendations provided to client and reviewed with daughter at end of session.

A: *Continued report of dizziness and habit of holding onto shower door during shower transfer indicate safety concerns with ADL and IADL tasks. Decline in dizziness rating (3/10) this session shows progress from initial evaluation rating (6/10). With consistent performance of HEP and continued balance and vestibular rehabilitation, client has potential to decrease dizziness and increase her safety in her independent living situation. Client would benefit from continued OT to address compensatory strategies during ADLs and IADLs.*

P: *Continue OT 1x/wk for 4 weeks to address safety concerns related to symptoms of L peripheral vestibulopathy. Sessions to focus on increasing client's tolerance of head movements without increased dizziness and client education regarding compensatory strategies for increased safety during ADLs and IADLs.*

Patricia D, OTR/L

TRANSITION PLANS

A transition plan is written whenever a client is preparing to transfer from one setting to another, particularly when services have been provided for an extended period of time and long-term needs are anticipated in the new setting. It is designed to provide current providers with a plan for maximizing client outcomes in the current setting and to give new service providers a clear picture of the client's background and current functional performance so that care is uninterrupted. Transition plans summarize the client's current occupational status, specify what service setting the client is leaving, state what setting the client is entering, and tell how and when the transition will occur.

Transition Plan: Early Intervention to Early Childhood Special Education

Name: *Kanisha G*   ***Expected Transition Date:*** *3rd birthday in May*   ***Diagnosis:*** *TBI, s/p MVA*

Precautions: *Seizure disorder*

Occupational History: *Kanisha experienced head and multiple orthopedic injuries following a MVA at 9 days of age. Since that time, she has had multiple cranial, hip, and leg surgeries. She is currently under the management of a neurologist as well as an orthopedist. Mom carries out a home program daily, which is designed to stimulate development.*

S: *Mom reports that although Kanisha's seizures, multiple surgeries, and illnesses have slowed her development, the family is hopeful that Kanisha will progress more rapidly through her developmental milestones now that the surgeries are finished and the seizures are under control.*

O: *Child received her first OT screening in the hospital 1 week post-injury. She received formal developmental assessments at 2, 4, 6, 12, and 24 months of age. Parents were given home program following the initial formal assessment. OT sessions were started twice weekly at 12 months of age and have continued to this date. Kanisha has also been followed every 3 months in the Birth-to-Three Developmental Clinic. She is approaching eligibility for Early Childhood Special Education (ECSE) services through the local public school as she will be turning 3 in a few months.*

Current Occupational Performance: *Current problems being treated in OT include visual regard and visually directed reach, midline orientation, postural symmetry, and motor overflow. Current goals for Kanisha include functional reach, grasp and release, rolling, and ability to sustain antigravity positions for ADLs and developmental play activities. Kanisha requires an adaptive chair to maintain upright positioning. She is dependent in all self-care tasks, including feeding. She requires hand-over-hand assistance to initiate play with toys. Kanisha's current motor and cognitive skills indicate functioning at approximately a 6-month level of development.*

A: *Low vision, low proximal tone, and increased tone of all extremities limit Kanisha's performance in self-care and play activities. Attentive family members and stimulating home environment are good indications for future progress toward goals. Kanisha would benefit from continuation of regular OT, PT, and speech therapy services to facilitate her ongoing progress through the developmental sequence.*

P: *Kanisha will receive her first ECSE evaluation in May. Parents have been given a home program, which has been updated as child has progressed in treatment. Home program will continue through the transition to ECSE services.*

Mia N, OTS
Kira S, OTR/L

Transition Plan: High School to Post-Graduation Plans

As noted in Chapter 13, a transition plan is part of a student's IEP. Each school may have its own format and content requirements for the transition plan. This example provides a SOAP note format for the transition plan of a student about to exit high school and transition to community services.

S: *Jordan communicates verbally in short phrases and voiced a basic understanding of upcoming transition as evidenced by statements "Almost done school" and "Get job." Parents no longer want him to remain in public school through his 21st birthday as originally planned, but they report concerns about maintaining a routine for Jordan during the day while they are at work. Parents report plan for Jordan to move into renovated basement apartment at their residence for increased independence while still receiving intermittent family supervision. They report no plan in the immediate future to explore alternative community living for Jordan as they believe he functions best in a familiar environment and do not want to overwhelm him with multiple changes at once. Parents would like to see Jordan walk across the stage during his graduation ceremony at the end of this school year.*

O: *Jordan has had an IEP in place since age 3 based on his diagnosis of autism spectrum disorder. A transition plan has been in place since age 16. Today's meeting to update transition plan included: Jordan, parents, special education teacher, 2 general education teachers, school life skills implementer, occupational therapist, Special Education Coordinator, support coordinator from County Family Resources Agency, vocational rehabilitation counselor, and representative from County Adult Day Services.*

School Services Summary: Jordan has received a combination of self-contained special education, general education integration, and occupational therapy services over the past few years with emphasis on development of basic life skills and supported employment skills.

Adaptive Behavior Summary: Jordan relies on a written calendar at home to know what is scheduled each day. He completes most ADLs with distant supervision. Jordan has progressed from following 1-step commands to following simple 2- to 3-step directions for IADLs and work simulation tasks and does best with a written list or picture schedule of the steps. When he is excited, Jordan continues to exhibit occasional self-stimulatory behaviors, including hand flapping and rocking, and needs verbal and tactile cues for redirection. When he is frustrated, particularly with an unexpected change in the day's planned schedule, he may slap his head and will repeatedly ask for confirmation about what is happening throughout the day.

Transition Services Summary: Vocational rehabilitation counselor confirmed eligibility of transition-related services to include vocational planning and on-the-job training with a work coach. Formal evaluation will be needed to determine exact level of services. Representative from County Adult Day Services confirmed that Jordan is on their wait list with anticipated opening in late May shortly after high school graduation. Support coordinator from County Family Resources Agency discussed funding options for continued 1:1 personal aide/therapy implementer up to 10 hours per week following graduation.

A: *Self-stimulatory behaviors and decreased frustration tolerance of unexpected changes limit Jordan's ability to perform IADLs and work tasks without visual cues and direct supervision. Improved ability to follow multistep directions indicates progress toward client and family goal of supported employment. Family support and availability of multiple community support services, including vocational rehabilitation, adult day program, and continued 1:1 aide/therapy implementer, are good indications for a successful transition from public school. Jordan would benefit from continued team collaboration to prepare for transition and to address family goals of graduation participation, supported employment, and supervised living.*

P: Continue to provide 60 minutes OT services weekly for remainder of school year with emphasis on the following:

- Working directly with Jordan and consulting with school staff to maximize inclusion in upcoming graduation ceremony.
- Consulting with County Family Resources Agency to provide home programming recommendations for continued 1:1 aide/therapy implementer. Also plan to provide recommendations to family for outpatient and community-based occupational therapists who can take over this role upon Jordan's transition out of public school.
- Consulting with vocational rehabilitation center regarding best fit for supported employment options based on current skill level.
- Consulting with County Adult Day Services staff regarding how best to support Jordan's upcoming transition from public school to part-time day program.

Marcus A, OTR/L

Transition Plan: Halfway House to Independent Living and Employment

Some occupational therapy practitioners seek out roles with community-based agencies that may have different job titles than occupational therapist or occupational therapy assistant. This transition plan note was written by an occupational therapy assistant who works at a local Community Action Center to connect clients with local, state, and federal programs and services to help them overcome obstacles and reach life goals.

Client: Jaci L

S: "I'm excited to move into my own place soon. I only have 2 more months before I leave the halfway house." Pt. reports she has maintained sobriety from all substances and has held the same job for 7 months.

O: Jaci completed 1:1 consultation with Community Action Professional (CAP) in community center conference room to develop transition plan from halfway house to independent living. Jaci has completed 10 of 12 months at ABC Halfway House and will exit the program in May. She has also participated in the Community Action Center skills development program and currently holds a part-time job at a local deli.

Housing Plans: Jaci has been approved for a housing choice voucher and was notified last week of an apartment available in May. She has saved enough money for the security deposit and first and last month's rent. Jaci received education regarding Community Action Center resources such as energy assistance program and gently-used furniture donation center to assist with expenses.

Transportation Plans: ABC Halfway House has been providing transportation to and from work. Jaci does not yet have a driver's license as she is still paying off fines for past driving infractions. Reviewed public transportation options between new apartment and current work location. Jaci completed bus pass voucher application online with guidance from CAP.

Work Plans: Jaci has already requested additional hours at her current job. Today she also explored job postings on the Community Action Center job board. She is interested in full-time work but understands that a significant increase in income will reduce her eligibility for some Community Action Center benefits. She wants to work on a budget to determine her best course of action with changing current level or place of employment.

Additional Services: Reviewed other Community Action Center resources to determine interest and eligibility. Jaci used Community Action Center computer to complete online application for Supplemental Nutrition Assistance Program (SNAP) benefits to assist with grocery costs. Also explored local food bank schedules.

A: Decreased awareness of eligibility for community resources previously limited client's plans for transition out of halfway house to community living. Continued sobriety, steady employment, and ability to save money shows good progress toward goals of halfway house program. Initiation of community resource applications following education on available programs indicates good potential for successful transition to independent living. Jaci would benefit from continued Community Action Center resource coordination and financial counseling to support her transition out of halfway house program.

P: Plan to follow up with Jaci in 1 month regarding energy assistance benefit eligibility and furniture needs for new apartment. Will also educate her regarding weatherization program (with landlord approval) to reduce energy costs and opportunity for participation in advanced skills training program to improve employment prospects. Plan to refer Jaci to Community Action Center financial counseling program.

Quierra J, COTA/L, CAP

DISCHARGE REPORTS

A discharge report is used to summarize the changes in the client's ability to engage in occupation and to make recommendations for referral or follow-up care if needed. Discharge reports often follow a format of their own, stating the date and purpose of the referral and giving a summary of the initial findings, the course of treatment, a summary of progress, and any recommendations for follow-up care. Discharge summaries may be done as SOAP or narrative notes, or the facility may have a particular form that is used. Some facilities use the same form for evaluation, re-evaluation, and discharge, making it quicker to prepare the discharge report.

Discharge Report: Inpatient Rehabilitation Facility

Name: Cindy C   **Age:** 71   **Dx:** L SDH

S: Client reports that she is very pleased with her progress and ability to take care of herself at home. She reports no steps to the front entrance of a one-story home, and no architectural barriers inside the house. She reports that she owns the following adaptive equipment already: wheeled walker, reacher, dressing stick, sock aid, long shoehorn, tub bench, raised toilet seat, and grab bars near the toilet and in the tub/shower. Family reports they have a plan to have someone with her 24/7 for at least 1 month.

O: Client participated in 20/20 OT sessions bedside and in rehab gym since admission on Feb. 6th.

	SECTION GG SCORE—ADMISSION	SECTION GG SCORE—DISCHARGE
Eating	3	6
Oral Hygiene	3	6
Toileting	2	5
Showering/Bathing	2	5
Upper Body Dressing	3	6
Lower Body Dressing	2	5
Put On/Take Off Footwear	1	6

Client completes all transfers and mobility with walker with supervision, except CGA needed for shower transfer. Client education provided in adaptive equipment techniques and HEP; client demonstrated ability to perform correctly. Client and caregiver provided with home modification recommendations.

A: Continued deficits in safety awareness limit client's independence in ADLs. Differences in admission and discharge abilities for ADLs show good progress. Since caregiver is available to provide SBA needed for safety in ADL tasks, all treatment goals have been met, and client is ready for discharge. Client would benefit from continued HEP for strengthening and endurance for functional tasks and home health OT to facilitate progress with ADLs and IADLs.

P: Client will be discharged home tomorrow with 24-hour supervision by family. Client to continue home exercise program. Adaptive equipment recommended: walker basket and reacher holder for walker. OT communicated with social worker to facilitate home health OT referral.

Taylor V, OTR/L

Discharge Report: Outpatient Lymphedema Clinic

S: Pt. reports decreased paresthesia (pins and needles) in affected R LE, improved sleep, and increased ability to complete lower body dressing with adaptive equipment. She reports consistent adherence to R LE compression garment wearing schedule and completion of home exercise program of affected R LE twice daily to improve lymphatic pumping. Pt. verbalizes understanding of risk reduction strategies to help maintain skin integrity.

O: Pt. has participated in 20 outpatient occupational therapy sessions over 12 weeks focused on complete decongestive therapy for secondary R LE lymphedema following surgery and radiation for uterine cancer. Interventions included manual lymphatic drainage, stretch bandage compression wrapping, fitting for compression garments, establishment of home exercise program, and education in skin care techniques and adaptive equipment use to improve independence in ADLs.

Circumferential Measurements:

	UNAFFECTED L LE—ADMISSION	AFFECTED R LE—ADMISSION	AFFECTED R LE—DISCHARGE
Upper Thigh/Groin	81 cm	103 cm	85 cm
Mid-Thigh	79 cm	88 cm	81 cm
Knee	68 cm	72 cm	70 cm
Calf	56 cm	60 cm	57 cm
Ankle	35 cm	39 cm	37 cm
Metatarsals	24 cm	28 cm	25 cm

Pitting Edema: At admission, 3+ pitting edema proximal R LE, 2+ pitting edema distal R LE. At discharge, 0 to 1+ pitting edema throughout R LE.

Lymphedema Life Impact Scale:

	ADMISSION	DISCHARGE
Physical Concerns	17	7
Psychosocial Concerns	19	6
Functional Concerns	15	6
Infection Occurrence Past Year	1x	1x

ADLs: At admission, pt. unable to don pants, sock, or shoe on affected R LE; was wearing only housedress and Velcro surgical shoe. At discharge, pt. independently able to don underwear and loose-fit pants independently using reacher, B socks with wide sock aid, and B open-heel slip-on shoes with reacher. Pt. does still require family assist to don R LE compression garment. Daughter lives with her and assists daily as needed.

A: R LE edema and paresthesias limited ADL performance and interrupted sleep at admission. Decreased circumferential measurements throughout R LE have resulted in improved sleep patterns and increased independence with lower body dressing. Adherence to compression garment wearing schedule and home exercise program are good indicators for continued home lymphedema management without further skilled intervention. Pt. would benefit from OT screening at next outpatient oncology follow-up appointment in 3 months to assess need for resumption of skilled direct OT services.

P: Plan to discontinue direct lymphedema OT intervention after today's visit. Pt. instructed to continue daily home exercise program, assess for skin integrity concerns, and contact referring physician if any issues arise prior to next follow-up with oncologist.

Mackenzie C, OTR/L, CLT

Discharge Report: Outpatient Pediatric Clinic

Occupational therapy services may be discontinued because the client has met all goals, the client has already received the maximum number of visits per year, the client is not showing enough progress to justify continuation of services, or for a variety of other reasons. In an ideal situation, the therapist will have time to plan and conduct a thorough reassessment to document progress from admission to discharge. In the note below, the therapist was surprised when the foster parent announced that this visit would be the child's last session due to beginning school-based occupational therapy and complex family issues limiting scheduling and transportation for outpatient services. Therefore, this discharge summary contains only a brief summary of the child's performance over time.

S: *Foster father requests discontinuation of outpatient OT services. "We just can't keep up with all these appointments with Nia in school all day now, my new work schedule, and my wife taking care of 3 new foster kids at home." He reports Nia will receive school-based OT 120 minutes/month to address classroom skills and self-care.*

O: *Nia has received outpatient OT services twice weekly for 3 months since placement with current foster family to address decreased L UE function related to spastic hemiplegia CP. She exhibits increased tone and decreased strength in L UE and has difficulty isolating finger movements of L hand. Interventions included L UE weight bearing while engaged in play activities, numerous repetitions of grasp/manipulation/release of various-sized items with affected L hand while dominant R UE was restricted, L hand strengthening exercises with therapy putty, and B UE coordination tasks.*

    Improvements Noted Since Admission: *Nia is now able to cut on a line with min A to stabilize paper in L hand. She can put on and take off slip-on shoes without assistance. She can place a straw into a juice box without assistance.*

    Ongoing Concerns: *Nia continues to demonstrate difficulty with B UE coordination tasks such as carrying large items with both hands, cutting out shapes, turning pages in a book, opening markers, manipulating clothing fasteners, and tying shoes.*

A: *Decreased strength and coordination of L UE result in delayed fine motor and self-care skills. Recent improvements in ADLs and cutting indicate progress and potential for continued functional improvement with ongoing direct OT intervention in the school setting. Nia would benefit from a re-evaluation in 6 months to determine whether supplemental outpatient services are needed again to address new concerns or update home activity program.*

P: *Per foster parent request, OT services will be discontinued at this time. Recommend follow-up with developmental pediatrician routinely to screen for future OT needs. Foster parent provided with list of home activities to facilitate B coordination including play activities that can be performed with new foster siblings.*

Elizabeth K, OTR/L

REFERENCES

American Occupational Therapy Association. (2018). Guidelines for documentation of occupational therapy. *American Journal of Occupational Therapy, 72*(Suppl. 2), 7212410010. https://doi.org/10.5014/ajot.2018.72S203

American Occupational Therapy Association. (2020). Occupational therapy practice framework: Domain and process (4th ed.). *American Journal of Occupational Therapy, 74*(Suppl. 2), 7412410010. https://doi.org/10.5014.ajot.2020.74S2001

American Occupational Therapy Association. (2022). *AOTA Occupational Profile template.* https://www.aota.org/

Boone, A. E., Henderson, W. L., & Dunn, D. (2022). Screening tools: They're so quick! What's the issue? *American Journal of Occupational Therapy, 76*(2), 7602347010. https://doi.org/10.5014/ajot.2022.049331

Shipp, M., & Havard, A. (2006). Documenting driver rehabilitation services and outcomes. In J. M. Pellerito, Jr. (Ed.), *Driver rehabilitation and community mobility.* Elsevier.

Suggestions for Completing the Worksheets

In this appendix, we offer suggestions for completing the worksheets throughout this manual. As a student or new therapist using this manual, you can work your way through the exercises and check your work against those in this appendix. Remember that your answer can be different and still be correct, as long as it contains the essential elements. As long as your information and protocol are correct, you should not sacrifice your own writing style to be more like someone else's.

COAST goals and SOAP notes are very difficult to write if there is no client or treatment session about which to write. Although there are many examples in this manual, there is no substitute for observing or working with actual clients. Only then will you be able to translate your treatment session into the health record in a meaningful way.

CHAPTER 5

Worksheet 5-1: Avoiding Common Documentation Errors

1. *Pt. stated my head really hurts this morning.*

    Pt. stated, "My head really hurts this morning."

2. *Resident reported "her right hand is working better today."*

    Resident reported her right hand is working better today.

3. *Student used right hand to cut with scissors. Student then switches to left hand for coloring tasks. Student did not demonstrate consistent hand preference.*

    Student used right hand to cut with scissors. Student then switched to left hand for coloring task. Student did not demonstrate consistent hand preference.

4. *The client's expressed excitement about the upcoming visit to the mall.*

    The clients expressed excitement about the upcoming visit to the mall.

5. *An occupational therapy referral was recieved from the childs' teacher.*

    An occupational therapy referral was received from the child's teacher.

Gateley, C. A. *Documentation Manual for Occupational Therapy, Fifth Edition* (pp. 239-262). © 2024 Taylor & Francis Group.

6. *The resident's were all in the dinning room weighting for there meal.*

    The residents were all in the dining room waiting for their meal.

7. *Client demonstrated appropriate social interaction by responding your welcome to another group member.*

    Client demonstrated appropriate social interaction by responding "You're welcome" to another group member.

8. *Pt. required moderate assistance to use dominate right hand in hygeine tasks.*

    Pt. required moderate assistance to use dominant right hand in hygiene tasks.

9. *Client does not demonstrate awareness of the affect of his mood on other member's of the group.*

    Client does not demonstrate awareness of the effect of his mood on other members of the group.

10. *Pt. expressed intrest in getting dressed. Pt. required verbal cues when doning pullover shirt to utilize adaptive teckniques due to right rotary cup injury.*

    Pt. expressed interest in getting dressed. Pt. required verbal cues when donning pullover shirt to utilize adaptive techniques due to right rotator cuff injury.

11. *The ot noticed assymetry in the childs sitting posture. Parents reports that the client is unable to sit independantly.*

    The OT noticed asymmetry in the child's sitting posture. Parents reported that the client is unable to sit independently.

12. *The OTR preformed a Cognitive Test on the client.*

    The OTR performed a cognitive test on the client.

13. *The Doctor called to check on the Patients status.*

    The doctor called to check on the patient's status.

14. *Pt. had right arm imobilized due to a clavical fracture.*

    Pt. had right arm immobilized due to a clavicle fracture.

15. *Client required several breif rest brakes during ADL's.*

    Client required several brief rest breaks during ADLs.

16. *The clinic employs three otr's and two ota's.*

    The clinic employs three OTRs and two OTAs.

17. *The students principle stated Jimmy is disruptive at school.*

    The student's principal stated, "Jimmy is disruptive at school."

18. *The childrens' mother has difficulty keeping all they're appointment's.*

    The children's mother has difficulty keeping all their appointments.

19. *Client needed a visual aide to help him learn how to preform self-catherization.*

    Client needed a visual aid to help him learn how to perform self-catheterization.

Worksheet 5-2: Using Abbreviations

1. *Client C/O pain in R MCP joint after ~15 min PROM.*

    Client complained of pain in the right metacarpophalangeal joint after approximately 15 minutes of passive range of motion.

2. *Pt. A&Ox4.*

    The client was alert and oriented to person, place, time, and situation.

3. *Client transferred w/c → mat with sliding board & max A x2.*

   Client transferred from his wheelchair to the mat using a sliding board and maximum assistance of two people.

4. *1° dx L BKA, 2° dx COPD, CHF, DM, & PVD.*

   Primary diagnosis is left below-knee amputation. Secondary diagnoses are chronic obstructive pulmonary disease, congestive heart failure, diabetes mellitus, and peripheral vascular disease.

5. *Pt. is S/P R THR. Orders received for OT 2x/day for ADLs & IADLs. WBAT R LE.*

   Patient is status post right total hip replacement. Orders received for occupational therapy two times per day for activities of daily living and instrumental activities of daily living. Weight bearing as tolerated for right lower extremity.

6. *Client has thirty degrees of passive range of motion in the left distal interphalangeal joint, which is within functional limits.*

   30° PROM in L DIP is WFL.

7. *Client is able to put on her socks with standby assistance but requires moderate assistance with putting on and taking off left shoe.*

   Client dons socks SBA but requires mod A to don and doff L shoe.

8. *The client requires contact guard assistance for balance during her morning dressing, which she performs while sitting on the edge of her bed.*

   CGA required for balance for AM dressing EOB.

9. *The patient participated in a bedside evaluation of activities of daily living. She was able to perform bed mobility with moderate assistance, but she needed maximum assistance to put on her adult undergarment. She was able to go from a supine position to a sitting position with minimum assistance and from a sitting position to a standing position with moderate assistance.*

   Pt. participated in bedside ADL eval. Mod A for bed mobility, max A to don adult undergarment. Supine → sit min A and sit → stand mod A.

10. *The resident came to the occupational therapy clinic via wheelchair escort. The resident was observed to lean toward his left. The resident needed verbal cues and minimum assistance in positioning his body in the wheelchair to maintain midline orientation and symmetrical posture. The resident transferred from his wheelchair to the toilet with moderate assistance of one person to help him keep his balance using a standing pivot transfer. He needed verbal cues and visual feedback from a mirror to maintain upright posture.*

    Resident to OT via w/c escort. Resident leans L and needs verbal cues, visual feedback from mirror, and min physical A to maintain symmetrical posture in midline. Standing pivot transfer w/c → toilet mod A for balance.

11. *The veteran participated in an evaluation in his room to determine relevant client factors. The veteran's short-term memory was three out of three for immediate recall, one out of three after 1 minute, and zero out of three with verbal cues after 5 minutes. The left upper extremity shoulder flexion was a grade of 4, shoulder extension was a grade of 4, elbow flexion was a grade of 4, elbow extension was a grade of 4, wrist flexion was a grade of 4 minus, wrist extension was a grade of 4 minus, and grip strength was 8 pounds. The left upper extremity light touch was intact. The right upper extremity muscle grades and sensation were within functional limits.*

    Veteran participated in eval. of client factors seated in w/c. Short-term memory 3/3 immediate recall, 1/3 after 1 minute, 0/3 with verbal cues after 5 min. L shoulder and elbow strength grade 4, wrist strength 4-, grip strength 8#. Light touch intact. R UE strength and sensation WFL.

CHAPTER 6

Worksheet 6-1: Identifying the Contributing Factors

1. **Area of Occupation = Work**
- _____ results in consumer's inability to sustain employment longer than 2 weeks.
  - ° *Use of inflammatory language at work*
  - ° *Need for frequent redirection to task*
  - ° *Drug-seeking behaviors at work*
  - ° *Inability to plan and sequence a task*
  - ° *Inattention to personal hygiene and social cues*
  - ° *Arriving late 3 to 4 times weekly following nightly excessive alcohol use*
  - ° *Lack of reliable day care*

2. **Area of Occupation = ADLs**
- _____ results in veteran needing 90 minutes to complete grooming tasks.
  - ° *Motor planning deficits*
  - ° *SOB on exertion and need for frequent rest breaks to regain O_2 saturation*
  - ° *<5 minutes activity tolerance before needing rest breaks*
  - ° *Inability to sequence task*
  - ° *Slowness in locating items due to low vision*
  - ° *Intention tremors and rigidity 2° Parkinson's disease*
  - ° *Decreased fine motor manipulation of L UE*
  - ° *Muscle weakness and limited AROM in B UEs*

3. **Area of Occupation = Education**
- _____ limits Avery's ability to complete grade-appropriate written worksheets.
  - ° *Increased tone in B hands 2° cerebral palsy*
  - ° *Attention span <2 minutes for seated classroom tasks due to sensory-seeking behaviors*
  - ° *Mod verbal cues required to sequence multi-step directions*
  - ° *Deficits in figure ground visual perceptual skills*
  - ° *Difficulty holding pencil due to multiple joint contractures related to idiopathic rheumatoid arthritis*
  - ° *Visual motor deficits*

Worksheet 6-2: Writing Occupation-Based Problem Statements

1. *The client has an acquired injury to his brain. As a result, he is not able to pay attention to task for very long at a time, and he is having trouble completing his morning routine. Typically, he can pay attention to what he is doing for about 2 minutes and needs to be redirected back to the task after that.*

   < 3-minute attention span 2° TBI interferes with ability to complete ADL tasks without redirection after 2 minutes.

2. *Jerrica is having trouble in school because she has difficulty staying within the lines when she is writing. She habitually grips her pencil in a gross grasp, although with help (someone's hand placed over hers) she can hold it with her thumb and two fingers.*

   Need for hand-over-hand assist to hold pencil in tripod pinch for writing tasks limits Jerrica's ability to complete writing tasks at school with expected level of neatness and accuracy.

3. *The resident is not very cognitively aware. About 40% of the time, she has trouble figuring out what to do first if she has to complete a self-care task, and she doesn't remember what she has just been told.*

   Memory and sequencing deficits result in need for mod verbal clues in ADL activities.

4. *Mr. J has recently sustained a R CVA. His L arm is flaccid, and he forgets that it is there. He needs physical and verbal help with ADL tasks about 60% of the time.*

   Flaccid L UE and L side neglect result in need for max A with upper body dressing.

5. *The consumer has had trouble finding a job. His appearance is unkempt, and he has a strong body odor, neither of which seem troubling to him.*

   Unkempt appearance and inattention to personal hygiene interferes with consumer's ability to find employment.

6. *The client is unable to transfer safely w/c to/from toilet without someone to remind him that he needs to follow his total hip precautions.*

   Unfamiliarity with hip precautions limits client's ability to complete safe toilet transfers without SBA.

Worksheet 6-3: Revising Problem Statements

1. *Trunk instability results in inability to complete LE dressing independently.*
   - **Tell what assist level is needed, if known, rather than saying not independently.**
   - **Say lower body rather than LE, since the client is dressing more than just the extremity.**
   - **Specify if there is one particular part of the task that requires assistance. For example:** *Trunk instability results in client needing mod A to maintain sitting balance EOB while dressing lower body.*
2. *Decreased activity tolerance results in child not tolerating much classroom activity.*
   - **Specify how much "very much" is.**
   - **Describe what kind of classroom activity. For example:** *Decreased activity tolerance limits child's ability to tolerate 30 minutes of desk work.*
3. *Consumer acts out.*
   - **Specify what is meant by "acts out."**
   - **Specify which area of occupation is affected by the acting out:**
     - **Inappropriate verbal and physical actions result in difficulty sustaining friendships.**
     - **Self-injurious behavior of cutting and burning extremities when upset affects relationships with spouse and is a safety concern.**

CHAPTER 7

Worksheet 7-1: Choosing Goals for Medical Necessity

- **Problem:** *Client unable to perform sewing due to 2+/5 strength in R hand musculature.*
  - **LTG:** *Client will perform embroidery independently for 20 minutes within 8 weeks.*
  - **STG:** *To improve performance of embroidery, client will use needle continuously for 5 minutes within 2 weeks.*

Other possible problem statements and goals:

- *Problem: 2+/5 strength in R hand musculature restricts client's ability to manipulate small items needed for grooming.*
  - *LTG: Client will complete grooming tasks independently within 1 month.*
  - *STG: Client will remove lid from toothpaste with min verbal cues for adaptive technique within 2 weeks.*

- *Problem: 2+/5 strength in R hand musculature limits client's ability to write more than 5 minutes.*
  - *LTG: Within 1 month, client will engage in handwriting tasks for 5+ minutes during monthly bill paying using adaptive pencil grip.*
  - *STG: Within 1 week, client will write first and last name using adaptive pencil grip.*
- *Problem: 2+/5 strength in R hand musculature results in client being unable to fasten ½" buttons on shirt.*
  - *LTG: Within 4 weeks, client will be able to fasten eight ½" buttons on shirt independently.*
  - *STG: Within 1 week, client will fasten two ½" buttons on shirt using button hook with min A for bilateral coordination.*

Worksheet 7-2: Evaluating Goal Statements

1. *By the time of discharge in 2 weeks, client will dress himself with min A for balance using a sock aid and reacher while sitting in w/c.*

   This goal has all of the necessary COAST components.

2. *Client will tolerate 10 minutes of treatment daily.*

   This goal lacks an occupation, an assist level, and a time frame. In addition, "tolerating 10 minutes of treatment" is not something the client will need to do after discharge. *Within 3 days, client will complete grooming activities with SBA for at least 10 minutes seated at sink with no rest break.*

3. *Client will demonstrate increased coping skills in stressful situations within 2 weeks.*

   "Coping skills" is far too broad. "Stressful situations" is also too broad. You need to set a goal for a specific situation. For example: *During family visit this weekend, client will maintain civil conversation with mother for 15 minutes, independently implementing anger management strategies when she experiences frustration.*

4. *Client will demonstrate 15 minutes of activity tolerance without rest breaks using B UEs to complete ADL tasks before breakfast each morning.*

   This goal lacks an assistance level and a time frame, and it needs to be rearranged to focus on the occupation rather than the specific condition. *By September 27th, client will complete dressing and grooming tasks with supervision in <15 minutes without rest breaks each morning before breakfast.*

5. *OT will teach lower body dressing using a reacher, dressing stick, and sock aid within 2 treatment sessions.*

   Most importantly, this goal is not client-centered. *Client will complete lower body dressing with SBA using reacher, dressing stick, and sock aid within 2 treatment sessions.* **(Remember, what the occupational therapy practitioner does is the intervention, not the client's goal.)**

6. *Patient will demonstrate ability to budget for the month.*

   This goal lacks an assistance level, a specific condition, and a time frame. *Within 2 weeks, client will create a written monthly budget with min verbal cues, using a calculator to calculate fixed and variable expenses.*

Worksheet 7-3: Writing Client-Centered, Occupation-Based, Measurable Goals

1. Ayana is not able to attend to task for more than a few minutes, which makes IADL activities difficult for her. Since she likes to cook and plans to return to cooking after discharge, you have been working with her in the kitchen. You would like to see her able to attend to a task for 10 minutes by the time she is discharged next week. Write a goal that addresses Ayana's attention span during cooking.

   Client will complete cooking activity with supervision, maintaining attention to task for least 10 minutes without redirection, within 1 week.

   or

   Within 3 treatment sessions, client will complete cooking activity with supervision, attending to task at least 10 minutes with 2 or fewer verbal cues for redirection.

2. Now write a goal for Ayana to be able to follow directions so that she can read the back of a boxed meal, and eventually a recipe, when she is cooking.

   Client will complete a cooking activity with min A to follow 3-step written directions within 3 sessions.

   or

   Client will follow simple recipe independently within 1 week.

3. Scott is having trouble dressing himself after his stroke. You have been teaching him an over-the-head method for putting on his shirt. Write a dressing goal for Scott.

   Client will don shirt independently using over-the-head method within 2 tx sessions.

   or

   Within 1 week, client will don shirt independently using one-handed techniques.

4. Nikki is very weak, and she wants to be able to go back to work as a receptionist. She also wants to be able to care for her 4-month-old child. Write a goal that addresses her activity tolerance during an occupation-based activity.

   Client will complete simulated infant-bathing activity with SBA, standing for at least 10 minutes, by discharge in 2 weeks.

   or

   Within 1 week, client will complete seated work simulation tasks independently using computer, telephone, and desktop office supplies for 20 minutes without rest breaks.

5. Demarco wants to live independently in the community, but he lacks basic money management skills. Write a goal for Demarco to improve his money management skills.

   Client will make change independently from $1.00 correctly 3/3 attempts within 2 weeks.

   or

   With min verbal cues, client will select 3 online ads for an apartment that rents for less than 1/3 of his monthly income within 3 weeks.

6. Taylor has become increasingly more depressed over the past several weeks and was admitted after a suicide attempt. You estimate that you will have her in group for 1 week. You would like to see her mood change in that week. Write an occupation-based goal that will indicate an improved mood.

   Within 1 week, client will follow her daily schedule independently, as demonstrated by attending at least 3 scheduled activities per day.

   or

   Client will verbalize interest in at least one future activity spontaneously within the next 2 days.

Worksheet 7-4: De-Emphasizing the Treatment Media

1. *Client will assemble a clock craft project independently using appropriate materials by anticipated discharge in 1 week.*

   Client will grasp/place/release objects of various sizes needed for IADL activities by independently assembling a craft project by anticipated discharge in 1 week.

   or

   Client will follow multi-step written directions for IADLs as evidenced by assembling a craft project independently from written instructions within 1 week.

2.   *Consumer will spend at least 30 minutes lacing a leather billfold during next 45-minute craft group session.*

Within 2 weeks, client will demonstrate attention to task required for sheltered workshop program by remaining seated and sustaining work on a desktop project for at least 30 minutes with min verbal cues.

3.   *Within 1 month, child will place 10 cotton balls into a jar independently to demonstrate improved dexterity for school activities.*

Within 1 month, child will place 10 pencils, markers, or other small classroom supplies into a zippered pouch independently.

CHAPTER 8

Worksheet 8-1: Choosing a Subjective Statement

1.   *Client was very cooperative and engaged in social conversation throughout the tx session.*

Even though the client may have been cooperative, and even though it may have been important in this treatment session, it is an assessment of the situation, and does not belong in the "S" category of the note. The client's social conversation might be important in some situations. However, there is a better choice for this particular note.

2.   *Client remarked that her grandson will be coming to visit later in the week, and that she will be very glad to see him.*

In this instance, a pending visit by the client's grandson is not really relevant to the treatment session or to how the client sees her progress. It might be important in another situation. For example, if the client was planning to go live with her grandson after discharge, it might be very relevant and might be a topic the occupational therapist wanted to explore further with the client.

3.   *Client reports that she feels "pretty good" today.*

Feeling "pretty good" today might be important because it might show progress or a change in her condition. In this case, however, it is not the best choice.

4.   *Client says she has difficulty moving R UE, although she does not know why it will not move. She reports, "It really doesn't hurt. It's just tight."*

The client's comments about her upper extremity seem most pertinent to this treatment session. Use of the R UE is relevant in all aspects of this treatment session.

5.   *Nursing staff report client is incontinent at night.*

This information should be documented in the nursing notes. The Subjective section of the note is generally used to document the client's views rather than views of the staff, except in rare instances. For example, if nursing staff had reported a safety concern with the client's ability to transfer to the toilet that was inconsistent with client report or occupational therapist observation, then that information would be relevant to this session. There is a better choice for this note.

Worksheet 8-2: Writing Concise, Coherent "S" Statements

1.   Mrs. P is recovering from a total hip replacement. During a treatment session, she makes the following statements:
     ◦   *"I used that dressing stick and sock aid like you showed me to get dressed without bending down this morning."*
     ◦   *"My hip doesn't hurt when I stand up or sit down, especially with that new toilet seat you got for me."*
     ◦   *"It's getting easier for me to get dressed now."*
     ◦   *"My daughter said they delivered all that bathroom equipment to her house yesterday."*

S: Client reports no difficulty using adaptive equipment to don pants and socks while maintaining hip precautions. She has not c/o pain with transfers and toileting using raised toilet seat. Family reports bathroom equipment ordered by OT has been delivered to daughter's home.

2. Tanner is a 14-year-old recently admitted to an inpatient adolescent psychiatric unit following an unsuccessful suicide attempt by overdose with his mother's sleeping pills. During a group session, he makes the following comments:

   ° *"I have nothing to live for."*
   ° *"I don't have any friends."*
   ° *"My family would be better off without me anyway."*
   ° *"The teachers at my school all hate me."*
   ° *"Maybe next time I should do it right and just use a gun!"*

   S: Client reports a lack of self-worth in both family and school situations and states that he does not have any friends. He continues to express suicidal ideation and suggested that he may use a gun in a future suicide attempt.

3. Wesley is at a SNF recovering from a recent R BKA. He makes the following comments during an ADL session:
   ° *Client told OT he has really bad arthritis in his R shoulder and L knee.*
   ° *Client rates pain at the site of his R BKA as 8 out of 10.*
   ° *Client said, "It hurts to stand on my left leg."*
   ° *Client stated, "It [sliding board] needs to be moved further up on the seat."*
   ° *When asked if he was okay after the transfer, he said, "I'm just tired."*
   ° *Client stated, "I'm through," and requested help to get closer to the bed.*
   ° *When client transferred to the bed for dressing tasks, he said, "This is the hardest part."*
   ° *Client stated he prefers to transfer toward the R side so he can push off with his L LE and avoid bumping his R BKA on the tire-rim of the w/c.*

   S: Client reports arthritis in R shoulder and L knee, pain on weight bearing. Pain at R BKA site 8/10. During transfer, client requested specific adjustments such as sliding board placement, proximity to bed, and approaching from R side. Fatigue reported after transfer.

4. Kira is a 3-year-old girl who recently transitioned from early intervention services at home into an Early Childhood Special Education (ECSE) classroom through her local public school. During your initial evaluation, you make the following notes for the "S" of your evaluation report:
   ° *Child cries for first 15 minutes after parent drop-off to classroom.*
   ° *Child does not use intelligible words.*
   ° *Child yells "Eee eee!" when she is happy about something.*
   ° *Kira does not use her augmentative communication device unless prompted by classroom teacher.*
   ° *Child attempts to get attention of peers by yanking on their clothing during play activities.*
   ° *Kira points to desired object when given a choice between two toys.*
   ° *Parent states, "I just don't know how I will be able to leave her. She's never been away from me for this long."*
   ° *Teacher asks for recommendations about calming activities to help Kira prepare for seated work and circle time.*

   S: Kira is nonverbal but does vocalize "Eee eee!" when excited. She cries during transition to classroom, and parent expresses concern about leaving her. Kira does not initiate use of her AAC device but does attempt to communicate via gesture. ECSE teacher has requested recommendations to help Kira be successful with classroom expectations.

CHAPTER 9

Worksheet 9-1: Using Categories

O: *Child participated in 60-minute OT session at day care to address feeding skills and reach/grasp/release during play. Child demonstrated strong R hand preference, flexed position of L UE, and did not spontaneously initiate use of L UE as a functional assist during self-care or play. With min A for facilitation of extension at elbow, child demonstrated ability to use L UE to reach, grasp, and release 5 objects with 1-2 verbal cues per object and* *restriction of R UE movement. Child was able to feed self independently with ~50% spillage, but demonstrated significant limitations in chewing action after ~3 rotary chews and swallowing ~90% of food without chewing. Child required verbal cues throughout session to maintain attention to task. Child wore soft spica thumb splint for entire session.*

Some or all of the following categories might be used to make this note easier to read:

- **L UE use or reach/grasp/release**
- **Feeding**
- **Attention/attention to task/attention span**
- **Splint**

Depending on the categories selected, the note might read like this:

O: Child participated in 60-minute OT session at day care to address functional use of L UE during play and self-care. Child demonstrated strong R hand preference, flexed position of L UE, and did not spontaneously initiate use of L UE as a functional assist during self-care or play. Child wore L soft spica thumb splint throughout tx session to facilitate functional grasp patterns.

Reach/Grasp/Release: With min A for facilitation of elbow, child used L UE to reach, grasp, and release 5 objects with 1-2 verbal cues per object and restriction of R UE movement.

Feeding: Child fed self independently with ~50% spillage, but demonstrated significant limitation in chewing actions with ~3 rotary chews and swallowing ~90% of the food without chewing.

Attention: Child required verbal cues throughout the session to maintain attention to task.

Worksheet 9-2: Being More Concise

O: *Pt. participated in 60-minute OT session bedside to complete morning ADL routine. Pt. presented with decreased standing balance and safety awareness. Pt. ambulated ~36 inches to shower with SBA for safety. Pt. instructed to complete shower while sitting. Pt. performed shower with SBA to manage IV line. Pt. able to wash upper and lower body with SBA and dry entire body with SBA after completing shower. Pt. required ~20 minutes to complete shower. Pt. then ambulated ~36 inches to chair and sat. Pt. needed verbal cues to remain seated while donning underwear and pants. Pt. able to dress upper and lower body with set-up after verbal cues to sit for safety. Pt. demonstrated good sitting balance but needed SBA for standing balance. Following shower, client was assisted back to bed for a nap.*

A more concise note might read:

O: Pt. participated in 60-minute OT session bedside for skilled instruction in self-care activities. Pt. presented with decreased standing balance and safety awareness. Ambulated ~3 ft. to/from shower with SBA to manage IV line while ambulating and showering for 20 minutes. Client showered with SBA and completed upper and lower body dressing with set-up after verbal cues to sit for safety. Client demonstrated good sitting balance but required SBA for standing balance. Client returned to bed with SBA at end of session.

Worksheet 9-3: Writing Good Opening Lines

1.   *Client seen in room for 45 minutes for self-care activities.*
   - *Client participated in 45-minute OT session in room to increase independence in ADL activities. Client has total hip precautions and demonstrates memory deficits and decreased safety with walker during ADLs.*
   - *Client participated in 45-minute OT session in hospital room for education on use of adaptive equipment and toilet transfer during morning self-care activities. Client does not consistently adhere to precautions during ADLs.*

2. *Client seen at sheltered workshop for 1 hr. to work on job skills.*
   - **Client participated in 1-hr. session at sheltered workshop to address skills needed for job task completion. Pt. has cognitive, sensory, and B integration deficits.**
   - **Client participated in 1-hr. session at sheltered workshop to improve efficiency of package handling work task. Session focused on sequencing, B coordination, concentration, and sensory awareness.**

3. *Client seen bedside for 30 minutes for morning dressing.*
   - **Client participated in 30-minute bedside session for morning dressing to improve safety and independence with ADLs to return home. Client exhibits decreased balance, B motor control, and functional mobility during ADLs.**
   - **Client participated in 30-minute bedside session to address balance and B UE motor control during morning ADLs. Client uses manual w/c for positioning and mobility and demonstrates decreased safety during ADLs due to poor balance and B UE coordination.**

4. *Client seen in kitchen for 1 hr. to work on independence in cooking.*
   - **Client participated in 1-hr. session in kitchen to address safety and independence during cooking tasks in prep for return home with limited caregiver supervision during the day. Client continues to exhibit decreased dynamic standing balance and inattention to affected L UE.**
   - **Client participated in 1-hr. session in kitchen to work on safety during cooking tasks. Session focused on attention to affected L UE positioning and dynamic standing balance.**

Worksheet 9-4: Being Specific About Assist Levels

__Yes__ *Child required HOH A* **to stay in the lines** *when following path with crayon.*

__Yes__ *Client needed mod verbal cues* **to participate in discussion** *during life skills group.*

__No__ *Resident needed min A to don socks due to pain.*

__No__ *Client required max A x 2 bed to bedside commode and bed to w/c transfers; dependent for toileting.*

1. *Client completed supine to sit with min A; bed to w/c with mod A.*
   - **Client completed supine to sit with min A to initiate activity; bed to w/c with mod A for balance.**
   - **Client completed supine to sit with min A to pull up using trapeze; bed to w/c with mod A to lift body weight.**
   - **Client completed supine to sit with min A to sequence movement; bed to w/c with mod A for postural control.**

2. *Client required SBA in transferring w/c to/from toilet.*
   - **Client required SBA for proper hand placement in transferring w/c to/from toilet.**
   - **Client required SBA for sequencing in transferring w/c to/from toilet.**

3. *Client retrieved garments from low drawers with min A.*
   - **Client retrieved garments from low drawers with min A to grasp drawer handles.**
   - **Client retrieved garments from low drawers with min A to release trigger on reacher.**
   - **Client retrieved garments from low drawers with min A to judge HALO placement in space.**

4. *Client required max A to brush hair.*
   - **Client required max A to reach back of head when brushing hair.**
   - **Client required max A to flex R shoulder past 35° when brushing hair.**

5. *Client completed dressing, toileting, and hygiene with min A.*
   - **Client completed dressing, toileting, and hygiene with min A to reach feet.**
   - **Client completed dressing, toileting, and hygiene with min A for activities requiring fine motor dexterity.**
   - **Client completed dressing, toileting, and hygiene with min A to adhere to hip precautions.**

Worksheet 9-5: De-Emphasizing the Treatment Media

1. *Client played catch using B UEs to facilitate grasp and release patterns.*

    Client practiced functional grasp/release patterns needed to manipulate household objects.

2. *Resident put dirt into pot to halfway point, added seedling, and filled remainder of pot with dirt transferred by cup. Resident completed 3 more pots while standing 8 minutes before requiring a 5-minute rest. Resident resumed standing position to water completed pots for approximately 5 minutes.*

    Resident demonstrated standing tolerance of 13 minutes during leisure activity with a 5-minute break after 8 minutes to increase standing needed for ADL tasks.

3. *Client painted some sun catchers in crafts group to be able to see that she could do something successfully.*

    Client completed a series of quick-success projects to increase self-esteem.

4. *Pt. cut out magazine pictures that indicated her emotions and glued them onto construction paper.*

    Client indicated how she feels in various daily situations through identification of pictures that represented those emotions.

5. *Child picked up beans with tweezers and placed them in pill bottle to work on tripod grasp in preparation for handwriting.*

    In prep for handwriting, child demonstrated sustained tripod grasp for 5 minutes using tweezers to grasp/ release small objects.

Worksheet 9-6: Revising the "O"

- An opening statement is needed, stating where, for how long, for what purpose the client was seen, and what the client's primary deficits are. One possibility is: *Client participated in 30-minute session in room for skilled instruction in compensatory dressing techniques and evaluation of splinting needs. Client presents with pain and limited function of dominant R hand.*
- The categories could be reduced to three: toileting, dressing, and splinting evaluation.
- It would be helpful to know what part of the task required assistance.
- The UE and LE wording is not inclusive enough since the client is dressing the upper and lower body rather than just the extremities.
- Under "hand status," there is no functional component, and "index finger greatest amount" is not very informative.
- The part about donning shoes could be condensed by saying *"Dons B shoes independently with elastic laces."*

CHAPTER 10

Worksheet 10-1: Differentiating Between Observations and Assessments

__O__ *Client is unable to don AFO and shoe independently for ambulation.*

__A__ *Inability to don AFO and shoe independently prevent client from completing IADLs required to live alone.*

__A__ *Decreased sensory tolerance limits the client's attention to task in the classroom.*

__O__ *Client required verbal cues to stay on task due to decreased sensory tolerance.*

__O__ *Client was unable to incorporate breathing and energy conservation techniques, requiring several prompts to complete task.*

__A__ *Inability to incorporate breathing techniques and energy conservation techniques into basic ADL tasks without verbal prompts limits her ability to live alone independently after discharge.*

1. *Client demonstrated difficulty with laundry and cooking tasks due to memory and sequencing deficits.*

   Deficits in memory and sequencing lead to difficulty with IADL tasks such as laundry and cooking necessary for independent household management.

2. *Client unable to complete homemaking tasks or basic self-care activities independently due to decreased endurance.*

   Decreased endurance limits client's ability to complete basic self-care and homemaking tasks safely and independently.

3. *Decreased level of alertness observed during morning dressing activities, requiring redirection to task.*

   Decreased level of alertness limits client's ability to complete basic ADL tasks.

4. *Client unable to follow hip precautions during morning dressing due to memory deficits.*

   Memory deficits limit client's ability to complete dressing tasks while adhering to hip precautions.

5. *Client problem solved poorly while performing lower body dressing, as evidenced by multiple attempts required to button pants and don socks successfully.*

   Decreased problem solving limits client's ability to dress herself without assistance and raises safety concerns with all ADLs.

Worksheet 10-2: Justifying Continued Treatment

__Yes__ Evaluation of a client

__No__ The practice of coordination and self-care skills on a daily basis

__Yes__ Establishing measurable, behavioral, objective, and individualized goals

__Yes__ Developing intervention plans designed to meet established goals

__Yes__ Analyzing and modifying functional activities through the provision of adaptive equipment or techniques

__Yes__ Determining that the modified tasks are safe and effective

__No__ Routine exercise and strengthening programs

__Yes__ Teaching the client to use the breathing techniques he has learned while performing ADLs

__Yes__ Providing individualized instruction to the client, family, or caregiver

__Yes__ Modifying the intervention plan based on a re-evaluation

__No__ Donning/doffing of a client's resting hand splint on a regular schedule throughout the day

__Yes__ Providing specialized instruction to eliminate limitations in a functional activity

__Yes__ Developing a home program and instructing caregivers

__Yes__ Making changes in the environment

__Yes__ Teaching compensatory skills

__No__ Gait training

___Yes___ Adding instruction in lower body dressing techniques to a current ADL program

___No___ Presenting informational handouts without having the client perform the activity

___Yes___ Teaching adaptive techniques such as one-handed shoe tying

Worksheet 10-3: Writing the Assessment—Ellie's Development

A: *Infant's inability to right head, roll, or push up to prone independently limits ability to engage in age-appropriate play skills and developmental exploration. Infant's decreased activity tolerance also limits her ability to engage in developmental play activities. Ability to maintain facilitated positions and decrease in need for oxygen indicate progress. Visual tracking and scanning by turning head indicates visual awareness and orientation and shows good potential for increased interaction with environment. Infant would benefit from continued facilitation of functional mobility during play as well as increasing strength and endurance through activities that facilitate typical development.*

or

A: *Decreased postural control and need for facilitation of weight shift limits infant's ability to perform early mobility skills needed for play. Limited mobility combined with her tolerance for less than 20 minutes of activity and the need for frequent rest breaks limit her ability to explore her environment and reach developmental milestones at a typical age. Ability to perform transitional movements with facilitation, orientation to black-and-white design, and ability to track in horizontal plane show good progress and potential for future developmental gains. Infant would benefit from continued OT services to stimulate developmental skills and from parent education in a home program.*

Worksheet 10-4: Writing the Assessment— Ms. D's Social Participation Skills

1. What problems do you see in the above "S" and "O"?
   - **Unkempt appearance**
   - **Interrupts when others are talking**
   - **Does not stay on topic of conversation**
2. What areas of occupation do these problems affect?
   - **Social participation**
3. What evidence of progress and/or potential do you see?
   - **Engages in conversation**
   - **States that she understands purpose of the group**
   - **Willingness to attend and participate in group**
   - **Spontaneously shared thoughts and ideas**
4. What would this client benefit from?
   - **Groups that focus on conversational skills**
   - **Skilled instruction in attending to social cues**
   - **ADL activities stressing hygiene and appearance**
5. Write a complete Assessment statement for this note.
A: *Client's unkempt appearance, interrupting behaviors, and need for redirection to topic of conversation interfere with her ability to engage in social participation with peers. Her expressed interest in groups and her willingness to engage in conversation and share her ideas show good potential to develop relationships and to express herself verbally in place of acting out. Client would benefit from participating in groups where conversational skills are stressed, from further facilitation of attention to social cues, and from instruction in ADLs stressing hygiene and appearance.*

Worksheet 10-5: Writing the Assessment—
Mr. Y's Functional Performance

- Problems:

  After reading through this note, several problems stood out for this occupational therapist:

  - Dynamic sitting balance
  - Weight shifting
  - Posture
  - Transfers

    (The four above are related to safety and functional mobility.)

  - Decreased AROM in R UE (mod A to reach)
  - Cognition

    Thinking a little further, the occupational therapist decided that the "cognition" problem might really be one of the following, because the patient does seem to understand the goal of the activity:

  - Short-term memory
  - Motor planning
  - Problem solving
  - Initiation

    Finally, the occupational therapist decided that the problem with initiation is probably some combination of problem solving and motor planning deficits.

- Progress/Potential:

  The therapist then groups the problems according to the impact they have on the client's occupational performance. She decides that the first four cause difficulty with functional mobility and are of particular concern because they create safety issues. The motor planning and initiation problem is a concern in the area of self-care, as is the problem with decreased AROM of the R UE. The need for continual instruction, whether it is a problem with short-term memory or with his ability to problem solve, is likely to require a lot of attention from a caregiver at home. The client does, however, understand why he is doing the task she has given him. As long as the goals are not set too high, he should be able to make good progress in rehabilitation. Her assessment and plan read as follows:

A: *Deficits in postural control, dynamic sitting balance, and weight shifting raise safety concerns during ADL transfers. Decreased AROM and motor planning ability negatively affect ability to perform self-care tasks. Need for continual instruction for safety will necessitate a high level of caregiver assistance during ADL tasks. Client's ability to understand treatment goals indicates good rehab potential for goals established. Client would benefit from continued skilled instruction in activities to increase balance, safe functional mobility, and independence in ADL tasks.*

Another occupational therapist might assess the situation a little differently. For example:

A: *Deficits in motor planning, movement initiation, cognition, and muscle weakness in R UE result in decreased safety and independence in ADL tasks and functional mobility during ADLs. Ability to tolerate 3 minutes of activity at a time indicates progress over baseline of 1 minute activity tolerance. Client would benefit from skilled OT to increase balance, functional mobility, and grasp/release activities with involved UE to increase independence in self-care activities.*

or

A: *Decreased functional use of R UE, decreased sitting balance, and difficulty with sequencing and problem solving limit ability to perform ADLs. Increased shoulder flexion and motor planning since initial evaluation and increased understanding of treatment activities indicate good rehab potential. Client would benefit from continued skilled OT to increase functional AROM, exercises in grasp, exercises in weight shifting to improve dynamic sitting balance, and evaluation of both cognitive status and ability to initiate activity to increase independence in ADL tasks.*

Worksheet 10-6: Writing the Assessment—
Marco's Visual Motor Skills

- Problems:
  - ° Decreased visual tracking and eye convergence
  - ° Low muscle tone/upper body weakness
  - ° Decreased bilateral coordination
  - ° Impaired fine motor skills
  - ° Poor handwriting
  - ° UE weakness
  - ° Proximal instability
- Progress/Potential:
  - ° Improvement in ability to form letters within lines
  - ° 90% accuracy from memory of some letters
  - ° Handwriting improvement

A: *Decreased upper body strength and proximal stability limit the child's ability to use his upper extremities in an accurate and coordinated manner in class. Lack of fine motor and bilateral coordination limit the child's accuracy in schoolwork (including handwriting, art, and play activities). Inaccuracy in visual tracking and eye convergence interfere with ability to form letters and numbers or to complete written work from a book or whiteboard at grade level. Lack of visual tracking and convergence skills also limit ability to perform age-appropriate games safely. Improvement in accuracy of letter formation since last note and ability to remember 6 letter shapes indicate good progress and good potential to meet IEP goals. Child would benefit from continued work on postural stability to support functional UE use, as well as from continued work on visual and motor skills needed for classroom activities.*

Worksheet 10-7: Writing the Assessment—
Mr. S's Social Participation Skills

- Problems:
  - ° Communication (changes subject rather than answer the question)
  - ° Assertion (does not define, and states he does not wish to use)
  - ° Nonresponsive to group role-play activity
  - ° Sitting with head down and eyes closed during group
  - ° Self-expression (verbal and nonverbal)
    These behaviors limit his appropriate social participation and his likelihood of leaving the institution.
- Progress/Potential:
  - ° Neat appearance
  - ° Attended group and was on time
  - ° Remained for duration of group

A: *Poor ability to define assertive behavior and the statement that he prefers manipulation and aggression as relational skills limit Mr. S's ability to resolve conflicts and relate to others effectively, thus limiting his ability to function independently in a community setting. Lack of participation in group activity limits ability to explore alternative ways of communicating with others. Ability to manage time, willingness to remain in group until the end, and good dressing/grooming skills indicate good potential to meet stated goal of moving to next level of least restrictive environment. Client would benefit from group and individual OT sessions to address social communication skills with emphasis on alternative conflict resolution skills.*

CHAPTER 11

Worksheet 11-1: Completing the Plan

Ellie's Development:

P: *Child will be seen in home twice weekly for 3 months for activities that encourage postural control needed for play and environmental exploration. Sessions to include parent education targeted at facilitating infant's development. Plan to formally reassess infant's developmental level using standardized testing in 3 months.*

Ms. D's Social Participation Skills:

P: *Client to continue social skills group 3x/wk for 1 week to improve conversational skills. Client will also be given individual feedback daily on her attention to appearance and social cues.*

Mr. Y's Functional Performance:

P: *Continue tx bid for ½-hour sessions for 2 weeks to work on R UE movement and cognitive retraining. Sessions will focus on improving independence in grooming, dressing, toileting, and bathing to work toward goal of returning home with spouse. Will consult with SLP regarding short-term memory strategies that can be incorporated during OT sessions.*

Marco's Visual Motor Skills:

P: *Continue OT twice weekly for 30-minute sessions for remainder of school year to improve functional performance in educational activities. Sessions to focus on improving postural control, bilateral coordination, and oculomotor control. Will consult with classroom teacher regarding classwork modifications to accommodate oculomotor deficits.*

Mr. S's Social Participation Skills:

P: *Client to participate in all regularly scheduled psychosocial skills groups for 1 month, in addition to weekly 1:1 session on unit to offer opportunities to relate effectively. Focus will be on increasing participation in group activities to improve effective communication skills with others.*

Worksheet 11-2: SOAPing Your Note

___**O**___ *Supine to sit in bed independently.*

___**O**___ *Client moved kitchen items from counter to cabinet independently using L hand.*

___**A**___ *Decreased coordination, strength, sensation, and proprioception in L hand create safety risks in home management tasks.*

___**S**___ *Client reports that his fingers are stiff this morning and that he is having trouble handling small items like buttons.*

___**A**___ *Increase of 15 minutes in activity tolerance for UE activities permits client to prepare a light meal with supervision.*

___**O**___ *Child participated in 60-minute eval. of hand function in OT clinic.*

___**A**___ *Decreased proprioception and motor planning limit independence in upper body dressing.*

___**P**___ *Continue retrograde massage to R hand for edema control.*

___**A**___ *Correct identification of inappropriate positioning 100% of time indicates memory WFL.*

___**S**___ *Client reports that she cannot remember hip precautions.*

___A___ *Veteran would benefit from further instruction to incorporate total hip precautions into lower body dressing, bathing, and toileting.*

___A___ *Client's improvement with repetition indicates good potential for successful access of augmentative communication device using eye gaze.*

___O___ *Client did not make eye contact during group session.*

___O___ *Client wrote check for correct amount to pay electric bill with 2 verbal cues.*

___A___ *Client's request to take breaks demonstrates awareness of her limitations in endurance.*

___O___ *Client completed weight shifts of trunk x 10 in each of anterior, posterior, left, and right lateral directions in preparation for standing to perform IADLs.*

___A___ *3+ muscle grade of R wrist extension this week shows good progress toward goals.*

___P___ *Continue OT 3x/wk for 2 weeks to address cognitive impairments that affect safe performance of IADLs.*

___A___ *Unkempt appearance in mock interview situation indicates poor judgment and self-concept.*

Worksheet 11-3: Identifying Areas for Improvement in a Note

- The "S" would be better if the therapist had asked pertinent questions, such as what the client's pain levels were.
- The occupational therapist is mixing the "O" data and the "A" data.
- There is nothing in the "O" to show that skilled occupational therapy is being provided. The list of observations of assist levels fails to provide the richness of skill used in treatment. The therapist erroneously puts some of that information in the "A" section, rather than assessing her data. In the "A" she tells us:

  Client independent in dressing EOB, but is min A in dressing when standing with a walker. L UE AROM is WFL, but R UE has deficits noted in shoulder flexion. Client needs SBA in bed mobility when rolling to unaffected side and min A in sit to stand 2° decreased UE strength. Client needs SBA for transfer to unaffected side in pivot transfer bed to w/c and min A w/c to toilet.

- Even if this information were moved into the "O," there is nothing to tell us what part of the task the assistance was for.
- The therapist used a nonstandard abbreviation of "VCs." She means verbal cues, but since VC is a standard health term meaning *vital capacity*, it is inappropriate in its usage here.
- The coordination deficits mentioned in the "A" section come out of the blue. There is no mention of coordination in the opening statement ("*to work on dressing and functional mobility during ADLs*"), nor is it mentioned anywhere else in the "O." Thus, the statement that coordination deficits are one of the problems noted and the statement that the client would benefit from coordination exercises are unsubstantiated. Remember not to introduce any new information in the "A" section of your note.
- There is no real assessment of the meaning of the data found in the "S" and the "O." There is a short list of problem areas, but no assessment of their impact on the ability to engage in meaningful occupation, and no assessment of the rehab potential shown by the client's willingness to "*do whatever it takes to get out of the hospital.*"
- The best thing for this therapist to do is to rewrite the "O" section, providing a more comprehensive picture of the treatment session. Then she needs to assess her data based on her observations. There needs to be an indication of how the observed data affect the occupational performance of the client, before the statements about what the client would benefit from.
- Depending on the assessment she makes, the plan to work on balance may be appropriate, but it is likely to be only one of the things to be addressed.

Worksheet 11-4: Revising a Note

Revisions for S:

- The first sentence is irrelevant unless the child usually resists attending.
- The fact that the grandmother came in is irrelevant because we have her report.
- The "S" could be much more concise yet still effective.

Revisions for O:

- Opening statement needs to indicate active client participation and needs to specify duration and purpose of session.
- Delete what the therapist did and reword to focus on the client.
- De-emphasize the treatment media in the first category and talk about the purpose. Keep this brief, since it is only prep for the sensory and oral motor work, or make it part of the introduction.
- In the opening statements, talk about sensory as well as oral motor to clearly indicate client's deficits.
- Avoid mixing "A" material into the observation.
- When talking about desensitizing, tell how much the client could tolerate, to measure progress.

Revisions for A:

- We do not see any indication of ability to concentrate on one activity at a time. This is not a problem with the "A," but a change that would need to be made in the "O" so that we can assess it in the "A."
- The second sentence is good with a little revision. It is a sweeping assessment statement and covers a lot of material. Is there more that could be said about the session than this? Are there any other problems? What about the problems tolerating the oral resistive exercises? Is there any progress?
- The third sentence needs to be changed to what she would benefit from rather than what the therapist hopes.

Revisions for P:

- There is no mention of frequency, duration, or purpose.
- There is no evidence of professional reasoning that upcoming sessions will address issues that continue to limit this child's functional performance.

Revised SOAP Note:

S: *Grandmother reports that Jenna now tolerates a few seconds of tooth brushing. Jenna asked for hands/arms to be wiped off and asked for oral ranging exercises to be stopped when her tolerance had been reached.*

O: *Child participated in 45-minute session in clinic to address sensory processing skills in preparation for accepting a wider range of textures during feeding and hygiene activities. Child presents with both oral and tactile defensiveness and demonstrates strong avoidance behaviors. Child tolerated 10 minutes of proprioception/deep pressure and vestibular input in preparation for engaging her attention in the therapy activities.*

Tactile: Child presented with foam, water, and foam stick-ups to desensitize her to textures used in feeding/hygiene but was hesitant to touch any of the objects. After prompting, child touched the foam but immediately wanted it wiped off.

Oral Motor: Child fed a baby doll as an intro to self-feeding. When putting the spoon to her own mouth, child began spitting. Child tolerated 45 seconds of oral resistive activities used to elongate and protrude the lips and stretch the cheek muscles for feeding.

A: *Child's reluctance to engage in sensory activities with wet or semi-wet media continues to interfere with eating and hygiene. Increased tolerance (from 8 to 10 minutes) of proprioceptive activities has resulted in an increased ability to concentrate on one activity at a time. Ability to tolerate 45 seconds of oral resistive activities, willingness to bring spoon to her mouth, and tolerance for a few seconds of tooth brushing also indicate progress. Client would benefit from continued desensitization and oral resistive exercises to decrease tactile defensiveness.*

P: *Child will continue to be seen for 45-minute sessions 2x/wk for 3 months to increase tolerance of certain tactile media and to decrease oral defensiveness. Focus will be on increasing tolerated food textures and improving oral range needed for self-feeding. Grandmother will be instructed in home activities to enhance Jenna's development of sensory processing skills.*

Worksheet 12-1: Choosing Intervention Strategies

STG (OBJECTIVE)	INTERVENTION	TYPE OF INTERVENTION
Client will manage finances independently within 3 weeks.	1. Complete worksheets with basic math skills (add, subtract, multiply, divide).	1. Activity
	2. Role play to make change correctly.	2. Activity
	3. Set-up task of reviewing fabricated bills to determine amount due and due date.	3. Activity
	4. Practice comparison shopping online using an electronic tablet or smart phone.	4. Activity
	5. Set up task of writing out a budget.	5. Activity
	6. Set up task of reviewing a fabricated banking statement to determine deposits, withdrawals, and purchases.	6. Activity
	7. Set up experience for deciding whether a given amount of money will be enough for living expenses once a set of fabricated bills has been paid.	7. Activity
	8. Have client make a purchase in the hospital cafeteria or gift shop.	8. Occupation
	9. Have family bring in credit card bill statements so client can pay bills online.	9. Occupation

Worksheet 12-2: Writing the Assessment and Intervention Plan— The Case of Georgia S

A: Decreased activity tolerance and standing balance, weakness in B shoulder flex/abd, and decreased problem-solving skills result in decreased safety and independence in dressing and grooming. Decreased standing balance impairs safety and independent functional mobility during ADLs. Weak grasp and pinch of R hand and decreased coordination impairs fine motor ADL tasks including donning sock and brushing teeth. Rehab potential is good for returning home with caregiver assistance. Client would benefit from continued OT to increase activity tolerance, dynamic standing balance, and safety for ADL tasks.

P: Pt. to be seen 60 minutes daily, 5x/wk for 2 weeks to increase independence in self-care activities. Client will be instructed in adaptive equipment/techniques. Interventions will also focus on increased activity tolerance, standing balance, and independence in functional mobility for ADLs, and increased R hand strength to complete dressing and toileting independently.

Strengths: Independence in self-care prior to CVA; able to ambulate with walker; intact sensation except R hand stereognosis; all UE AROM WNL or WFL.

Functional Problem Statement #1: Impaired problem solving, decreased coordination, decreased stereognosis, and decreased standing balance impair ability to perform self-care tasks independently.
LTG #1: Client will complete all dressing and grooming tasks independently using walker for task set-up by anticipated discharge on 8/18/2023.

STG (OBJECTIVE)	INTERVENTION
STG #1: Client will don/doff gown and robe with min A by 8/4/2023.	1. *Instruct client in upper body dressing techniques and have client demonstrate over-the-head and button-up methods, first in sitting, then progress to standing.* 2. *Provide tactile cues to use alternative techniques.* 3. *Have client problem solve next step of dressing or grooming tasks in sequence using visual aid and then verbal cues as needed. Ask client what to do next or why this is not working now.* 4. *Engage client in reaching activities that provide a graded challenge to balance.* 5. *Engage client in activities that increase AROM and fine motor tasks such as buttoning and zipping that are graded for level of difficulty in coordination.*
STG #2: By 8/11/2023, client will complete grooming tasks standing at sink for at least 10 minutes with CGA for balance and one 30-second rest break.	1. *Educate client on identifying signs of fatigue. Plan rest breaks as needed to decrease fatigue.* 2. *Perform tabletop activities including self-care tasks with time increasing as tolerated.* 3. *Perform deep breathing exercises and instruct in energy conservation techniques.* 4. *Instruct client in therapy putty exercises to be performed in room in between OT sessions to increase grip and pinch strength.* 5. *Gradually introduce standing components during morning ADLs such as standing to retrieve clothes from closet or standing to complete one grooming task.*

Functional Problem Statement #2: Fatigue during ADLs and decreased dynamic balance during toileting raise safety concern for being home alone during the day.
LTG #2: By discharge on 8/18/2023, client will perform toileting independently using a walker and bedside commode.

STG (OBJECTIVE)	INTERVENTION
STG #1: In 1 week, client will complete toileting using 3-in-1 commode frame over toilet with min A to manage clothing.	1. *Instruct client in safe transfer techniques; reinforce compliance when transferring to/from bed, armchairs, commode, and mat for therapeutic activities, strengthening exercises, toileting, or dressing activities.* 2. *Provide R UE strengthening and AROM through reaching and weight bearing activities such as reaching at sink for grooming and dressing items in graded challenging positions, pushing up from armchair and bedside commode, and tabletop activities of interest that require alternating support on one arm while actively reaching with the other.*
STG #2: In 2 weeks, client will complete toileting with SBA using 3-in-1 commode frame over toilet with SBA for safety while adjusting clothing.	1. *Continue with transfer education and practice.* 2. *Interview client and daughter regarding home environment; explore and discuss equipment use and placement in home; discuss support services needed if discharge to home is warranted.* 3. *Collaborate with social work to schedule home safety assessment via home health at time of discharge from rehab if discharge home ends up being the family's plan.*

Discharge Plan: To home if environmental adaptations and support of caregiver and/or agency services are available. If client is not independent in self-care activities by 8/18/2023, the recommendation will be to discharge to a skilled nursing facility for 2 to 3 weeks until self-care goals are met.

Worksheet 12-3: Planning Interventions Using Groups— Complex Mental Health Needs

> With the introduction of new psychotropic medications and the ongoing effort by third-party payers to shorten inpatient hospitalizations, patients with mental health diagnoses are often admitted for just a few days with an emphasis on crisis stabilization and connecting the patient with community resources. Planning interventions for a group of people who all have very different needs can be complex. You need to remember that your therapeutic use of self is the most important part of the group. It is the creation of a supportive situation, rather than the task itself, that is the goal.
>
> In an intervention plan for a client with a physical diagnosis, you might carry out all the interventions listed on the plan. You would not have the time or capacity to carry out every intervention listed below. These are just ideas to get you started. You will choose an activity for your group and then customize your interventions to meet each client's needs.

Problem #1: *Exacerbation of depressive symptoms resulting in a suicide attempt.*

LTG #1: *By anticipated discharge in 4 days, Heather will verbally identify strengths, care for her appearance, make eye contact when interacting with others, and develop a plan for coping with suicidal thoughts, all as evidence of improved self-esteem.*

GROUP	INTERVENTION
Goals Group	1. *Listen attentively to Heather when she shares her goal.* 2. *Offer eye contact and offer Heather the opportunity to make eye contact in return before cueing her.* 3. *Help Heather identify the relationship between her values and her daily goals (i.e., a goal to wash her hair if related to valuing a neat and clean appearance).* 4. *Help Heather break down larger goals (such as "be happy") into smaller accomplishable and measurable increments.* 5. *Show respect for Heather's choices.* 6. *Provide feedback on Heather's successes in meeting her daily goals.* 7. *Facilitate goal choices that show increased self-esteem.* 8. *Compliment Heather on her appearance when any part of her appearance shows more attention to her self-care.* 9. *Facilitate goal choices that involve taking care of herself.*
Stress Management Group	1. *Welcome Heather by greeting her warmly, sitting by her, or smiling.* 2. *Offer opportunities to identify strengths through visualization and imagery.* 3. *Help Heather identify stresses that led her to recent suicide attempt.* 4. *Help Heather identify stresses that occur frequently.* 5. *Help Heather identify physical and behavioral changes that occur when she experiences stress.* 6. *Help Heather identify both successful and unsuccessful stress relief strategies that she has used in the past.* 7. *Brainstorm ways of handling stressful situations that seem overwhelming before those situations become life-threatening.* 8. *Use positive affirmations.* 9. *Provide practice for a variety of stress management strategies.* 10. *Develop a plan for managing stress when feeling overwhelmed.*

IADL Group	
	1. *Identify strengths about each person through group discussion, art activities (draw your best quality, personality collage, etc.), and games.*
	2. *Use a peer feedback activity that gives group members opportunities to identify and recognize each other's strengths.*
	3. *Offer quick success projects, such as putting together jewelry, making bookmarks, or completing small kits.*
	4. *Ask Heather for her ideas about how best to use the group time.*
	5. *Note aspects of Heather's work that are executed with competence.*
	6. *In a group of interested clients, learn to apply makeup or style hair.*

Problem #2: *Stress related to recent role changes results in Heather's inability to concentrate and make decisions for her daily life.*

LTG #2: *Heather will apply a decision-making strategy to her two most important current life decisions by discharge in 4 days.*

GROUP	INTERVENTION
Goals Group	1. *Identify a small accomplishment goal for the day.*
	2. *Help Heather identify what is realistic to accomplish in 1 day.*
	3. *Help Heather make her goal measurable.*
	4. *Write that goal on a card for Heather to carry with her throughout the day.*
	5. *Make a verbal contract with Heather to accomplish her goal.*
	6. *Teach the relationship between setting daily goals and making larger life decisions.*
	7. *Follow up daily on Heather's goal for the day.*
	8. *Encourage Heather to make goals related to major life stressors.*
Stress Management Group	1. *Help Heather identify triggers in her environment that cause a stress reaction.*
	2. *Help Heather identify negative thoughts that increase her stress level. Instruct Heather on how to replace them with more positive and realistic thoughts.*
	3. *Help Heather bring her thoughts to the present moment and to come back into the present moment when she drifts into the past and future.*
	4. *Use movement, such as stretching or progressive relaxation, to help Heather focus on the task at hand.*
IADL Group	1. *Ask Heather what strategies she uses to focus her mind.*
	2. *Plan group topics around Heather's current issues, such as ways of getting to sleep, overcoming loneliness, and feeling worthwhile.*
	3. *Use a cognitively stimulating activity to help Heather focus.*
	4. *Instruct Heather on a problem-solving strategy and practice applying it to sample problems.*
	5. *Brainstorm strategies for making good decisions and rank these in effectiveness.*
	6. *Ask Heather to identify one major decision needing to be made, and list pros/cons of each possible course of action.*
	7. *Role play a decision-making situation.*
	8. *Use games that require decision making.*
	9. *Adapt tasks so that Heather will be able to concentrate on a task long enough to complete it.*

Problem #3: Inability to manage anger constructively resulting in behaviors that damage self, relationships, and property.

LTG #3: By anticipated discharge in 4 days, Heather independently will identify potential anger triggers, identify her physical reactions to being angry, and develop a plan to prevent escalation and destructive behaviors.

GROUP	INTERVENTION
Goals Group	1. *Use active listening to help Heather identify feelings related to her goals.* 2. *Ask Heather about daily incidents involving anger and encourage goals for useful solutions if incidents arise.*
Stress Management Group	1. *Use stress management techniques that focus on body sensations.* 2. *Teach Heather to focus on the breath to bring her to the present moment, to relax, and to enhance sleep.* 3. *Invite Heather to identify and express feelings that arise during the exercises.* 4. *Use sounds and recordings that activate the parasympathetic nervous system.* 5. *Identify strategies for restful sleep and encourage her to practice these at night.*
IADL Group	1. *Teach anger management strategies.* 2. *Help Heather identify potential anger-provoking situations.* 3. *Help Heather identify early physical signs of escalating anger.* 4. *Help Heather develop a plan for what to do when she notices her anger beginning to escalate.* 5. *Help Heather identify safe outlets for anger to prevent it from escalating.* 6. *Instruct Heather on constructive ways to communicate her anger to others.* 7. *Help Heather identify feelings that arise during the group.* 8. *Use sounds and language to elicit feelings.* 9. *Use art activities to explore and express feelings.* 10. *Identify stressors that trigger anger through group discussion, adapted games, or art.* 11. *Role play situations around anger and frustration.* 12. *Identify social supports (friends, family, support groups, crisis lines) to use when angry.* 13. *Teach and role play problem solving.* 14. *Coach Heather as she practices managing anger with phone calls and visitors.* 15. *Teach the use of an "anger continuum" to recognize varying degrees and experiences of anger.*

INDEX

Printed in the United States
by Baker & Taylor Publisher Services